Allergy and Asthma Relief

READER'S DIGEST

Published by
The Reader's Digest Association Limited
London • New York • Sydney • Montreal

Allergy
and
Asthma
Relief

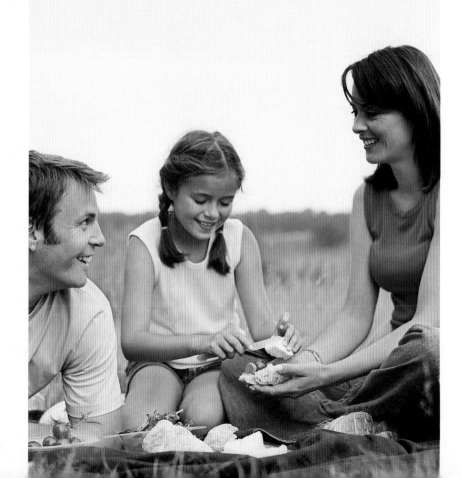

Consultants

Dr Chris Corrigan MA MSc PhD FRCP
William E. Berger MD
Sheena Meredith MB BS
Maureen Jenkins RN BSc(Hons) NP Dip. DPSN Asthma Dip. Intensive Care Dip.
Pamela Mason BSc MSc PhD MRPharmS

Note to Readers While the creators of this work have made every effort to be as accurate and up to date as possible, medical and pharmacological knowledge is constantly changing. Readers are recommended to consult a qualified medical specialist for individual advice. The writers, researchers, editors and publishers of this work cannot be held liable for any errors and omissions, or actions that may be taken as a consequence of information contained within this work.

About the consultants

Dr Chris Corrigan is Reader and Consultant Physician in Allergy and Respiratory Medicine at King's College London School of Medicine, which incorporates Guy's, St. Thomas' and King's College hospitals. He has spent over 20 years researching into the immunological mechanisms of asthma and allergy, particularly the role of T lymphocytes, and the implications for new treatment. In collaboration with the leading asthma charity Asthma UK and Imperial College London, the College has recently won funding from the Medical Research Council to set up the UK's first centre dedicated to asthma and allergy research.

Dr Corrigan is also Secretary of the Royal College of Physicians Joint Committee on Higher Medical Training in Allergy and Immunology, and Secretary of the British Society for Allergy and Clinical Immunology, the professional society for allergy practitioners, which has been actively lobbying the government for a better network of allergy services across the UK.

Dr William E. Berger is a clinical professor in the department of paediatrics, division of allergy and immunology, at the University of California, Irvine, College of Medicine. He is the founder of the Allergy and Asthma Associates of Southern California Medical Group, where he treats both adult and paediatric allergies. He is a past president of the American College of Allergy, Asthma and Immunology, a professional organization that represents more than 4,000 allergy and asthma specialists in the USA and elsewhere. Dr Berger is the author of many academic papers on allergies, asthma and the immune system, has written articles for newspapers and magazines and is the author of a top-selling book on allergies and asthma.

Sheena Meredith has a medical degree and a postgraduate qualification in medical law. She is an established medical writer who has contributed to publications as diverse as *The Daily Telegraph* and *Doctor* magazine. She was formerly Medical Editor of *Medical News*, a weekly magazine for GPs, and Health Editor of *Company* magazine. She has written or contributed to numerous books on health, medicine and law, including the Reader's Digest *Complete A-Z of Medicine and Health* and *Family Guide to Alternative Medicine*, and has written extensively on respiratory diseases and allergies, including articles in *Respiratory Disease in Practice* and a book on eczema (Vega 2002).

Maureen Jenkins is an Allergy Nurse Consultant for Sussex Allergy Service, which she set up in 1997 as a community referral service for primary care assessment and management of patients with all types of allergy. She also undertakes immunotherapy clinical and research work in Portsmouth and is a Trustee of Allergy UK (formerly The British Allergy Foundation) on whose behalf she set up and managed a university accredited allergy diploma course for GPs and nurses in 2000, with funding from the Department of Health. Maureen has written papers and taken part in many media and professional presentations on allergy.

Pamela Mason is a pharmacist and nutritionist with a particular interest in nutritional supplements and other complementary medicines. Her publications include numerous articles, training programmes and a book on dietary supplements. She speaks at international conferences, is an occasional lecturer at UK schools of pharmacy and a consultant for the Health Supplements Information Service (HSIS).

Contents

PART THREE
The Breathe Easy Plan

PART FOUR
Special situations

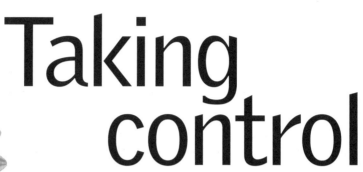

Taking
control
of allergies and asthma

Controlling the symptoms of asthma and allergies might sound straightforward, particularly to anyone who has never experienced them. Yet, in surveys of people receiving treatment, 75 per cent wish that their disease was better controlled and say that it affects their quality of life. A sixth of people with severe asthma report weekly attacks so severe that they cannot speak.

Asthma costs the NHS nearly £900 million annually, but it has been estimated that up to 75 per cent of hospital admissions for asthma are avoidable. Each year over 12 million working days are lost to asthma and on average 1,400 people die (that is one person every 6 hours). It is a disease that affects so many families. In the UK around 5.2 million people are currently receiving asthma treatment – that is, someone living in one in five households.

The situation with allergic diseases is no less disturbing. Severe hay fever causes more lost days at work and school than asthma and is the commonest chronic debilitating disease in the UK. Many sufferers don't know about the value of proper allergy diagnosis and treatment and put up with unnecessary symptoms, which have a major and distressing impact on aspects of their life including sleep, exercise tolerance, performance in examinations and at work or school, playing sport, a good sex life, and many others. Disease caused by asthma and allergies is a major sociological and economic problem worldwide.

Given the statistics, it is hard to believe – but true – that most sufferers do not consider their condition serious, and many do not consult their doctors for help. But it is also true that there is a poorly developed network of NHS care for allergy sufferers and little government funding for asthma research. The British Society for Allergy and Clinical Immunology, the professional association of allergists in the UK, is working hard to persuade the Department of Health to rectify this, while charitable organizations such as Asthma UK, Allergy UK and The British Lung Foundation campaign to raise awareness.

Fortunately, there is much you can do to help yourself and *Allergy and Asthma Relief* – featuring the Breathe Easy Plan – has some practical solutions that can make an immediate difference. The book tells you how to evaluate the severity of your disorder, what questions to ask doctors and when it is important to seek more specialist advice from an allergist. It explains the causes of asthma and other allergic diseases, discusses which specific allergens might be involved, how changes to lifestyle and environment can help and the different types of medicine available.

Armed with this knowledge, allergy and asthma sufferers can talk more knowledgeably to their doctors and embark on the book's Breathe Easy Plan. The instructions are specific and clear, though some of the changes may be easier than others to implement. It takes a lot of motivation to modify your eating habits, home environment, reactions to stress and attitudes towards taking medicines. But for asthma and allergy sufferers who feel trapped by their disease, a better quality of life is a powerful incentive.

There are no deadlines and while many of the steps are best taken sequentially, readers can accomplish them at their own pace. Sit back, read, learn and enjoy the book. The knowledge it contains is the first step to allergy and asthma relief: the rest is up to you.

Dr Chris Corrigan

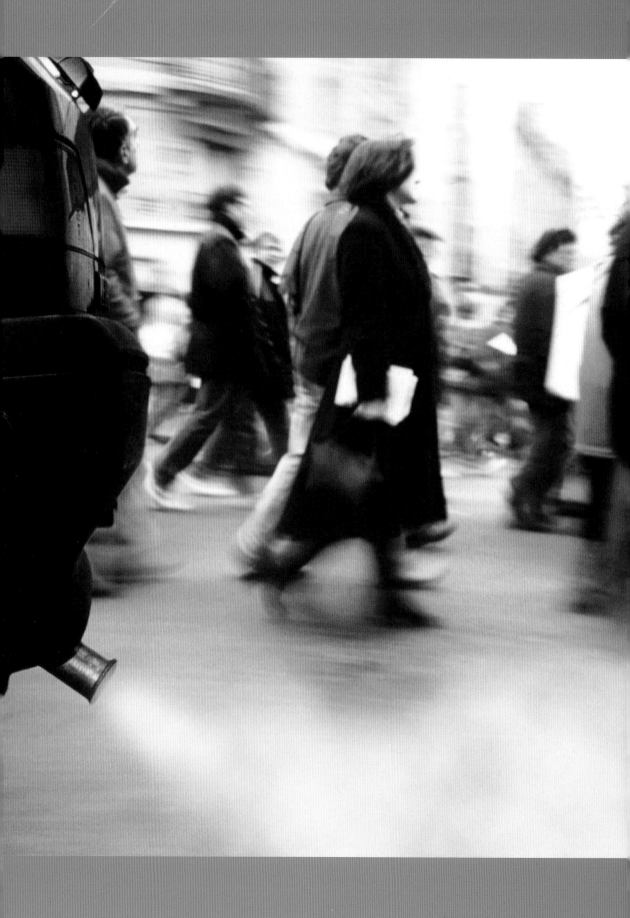

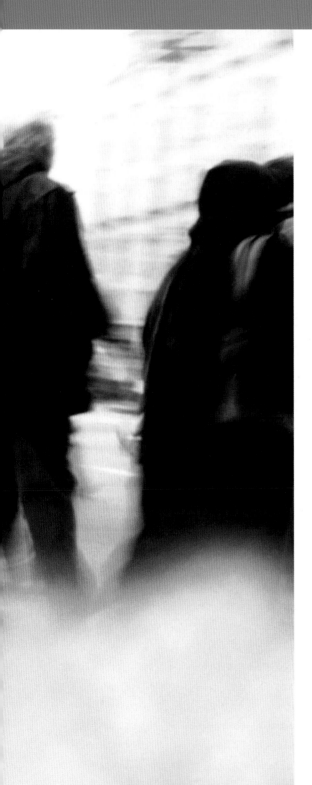

PART ONE

The **problem**

Is *epidemic* too strong a word
to describe the rise of allergies
and asthma in our modern world?
Probably not. An astounding
number of people today struggle
with the sneezing, wheezing
and discomfort of allergies and
asthma. The reasons are complex
and conflicting, but also fascinating.

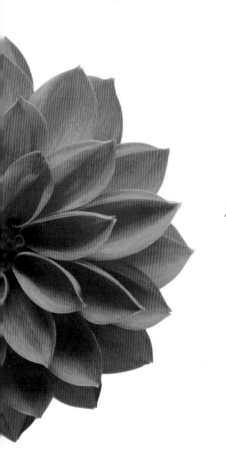

Chapter one

An epidemic
in the air

Augustus Caesar. Peter the Great. Ludwig van Beethoven. Charles Dickens. John F. Kennedy. Leonard Bernstein. Liza Minnelli. Paula Radcliffe. All famous people whom you probably never knew were afflicted with asthma, allergies, or both.

Of course, you don't have to be a great leader, a creative genius or a world class athlete to suffer from these disorders; you just need to be human. These days, asthma and allergies are reaching epidemic proportions in the UK and other countries, burdening already overloaded health care systems, putting children's long-term health at risk and costing employers billions in lost work days and productivity.

The diseases themselves are not new. More than 1,000 years ago, the Persian physician Ali Razi wrote 'An Article on the Reason Why Abou Zayd Balkhi Suffers from Rhinitis When Smelling Roses in Spring'. In it, he reported on his philosophy teacher, who complained annually of sinus pain and inflammation 'when the smell of flowers amplifies the illness'. The treatment recommended in those days is unlikely to be considered acceptable now: in cases of severe nasal pressure, Ali Razi wrote, the patient's hair should be cut and his head covered with mustard.

In the early 1800s, London physician John Bostock, who studied his own affliction, provided the first detailed account of seasonal allergies. He coined the phrase 'hay fever' because his condition typically worsened during the hay-making season. At that time the condition was so rare that Bostock wrote, 'I have not heard of a single unequivocal case among the poor.'

Now, of course, the condition is the opposite of rare. Although accurate statistics are hard to come by, professional estimates maintain that allergies and asthma together affect roughly 20 million adults, making them the most common chronic health problems in the UK (high blood pressure is number two). Asthma and other respiratory diseases (including allergic rhinitis, or hay fever) are the most common chronic conditions among children, with asthma alone affecting about 1.1 million children, or one child in every 10.

Given those statistics, the chances are that you or someone you know suffers from the itchy eyes, sneezing, wheezing, runny nose and general misery of allergies or from the choking, can't-get-a-breath suffocation of asthma. That is why you're reading this book. You know how miserable it is to live your life dependent on an inhaler and stuck indoors on beautiful summer days.

What you probably don't know is how simple it is to live a complete and active life even if you have allergies or asthma. That's what this book and our Breathe Easy Plan will show you.

A pervasive problem

Look around you. One in four people in the UK now has an allergy-related problem at some time during their life and the number of allergy sufferers is increasing by almost 5 per cent a year. The figures include those with skin, food, insect and medication allergies as well as respiratory allergies.

Asthma is one of the main reasons that children undergo hospital treatment, with pre-school children three times more likely than older children and six times more likely than adults to be hospitalized.

Asthma-related GP consultations increased almost five-fold between 1976 and 1994. There are now around 74,000 emergency hospital admissions a year due to asthma, a quarter of which are children under the age of four.

asthma by **numbers**

- Asthma now costs the NHS an average of £890 million per year.
- More than 12.7 million working days are lost to asthma each year.
- Each week 14,500 first or new episodes of asthma are presented to GPs in the UK. Respiratory disease is the most common illness responsible for an emergency admission to hospital.
- Around 1,500 people die from asthma in the UK each year – that's equivalent to more than four a day.

Thirty or forty years ago, few if any hospitals or medical centres employed allergists and far fewer people were admitted to hospital suffering from asthma. Cases of food anaphylaxis (severe, life-threatening allergic reactions to food) were extremely rare; now most casualty departments have admitted patients suffering from anaphylaxis related to food, latex, drugs or insect allergies.

The past five decades have seen a surge in the incidence of all immune-based diseases. For instance, in the UK potentially life-threatening, but previously rare allergies such as peanut allergy, now affect as many as one in 70 children. Atopic dermatitis (itchy rash, or eczema) is the most common skin condition in children aged under 11, with 20 per cent of children now living with the condition compared to just 7 per cent in the 1970s.

According to the Royal College of Physicians, one in three 13 to 14-year-old children report symptoms of asthma, 9 per cent have eczema and 40 per cent have allergic rhinitis. Between 1990 and 2001 in England hospital admission rates for anaphylaxis rose sevenfold and there was a 500 per cent increase in food allergies. Cases of skin rashes (urticaria) doubled and hospital admissions for allergic swelling (angio-oedema) rose by 70 per cent.

As for asthma, a recent survey by the European Commission showed that the UK has the highest rate of asthma in the EU. According to an Asthma UK report in 2005, Wales, with 260,000 asthmatics, is top of the world league.

Top five allergy and asthma myths

1 Some dog breeds, such as Chihuahuas, are better for people with asthma and allergies

REALITY: it's the protein in the pet's saliva, dander and urine that causes allergies, not the hair. Since all dogs have dander, saliva and urine, there are no particular breeds that are better for people with asthma and allergies.

2 Asthma can be cured

REALITY: there is no cure for asthma. However, with the proper diagnosis and treatment, people with asthma can lead normal, active lives with little disturbance to quality of life.

3 Moving to a different area will cure asthma and allergies

REALITY: moving to the coast or an upland area may relieve allergies for a few months but new allergies – to new local plants, for instance – can develop within a short period. Moving house does not offer an escape from allergies and asthma.

4 Children outgrow asthma

REALITY: asthma is a chronic state of hyper-responsiveness. Some children have asthma symptoms that clear up during adolescence, while others worsen, but the tendency towards over-sensitive airways remains. Unfortunately, there is no way to predict a child's clinical progress.

5 Allergies are a harmless problem

REALITY: allergies are serious and should be treated effectively. Left untreated, they may lead to poorer quality of life, including impaired sleep and learning ability and absences from school and work. Untreated allergies may also result in chronic respiratory problems, such as asthma and sinusitis, and skin disorders such as eczema and urticaria (hives). Some allergies, such as those to foods, drugs and insect stings, may even lead to life-threatening anaphylaxis – an allergic reaction affecting major body systems that can be fatal.

Compared with 30 years ago, the weekly incidence of asthma episodes in the UK is now three to four times higher in adults and six times higher in children. Death rates from asthma in the UK have not fallen greatly over the past 20 years and the decline in the death rate appears to be slowing despite medical advances during this time that have improved the management and treatment of asthma.

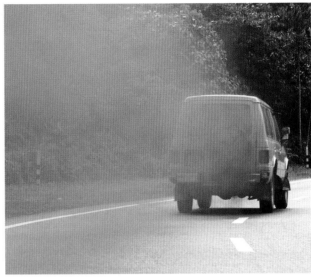

The worrying thing about this boom in allergies and asthma is that no one really knows why it is happening. There are plenty of theories. Some blame it on genetics, but while genetics play a role in asthma and allergies, our genetic traits change far too slowly to account for such a sudden increase. And some allergic reactions, such as those produced by plants, dyes, metals and chemicals, have no genetic basis. Other theories include:

If airborne waste from car exhausts boosts allergic responses, as Japanese research suggests, the UK's bid to cut emissions could have a very positive effect.

▍ **We are spending more time indoors** and are thus exposed to more indoor allergens and air pollutants.

▍ **Our world is too clean,** preventing our immune systems from doing their jobs properly (see 'Are we too clean?' on page 18).

▍ **An epidemic increase in obesity rates,** coupled with a dramatic drop in fruit and vegetable consumption, is playing havoc with our immune systems.

▍ **Airborne waste materials from fossil fuel combustion** (for example, exhaust fumes from cars and other vehicles, or smoke from factories and power plants) could be affecting the mucous membranes in the lungs and nose, boosting allergic responses, Japanese research suggests.

▍ **Complications during pregnancy,** particularly those related to the uterus, such as pre-eclampsia, haemorrhage after birth or pre-term contractions, could be resulting in a higher risk of allergies and asthma for the children born of those pregnancies.

▍ **Immune system defects** resulting in allergies and asthma are set early in life, probably in the foetal stage, and are locked into one's 'immunological memory', researchers say. In recent years, scientists have mapped several allergy-asthma genes, finding that genes do play a role in determining who will develop asthma but also how severe the disease will be once it develops.

Yet despite decades of research and data, a report issued in March 2002 found that researchers were no closer to understanding the roots of the asthma epidemic than they were when it first began 20 years earlier. They are hampered by the absence of a standardized system for monitoring trends, as well as flawed and inconclusive data.

The very complexity of diseases such as asthma and allergies also makes it difficult to identify a cause or causes. In fact, it's quite likely that there is no single disease called 'asthma' but rather multiple diseases that fall within the realm of asthma, just as there are multiple forms of headache. Also, as with any complex chronic disease, such as heart disease, diabetes or arthritis, there will never be a single cause or only one treatment. Instead, as we learn more about the genetics of individuals, it's likely that treatments will become more individualized.

Defining allergies and asthma

Whether it's a pollen, dust mite or pet dander allergy, a life-threatening food allergy, disfiguring and endlessly itching eczema, or chest-tightening asthma, these are all real diseases, not simply irritating annoyances that will go away if you stop thinking about them. Yet that is how they were once viewed; in the past, some doctors believed that allergies and asthma were conditions of the mind caused by anxiety or even hysteria. Today we know they are the result of biochemical changes involving your immune system, the environment and your genes. We will cover that in more detail in later chapters.

Allergies and asthma are two different diseases but they are often linked, and asthma may have a strong allergic component. The name for the close connection between the two is allergic airway syndrome, or rhinobronchitis. Although allergies may contribute to asthma (about 80 per cent of people with asthma also have allergies, and people with allergies are three times more likely than those without to develop asthma), asthma doesn't cause, or even contribute to, allergies. Often, people with allergies have no symptoms of asthma, but if they are exposed to cold air, exercise or infection, they show significant bronchial 'hyper-responsiveness', or asthma-like symptoms. They don't have asthma per se, but their lungs do have a greater tendency to react to these situations in an asthma-like manner than those of someone who has no allergies.

Researchers suspect several reasons for the close relationship between allergies and asthma.

Similar anatomy The microscopic anatomy of the tissues in the nose and lungs are almost identical, with very similar cells. Both are exposed to the same allergens and irritants, and they respond similarly.

How the respiratory system works

While the process of respiration sounds simple – provide your body with oxygen and rid your body of carbon dioxide – it is quite complex. Here are the key elements of the respiratory system and what they do.

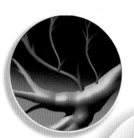

TERMINAL BRONCHIOLES Like the tiny twigs that provide nourishment to the leaves of a giant tree, these ultra-thin branches are the last in a line of bronchial tubes that transport gases to and from the alveoli.

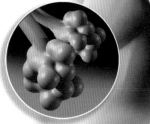

ALVEOLI These clusters of hollow sacs are where oxygen and carbon dioxide are exchanged between the lungs and the bloodstream.

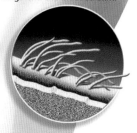

CILIA Millions of these tiny hairs line the respiratory tract. Beating at between 12 and 16 strokes per second, they create waves that move germ-catching mucus up and out of the lungs.

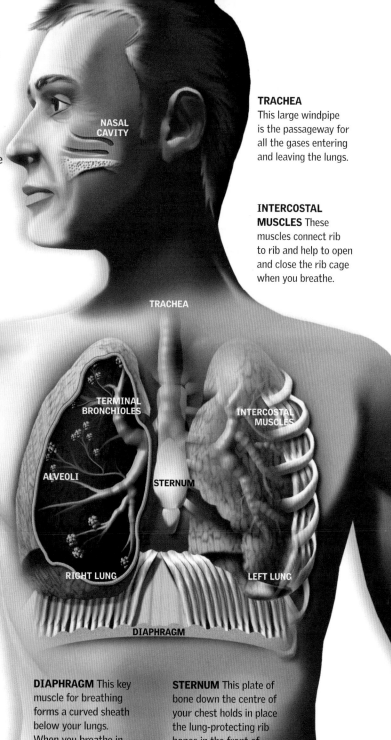

NASAL CAVITY

TRACHEA

TERMINAL BRONCHIOLES

ALVEOLI

STERNUM

INTERCOSTAL MUSCLES

RIGHT LUNG

LEFT LUNG

DIAPHRAGM

TRACHEA This large windpipe is the passageway for all the gases entering and leaving the lungs.

INTERCOSTAL MUSCLES These muscles connect rib to rib and help to open and close the rib cage when you breathe.

DIAPHRAGM This key muscle for breathing forms a curved sheath below your lungs. When you breathe in, your diaphragm drops, increasing the size of your lungs.

STERNUM This plate of bone down the centre of your chest holds in place the lung-protecting rib bones in the front of your body.

Are we too clean?

Although no one knows why the incidence of allergies and asthma is skyrocketing, a leading theory holds that our world (at least the Western world) is simply too clean. Some researchers call this the hygiene hypothesis. One researcher, Dr Marc E. Rothenberg PhD, section chief of allergy and clinical immunology at the Children's Hospital Medical Center of Cincinnati, calls it the delinquency theory, based on the notion that the immune system has so little to do that it turns into a kind of physiological juvenile delinquent, itching to get into trouble.

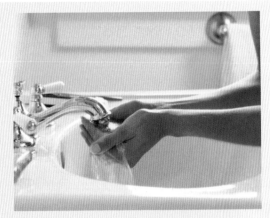

It is a much-studied hypothesis. Since 1997, scientists have published more than 6,000 research reports examining the apparent links between civilized living and allergies and asthma.

The problem stems from the tremendous advances we have made in the past 50 years in combating infectious diseases, parasites and other pathogens. With vaccines eliminating many previously common childhood diseases, antibiotics vanquishing others, and our enthusiasm for cleanliness (just think about the tremendous explosion in sales of antibacterial wipes, soaps and lotions), a germ doesn't stand a chance.

This means that the immune system is left twiddling its virtual thumbs. Its entire function is to recognize the difference between 'self' and foreign bodies. Self is fine, and some foreign bodies (such as HIV and the common cold virus) are bad. Yet many foreign bodies you come in contact with (such as the hundreds of food proteins you eat and

■ **The nasal-bronchial reflex** Nerve fibres originating in the upper airway connect to the lungs, allowing allergic reactions in the nose to cause a reflex in the lungs.

■ **Nasal blockage resulting in increased mouth breathing** This, in turn, means that air taken in is not warmed or filtered as it is when it's breathed through the nose, possibly triggering spasms as it moves into the lungs.

■ **Postnasal drip of inflammatory material** Inflammatory chemicals commonly found in the noses of people with allergic rhinitis drip into the lungs while they sleep, causing asthma to worsen.

As we said, however, allergies and asthma are two different conditions. So let's start with allergies. Simply put, if you have allergies, you have a hyper-sensitive immune system, one that responds entirely inappropriately to things such as plant pollen, other grasses and weeds, certain foods, latex, insect bites or certain drugs, all of which are known as allergens.

The most common of these allergic conditions is allergic rhinitis, which is an inflammation of mucous membranes that occurs when allergens touch the lining of the nose. Allergic rhinitis is characterized by sneezing, congestion, the thousands of molecules you breathe in daily) are also fine. The immune system has to learn at an early age how to distinguish the good foreign bodies from the bad, just as a toddler has to learn what 'hot' means. One way in which the immune system does this is through its encounters with endotoxins, molecules that occur naturally in every bacterium's outer envelope and are released into the environment whenever bacteria die.

The fewer endotoxins your immune system encounters in childhood, the less likely it will learn that important distinction. Instead, it may simply start attacking *all* foreign bodies – as well as your own body. The result is diseases ranging from allergies and asthma to autoimmune conditions such as multiple sclerosis and rheumatoid arthritis.

Some evidence supporting this theory can be found in the disparate rates of allergy and asthma within a country. In studies in Europe and the USA people living in rural and farm homes tended to have far less atopy (genetic risk of allergies) and asthma, even though they had much higher exposure to endotoxins from living near animals. For instance, a study in Basel, Switzerland showed that children of part-time farmers had a 76 per cent higher risk of hay fever and other allergies than those of full-time farmers, suggesting that greater exposure to the farm environment can be more protective. Another study of asthma prevalence in children living on the Pacific atolls of Tokelau and in Tokelauan children living in New Zealand, a more modern environment, found that only 11 per cent of the children living on the atolls had asthma, compared with 25 per cent of Tokelauan children in New Zealand.

Several recent studies showing that children who have pets when they're young are less likely to develop allergies when they're older lends credence to the theory.

Obviously, this doesn't mean you should send your children out to the woods and let them fend for themselves, but maybe you could consider allowing them a pet (see page 45). Remember, a little dirt won't kill them – and it may even help.

itching and dripping of the nose, and itchy, watery eyes. It can be seasonal; this condition affects up to 25 per cent of adults and up to 40 per cent of children in the UK – or it may be perennial, meaning that it never goes away.

Not sure if you have allergies? Well, if you're constantly sneezing, sniffling and clearing your throat, if your head feels stuffed full, if the skin under your eyes looks as if you've been in a brawl, or if the sight of peanuts can make your skin break out in hives, you probably do. Allergies are rarely fatal, and the handful of deaths that occur each year are from food, medication or insect allergies, not from the most common type of allergic rhinitis. You'll learn much more about rhinitis and find a questionnaire to help you to diagnose the condition, in chapter 3.

Asthma, on the other hand, can make you really ill extremely quickly. A chronic – meaning long-term – disease of the pulmonary system, or lungs, it is made worse by that overactive immune system. Symptoms include coughing, wheezing and shortness of breath. During an asthma attack, the airways (bronchial tubes) in your lungs react to some stimulus, or trigger. They become inflamed and produce more mucus than usual. At the same time, the muscles around the airways tighten, making it difficult to breathe. People with asthma

Blame it on Mum

Are you wondering whether you have allergies? Ask your mother when she started menstruating. Researchers in Finland reviewed a study of 5,000 pregnant women who had been asked when they began to menstruate. They then gave the women's now-30-something children allergy tests for various types of grasses and house dust mites. They found that mothers whose periods started when they were younger than 12 were almost 1.5 times more likely to have children who later developed allergies than those who started menstruating at 16. Why? Well, the researchers don't really know, but they do have their theories. One is that differences in the maternal oestrogen environment, which manifested itself in the varying ages of menstruation, somehow programmed the immune systems of the foetuses.

describe an attack as feeling as if they are 'breathing through a straw' or are drowning. In a sense, they *are* drowning as their airways squeeze shut and their lungs become starved of air. Although there is no cure for asthma, it can be treated and controlled. You'll learn more about asthma in chapter 4.

Both allergies and asthma can strike regardless of sex, race, socio-economic status and overall health. They don't care if you're an 8-stone weakling or a professional football player. You can develop allergies and asthma in childhood or in your sixties, and in rural or urban areas. However there is evidence that, your age, sex, race and socio-economic status may play a role in both your *risk* of developing these diseases and in their severity.

For instance, research carried out at Edinburgh University among three ethnic groups found that black people had only slightly higher rates of asthma than white people, but were twice as likely to have hospital admissions because of it. The study also showed that south Asian children had the fewest asthma symptoms, and diagnosis rates among black people were almost double those of Asian people.

Possible reasons for the disparity in results include differences in the way that ethnic groups used health services and a lack of understanding about asthma and about self-management of the condition that led to south Asians being more likely to seek medical help only at crisis point.

Recent figures suggest that women are about three times more likely than men to have severe asthma and are more often admitted to hospital because of their condition. Throughout childhood, asthma is generally more common in boys than in girls. This trend reverses during puberty, when more girls develop asthma for the first time, and by the age of 18 asthma is more common in girls. However, a 2005 study at Aberdeen University found that girls and boys were equally likely to suffer from the condition.

After this brief description of *what* asthma and allergies are, it's time to think about the *whys*. What is going on in your body that can make something as simple as a grain of pollen wreak so much havoc? You'll find out in chapter 2.

Chapter two

Why your
immune
system falters

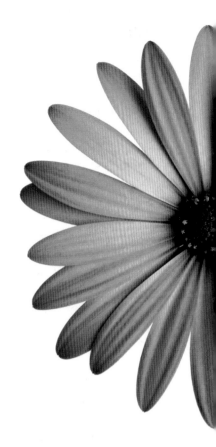

When it comes to the causes of allergies and asthma, you can forget the usual suspects. They are not infectious diseases, so viruses and bacteria can't be blamed. Nor can you blame working too hard, standing in the rain, eating too much fat, or being attractive to mosquitoes.

Instead, blame yourself – or more specifically, your immune system, the same one that is designed to protect you from harm. When you have allergies or asthma, it acts like a cat on speed: hyperalert to any potential invader, seeing enemies where it should see friends, and ready to fly into action at the slightest provocation or even a peaceful interaction.

To understand why your immune system sometimes goes into overdrive you first need to understand how things are *supposed* to work.

The guardian of health

If you have read anything about the immune system, you have doubtless seen it portrayed as a miniature army that is constantly on the defence against attack, equipping its 'soldiers' with the weapons necessary to fight evil germs, and

What's the difference between atopy and allergy?

If your doctor says you are atopic, it doesn't mean you're losing your hair or your train of thought. Atopy is simply a genetic predisposition to some forms of allergy or, more specifically, to produce IgE in response to certain allergens. It classically comprises asthma, allergic rhinitis and eczema – not food and drug hypersensitivities, for which there isn't the same kind of genetic predisposition.

To put it another way, someone who is allergic reacts adversely to exposure to allergens; someone who is atopic is genetically predisposed to developing allergies. Thus, you can be atopic without being allergic. People with an atopic tendency are simply more at risk of other allergies, such as latex allergy (for which there are numerous risk factors), than someone without atopy.

How do you find out if you are atopic? The simplest way is to consult your mother – or your father, brother or sister, aunts, uncles and cousins. If they had any form of allergy, you are probably atopic. In this case, you should follow the Breathe Easy Plan in part 3 – even if you haven't yet developed any full-blown allergies. It may reduce your exposure to common allergens enough to prevent your immune system from becoming hypersensitive.

always girding itself in readiness for battle. You can almost feel tiny spears being thrown around inside your body.

The reality is far less warlike. A better analogy would be the security operation at a busy airport. Here's the reason why. With every breath you take, with every bite of food you eat, with every touch on your skin, your body encounters and processes millions of foreign cells and alien molecules. As with the tens of thousands of people passing through airport corridors each day, the vast majority of substances passing through your body are welcome and harmless. But every now and then something harmful slips through – an airborne virus, a splinter in your finger, an unseen bit of mould on a piece of bread. A well-functioning immune system, using a broad array of covert tactics and screens, identifies and disposes of unwelcome substances, usually unnoticed by the rest of your body.

Just as for airport security, the greatest challenge for the body's immune system is discriminating between the good and the bad. Maintaining that ability to discriminate is crucial. A weak immune system can allow viruses and bacteria to proliferate inside your body or make healing from injury difficult and slow. That is why diseases that suppress immunity, such as AIDS, are so dangerous.

At the other extreme, an overactive immune system is also problematic. An overactive immune system can attack the very thing that it is supposed to protect – you. For example, rheumatoid arthritis is a disease in which your immune system attacks one or more of your joints. An overactive immune system can also view foreign bodies that are generally safe and benign, such as the proteins in food, as potential terrorists that need to be eliminated. It is this state that you have to worry about with allergies and, to a lesser extent, asthma. Understanding how the body's immune system differentiates between welcome and unwelcome cells is the key to understanding the causes of allergies and asthma. That's what we'll explain in the following section.

Telling self from non-self

The immune system operates on one fundamental truth: there is 'self' and there is 'non-self'. Ideally, immune system cells go after only non-self molecules, such as bacteria, viruses, fungi, parasites and even tumours, and leave self cells, such as nerve, muscle and brain cells, alone. In most cases, that is exactly what happens.

The immune system knows which are 'good' cells and which are 'bad' cells because the surface of every cell in your body sports special proteins called human leukocyte antigens, or HLAs. Immune cells also identify intruders by characteristic shapes, called epitopes, that protrude from them. Think of HLAs and epitopes as a cell's ID badge, proclaiming its right to be in your body – or its alien nature. As immune cells circulate, looking for foreign bodies to eliminate, they are constantly scanning the landscape for any HLAs they don't recognize. If they see a cell without the appropriate identification, a complex series of events begins, eventually ending with the destruction of the invader.

These intruders include everything from the bacteria and viruses mentioned above to grains of pollen. Even chemicals, drugs and particles (such as latex powder) count as foreign. They are all called antigens, and they're the alarm bells that startle the immune cells into action.

The cells doing the detect-and-destroy work are white blood cells. Millions of them circulate in blood and tissues, helping to defend your body from infection. There are five main types.

Lymphocytes Think of these cells as the surveillance team, constantly circulating throughout your body on the lookout for antigens. When they find any, they develop plans for attacking the invaders and convey those plans to other members of the immune system team. They also form the institutional memory of the immune system, storing those plans of attack on what amounts to a cellular hard drive, then calling it up again if the antigens reappear. There are two types of lymphocytes:

T lymphocytes, or T cells, secrete potent substances to attract the immune system cells that do the actual destruction work. Then they serve as a kind of cheerleading squad to keep the defence team at its job. Certain T cells do more than simply mark the antigens: they also attack and destroy diseased cells.

B lymphocytes, or B cells, are immune cells that actually produce antibodies, specialized fighter proteins that help your immune cells to do their job. B cells have long memories for their enemies and may remain in your body for years, ready at any time to turn into little antibody factories whenever an antigen that they recognize appears. This is how vaccination works. A tiny bit of a (usually) killed virus, or antigen, such as polio, measles or flu, is injected into your bloodstream, provoking your B cells to create antibodies. Then, if you ever encounter the fully functional form of the virus, your body can quickly marshal its defences and produce millions of the required antibodies without delay. If your B cells had never come across that particular antigen before, the antibody response would be much slower, and the intruder could gain the upper hand.

2 Macrophages These large cells engulf and destroy large particles such as bacteria or yeast.

3 Neutrophils The most numerous white blood cells, neutrophils are the first to arrive on the scene after an injury occurs. Their favourite food is bacteria and one neutrophil can eat about a dozen bacteria, destroying them with a substance similar to household bleach. The cells don't live long – about 12 hours – and if they eat their fill before then, they die sooner. Even in death, however, they have a mission to fulfil: releasing little chemical 'SOSs' that alert and attract more neutrophils.

4 Eosinophils These white blood cells secrete chemicals that trigger the inflammatory process (see page 26) and help to destroy foreign cells. They work together with lymphocytes and neutrophils, both of which release certain

---

The white blood cells

Circulating in your blood and scattered through all the tissues of your body is an army of defensive cells collectively known as white blood cells, or leukocytes. Their name is derived from their appearance under a microscope, which is colourless compared to the red blood cells with which they circulate in the bloodstream. Here are the five main types.

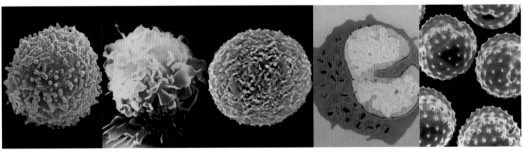

LYMPHOCYTES Found mostly in the lymphatic system, these search your body for cells that don't belong there and alert other cells to their presence.

MACROPHAGES These engulf and destroy large cells, such as bacteria or yeast, as well as the debris from natural cell formation in a growing body.

NEUTROPHILS The most common type of white blood cells in the bloodstream, they are first to appear at the site of an injury. Their job is to destroy unwelcome cells.

EOSINOPHILS These make up 4 per cent or less of active white blood cells. They attack larger cells, in part by secreting toxins that trigger inflammation.

BASOPHILS When they find damaged tissue, these cells release granules of germ-killing toxins and histamine, a substance that triggers inflammation.

substances that attract eosinophils to a particular site so they can release parasite-killing toxins. Eosinophils can play a big role in asthma. When they are called to a site during an allergic or asthmatic attack, they release toxins inappropriately, damaging the lining of air passages. Thus, one focus of asthma treatment is to stop eosinophils from accumulating in the lungs and prevent those already there from causing damage. That is the goal of steroid inhalers.

5 Basophils Also called granular leukocytes, these white blood cells are filled with granules of toxic chemicals that can digest micro-organisms. Basophils are also implicated in allergy attacks because, like eosinophils, they release a host of chemicals that contribute to the inflammatory response, including histamine (hence the use of *anti*histamines to treat allergies).

The lymphatic system

The immune system is much more than a mishmash of cells, however; it's a true system, with its own transportation network and rest stops, known as the lymphatic system. This pipeline of lymphatic vessels, similar to blood vessels, runs throughout your body. It collects lymph fluid from the spaces around cells and returns it to the bloodstream. Throughout this transportation network are way stations called lymph nodes – small, bean-shaped masses found in places such as your neck, groin and armpits. They are filled with lymphocytes and act as filters for the lymph fluid, removing micro-organisms and other pathogens so that the lymphatic cells can destroy them on the spot. That's why your neck and underarms feel tender when you are ill; the lymph nodes there are working overtime, filtering and destroying the antigens responsible for your illness.

The spleen is part of this system, functioning like a super-size lymph node. Lying in the upper left side of your abdominal cavity just under your diaphragm, it serves as a truck stop for immune cells, which wait there until they are required. It also filters blood, which is why, although you can manage quite well without a spleen (it is often injured in traumatic accidents and subsequently removed), you may be more prone to infections if your super-size filter is gone.

Your tonsils and adenoids, small organs found at the back of your throat, also play a role. They are the birthplace of phagocytes, immune cells that target bacteria that enter the mouth.

The third and final major player in the body's immune system is the thymus gland. Located just above and in front of your heart in the upper centre part of your chest, it acts like a boarding school for T lymphocytes, secreting a hormone that helps the T cells to mature into their different types.

Inflammation

Remember the two types of white blood cells called basophils and eosinophils? They're the immune cells that trigger the inflammatory reaction. Inflammation is a cornerstone of the immune system, but it can be a double-edged sword, especially when it comes to allergies and asthma.

Inflammation, in simple terms, is what happens when a part of your body swells and heats up. It is your body's response to a host of insults: invasion by bacteria or viruses, injury or reaction to your own tissues. When tissues are injured, they and the cells that flock to the injury release a barrage of chemicals, including histamine, bradykinin, serotonin and others. These chemicals cause blood vessels to leak fluid into the tissues, leading to swelling, redness and heat. This in turn throws a kind of barrier around the foreign substance, preventing

How inflammation works

To most of us, 'inflammation' means that a body part has become red, hot and swollen. That is true, but the fascinating story lies in the 'how' and 'why'. In fact, inflammation is your body's rapid response mechanism for repairing tissue that is injured or infected.

1 A foreign body (germ, splinter or allergen) is detected by white blood cells, which release several chemicals to launch a healing response.

2 Small blood vessels near the site leak fluid (causing swelling) and other white blood cells (which attack the foreign body). In addition, blood flow to the area increases, causing it to redden and heat up.

3 Tissue damage and signals from white blood cells trigger nerve pain receptors, increasing the pain of the injury. The aim is to dissuade you from using the injured body part until it heals.

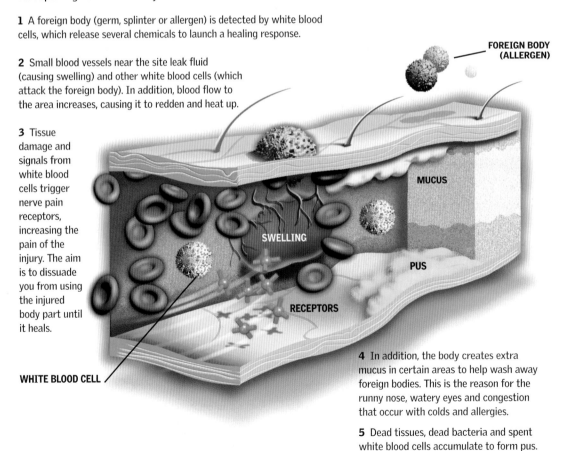

FOREIGN BODY (ALLERGEN)

MUCUS

SWELLING

PUS

RECEPTORS

WHITE BLOOD CELL

4 In addition, the body creates extra mucus in certain areas to help wash away foreign bodies. This is the reason for the runny nose, watery eyes and congestion that occur with colds and allergies.

5 Dead tissues, dead bacteria and spent white blood cells accumulate to form pus.

it from escaping into the body and infecting other tissues. The chemicals also attract white blood cells that 'eat' the foreign substance as well as dead or damaged cells. The pus that often forms after an injury, then, is a mixture of dead tissue, dead bacteria and live and dead macrophages.

Inflammation also increases mucus secretions, resulting in the runny nose, watery eyes and congestion that are associated with allergic reactions. It can also cause the smooth muscles of your airways to constrict, resulting in the tightening sensation and gasping for air so common during an asthma attack. Inflammation is usually a beneficial healing process but, when it continues unabated, problems develop because it can harm tissues.

Understanding antibodies

Now on to the antibodies, bringing us closer to how this whole system fits with allergies and asthma. As noted earlier, the white blood cells known as B lymphocytes secrete proteins called antibodies. Your blood contains more than 1 *trillion* antibodies, and with every new threat – even previously unseen viruses such as the one responsible for severe acute respiratory syndrome (SARS) in the winter of 2003 – the B cells secrete new forms of antibodies. Most antibodies don't actually destroy the foreign invaders; they latch onto them and mark them in some way so other immune system cells can do the dirty work, or they send out chemical signals calling other white blood cells to action.

Antibodies are made up of chains of molecules that form a Y shape. The sections that make up the tips of the Y's arms vary greatly from one antibody to another; this is called the variable region. It develops a unique shape based on that of the antigen it was created to react to, so that it can 'lock' onto that antigen just like a key fitting into a lock. Sometimes this locking neutralizes the antigen, thereby rendering it harmless; sometimes it ruptures the cells of the foreign body; and sometimes it forces antigens to clump together, creating a sitting-duck target for other immune cells to attack.

Your blood contains 1 trillion Y-shaped chains of molecules called antibodies and with every new threat encountered, your immune system creates new antibodies.

The stem of the Y links the antibody to the white blood cells that may be required to destroy the pathogen. This stem is identical in all antibodies of the same class and is called the constant region.

There are five classes of antibodies, each with a slightly different function and operating method. Scientists call them immunoglobulins, or Igs for short.

Of the five, IgE is the one we could call the 'allergy antibody', since IgE antibodies are the main culprits contributing to allergies. Normally, they are present in tiny quantities in the body and are produced in response to relatively large invaders, such as parasites like ringworm and fluke. That is one reason why allergies are far less prevalent in less developed parts of the world and why some researchers think our predilection for cleanliness has gone too far. They theorize that when people come into contact with these parasites, IgE goes out and does its job. If it never gets a chance to do its job, it begins to behave erratically. Instead of attacking parasites as it is supposed to do, it starts to attack proteins and molecules that it *should* recognize as perfectly harmless, such as dust and peanuts and pollen.

When that happens, the IgE binds the allergen molecule either to basophils – the white blood cells described earlier – or to cells called mast cells, which are found in the mucous linings of tissues throughout the body, such as the mouth, throat, nose, lungs, skin or intestinal tract. This binding triggers the mast cells or basophils to release large amounts of inflammatory chemicals, such as histamine, prostaglandins and leukotrienes.

A brief summary

Are you getting confused? Here's a crib sheet on the science of allergies, as described in this chapter.

A White blood cells are a major component of the immune system. These cells float freely in the bloodstream, seeking out and destroying viruses, bacteria and other things that shouldn't be there.

B There are five types of white blood cells.

- Lymphocytes
- Macrophages
- Neutrophils
- Eosinophils
- Basophils

C There are two main types of lymphocytes: T cells and B cells.

D B-lymphocytes create antibodies, which are proteins that latch onto pathogens, marking them for destruction by the other white blood cells.

E There are five types of antibodies: IgA, IgD, IgG, IgM and IgE.

F IgE is the antibody involved in allergic reactions. It binds to mast cells in moist tissues in the body, sensitizing them to an allergen. When the allergen comes along, it interacts with the IgE antibody, which then prompts the mast cell to release chemicals that cause the allergic reaction.

G Basophils and eosinophils are also involved in allergic reactions. These white blood cells, like the mast cells, release chemicals that also contribute to the inflammatory reaction.

H The result is an allergy attack: coughing, runny nose, itchy eyes, and so on.

It is these chemicals – not the actual dust mites or cat dander – that are responsible for the miserable coughing, wheezing, runny nose, itchy eyes and itchy skin of an allergy attack. Because the mast cells are constantly calling up new recruits in the form of additional basophils and eosinophils, the attack can continue long after the allergen has been removed. In fact, one way that doctors screen for allergies is to measure the levels of IgE and eosinophils in your blood; if they are high and you haven't just returned from Africa or some other place where you could have been infected with parasites, the likelihood is that you have allergies.

How allergies happen

The immune system can fail – and fail quite spectacularly, at that – in three main ways.

First, there's the failure most people are familiar with: weakened immunity. This is what occurs as a result of chronic, or long-term, illness. For example, cancer (as well as cancer treatments) can greatly weaken your immune system.

Stress also weakens immunity. It turns out that the very chemicals released when you're under stress, such as adrenaline, are the same chemicals that keep your immune system in check so it doesn't get out of control. If you're under the kind of chronic, grinding stress that comes with a job you hate, money issues, too many deadlines, problems with your children, an overcommitted life or concerns about relationships, your body releases these chemicals non-stop. They in turn suppress your immune system, leading to a host of problems, ranging from colds and other viruses to cancer and heart disease.

HIV, which causes AIDS, also suppresses the immune system. The virus does this by deliberately attacking certain T cells, causing vulnerablity to numerous infections from very basic pathogens that we live with all the time. People with AIDS eventually die not from the virus itself but from some ancillary disease that has taken advantage of their weakened immune systems.

The second category of immune system failure is overactivity. Autoimmune diseases such as multiple sclerosis, Crohn's disease, lupus and Type 1 diabetes fall into this category. These diseases occur because the immune system fails to recognize 'self' cells as safe and attacks them as invaders. In Crohn's disease, for instance, it attacks cells in the gut; in diabetes, it kills off insulin-producing cells in the pancreas; and in multiple sclerosis, it attacks the coatings of nerves.

The third category of immune system breakdown is the one that results in allergies and asthma. It has some characteristics of overactive immunity in that the immune system reacts to the wrong thing. Instead of attacking your own cells, though, it attacks normally harmless molecules such as food proteins and

Inside an allergic reaction

Allergens are foreign substances that are not harmful to your body but which your immune system has learned to attack anyhow. Once an allergen is detected by your immune system, a fast but complicated process begins that leads to the sneezing, congestion and other symptoms of allergies.

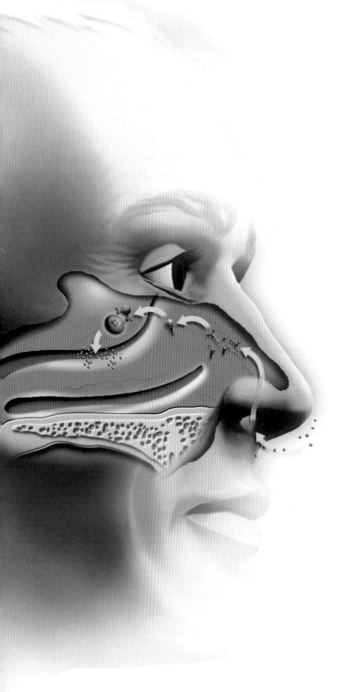

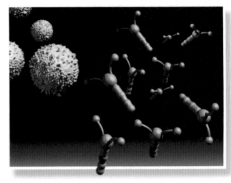

1 Initial exposure to an allergen causes your body to create Y-shaped antibodies unique to that allergen. These antibodies then stay in your body, ready to pounce if the allergen shows up again.

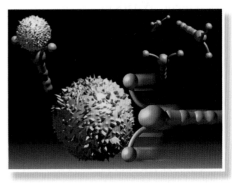

2 On the next exposure to the allergen (which could occur years or even decades later), the antibodies discover it and immediately lock onto it.

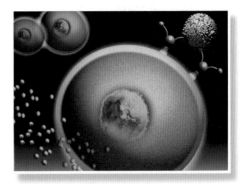

3 The antibodies then attach to a mast cell lining your nose, throat, lungs or elsewhere, which in turn triggers the release of inflammatory chemicals. The inflammatory process begins, with swelling, creation of mucus, reddening, heat and vessel constriction – and there's your allergic reaction.

pollens in an overreaction that is tantamount to using a fire hose to put out a match.

Most people with allergies have some genetic predisposition to them, a code deep within their ancestral material that presents the *possibility* of allergies or asthma. But just because you have a genetic recipe for a condition doesn't always mean you will develop that condition, and with allergies and asthma it takes the right environment to provide the final ingredient. What's more, you can develop an allergy even with no genetic predisposition if you are exposed to the substance frequently enough. For instance, latex allergies have risen quite steeply since the 1980s, when the AIDS epidemic resulted in health care providers and emergency personnel using dozens of latex gloves a week to protect against all body fluid encounters.

Beyond the usual allergies

Although the majority of allergies are provoked through the IgE-mediated response, called Type I response, there are three other hypersensitivity immune responses.

- **Cytotoxic reactions (Type II)** This type of hypersensitivity involves cell destruction, particularly red blood cells and platelets, which can affect the ability of your blood to clot. These reactions typically occur with mismatched blood transfusions.

- **Immune complex reactions (Type III)** This type of reaction often occurs three weeks or so after you have taken the final dose of a drug such as penicillin, and it plays a role in the development of autoimmune diseases. With a Type III reaction, you usually feel as if you have flu, with fever, skin rashes, hives and swollen, tender lymph nodes. It can result in lung or kidney damage.

- **Cell-mediated reactions (Type IV)** This type of reaction results in allergic contact dermatitis, a skin rash that occurs when you touch something to which you are allergic. More on that in chapter 14.

The allergic response works like this. An initial exposure to an allergen, such as pollen, dust mites, pet dander or shrimp protein, causes your body to increase production of IgE. Each IgE is specific to an allergen; therefore, a person with multiple allergies will have different IgEs for each allergen. The IgEs stick to mast cells or basophils, thus sensitizing you to a particular allergen.

This initial exposure could happen years before an allergy actually occurs – even in the womb. Some researchers suspect that peanut consumption by pregnant or breastfeeding women could be a major reason for the growing number of peanut allergies in US children. When they start eating peanut butter at age two or three, the reaction is triggered. Or a child who is stung by a bee may have no allergic reaction until she is stung again, a year later. Or perhaps you've been overexposed to penicillin. One day, you get a throat infection and your doctor again prescribes penicillin. This time it is the final straw, tipping your sensitivity into a full-blown allergy.

When this happens, the IgE molecules go wild. Now they recognize the allergen as a foreign substance, lock onto it in that lock-and-key manner, and tie it to a mast cell or basophil, which in turn triggers the release of inflammatory chemicals such as histamine, prostaglandins and leukotrienes and leads to symptoms such as bronchial constriction, coughing and wheezing.

That initial reaction is called the early phase reaction. It can be followed several hours later by another reaction (late phase) in which chemicals released by the mast cells send out another call for inflammatory cells (basophils and eosinophils). In some people with perennial allergies, the tissue never returns to normal and can be inflamed and sensitized even by a trigger such as cigarette smoke or perfume (to which you don't have an actual *allergy*).

Allergic reactions are usually localized – that is, they happen right at the spot in which the allergen is detected. Get an allergen on your skin, and your skin reacts. Get an allergen such as pollen in your nose, and your nasal lining becomes inflamed.

However, if an allergic reaction is severe enough to occur throughout your body, you get anaphylaxis (see page 274), in which your entire body goes into shock. This is a potentially deadly situation that can be halted only with emergency doses of adrenaline, which puts the brakes on the immune reaction.

Putting it all together

So what does all this have to do with asthma? A lot, as it turns out. Although asthma is defined more as a respiratory condition than an immune system disorder, it has its roots in the immune system. For instance, an initial 'trigger' in asthma may be the release of inflammatory chemicals from the immune system. These cells lead to the production of too much mucus and increase the responsiveness of the smooth muscles in the airways, making them more likely to close up.

Asthma is a chronic, or long term, condition, as you'll discover in chapter 4. Asthma attacks are only the acute phase of the disease. For all that we *do* know today about the role of the immune system in asthma and allergies, there is still more that we *don't* know about these diseases, particularly asthma.

Ironically, the devastating AIDS epidemic has had one silver lining. It has resulted in an explosion of knowledge and understanding about the immune system. That understanding is leading to new treatments for everything from cancer to allergies and may well change the very nature of how we diagnose and treat these diseases.

The next three chapters explain the nature and treatment of allergic rhinitis, the most common form of allergy; asthma; and one of the most dangerous forms of allergy – food allergies. As you read through those chapters, this brief explanation of the immune system should prove useful background knowledge.

Chapter **three**

All about
allergies

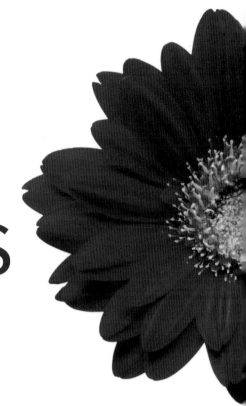

You're sneezing, your throat is scratchy and your eyes itch. Or you have a strange rash on your arms that just won't go away. Or raised red wheals have appeared on your chest and back. Or every time you eat prawns, your lips and mouth swell and you begin wheezing.

All of these are symptoms of allergies. In fact, as you'll discover in this book, the forms and types of allergy are many and varied. Later, you'll learn more about some of the less common types, such as food, insect, medication and skin allergies. This chapter focuses on the form of allergy responsible for the greatest misery in the most people: allergic rhinitis, often in the form of hay fever.

Allergic rhinitis usually becomes apparent before the age of 20, but it can develop at any age. In fact, it may be diagnosed as early as the first year of life. Today the condition affects 40 per cent of children and 10 to 25 per cent of adults. Its prevalence has almost tripled in the past 20 years, and it accounts for some 3 per cent of all GP consultations.

At one time, allergic rhinitis was viewed as nothing more than an annoyance, not really worth treating seriously and certainly not capable of inflicting the kind of economic and physical toll that we now know it does. In recent decades it has been recognized that the condition is associated with several other respiratory illnesses, including asthma, and that it can significantly affect your ability to work or study. In fact, a survey conducted in 2005 by the European Federation of Allergy and Airway Diseases Patients' Associations confirmed that the condition has a substantial effect on people's lives, with 92 per cent of patients saying that they suffer symptoms for more than two months a year. Half of the patients said their symptoms affect their school and work moderately to severely; three quarters said that it limits their choice of outdoor activities; and 85 per cent reported that their symptoms disrupt their sleep.

The survey also showed that not all allergic rhinitis is the same. Of those surveyed, seven in ten people suffer symptoms for at least four days a week, that last for at least four consecutive weeks. These people experience far worse symptoms and allergic rhinitis has a far greater impact on their daily life and emotional well-being.

'The message to sufferers of allergic rhinitis is clear,' says Dr Erika Valovirta, the association's medical committee co-ordinator. 'Visit your doctor for a proper diagnosis and for prescription medicines, which should be taken as directed at the right dose and the right frequency. That way people get the maximum benefit. In addition, while decreasing exposure to allergens is a sensible step, it should be undertaken in conjunction with a doctor's diagnosis and advice.'

The allergy ripple effect

The primary symptom of allergic rhinitis is a stuffed and/or runny nose. This is due to inflammation of the nasal lining; if it persists, the moist, damp environment provides the perfect breeding ground for viruses and bacteria, which can lead to many other problems, such as ear infections, sinus infections (sinusitis) and asthma. If you are prone to sinus infections, ask your GP if you might have allergies.

Sinusitis affects 15 per cent of the UK population. It is defined as an inflammation of the lining of the nasal sinuses, the hollow cavities within the cheekbones around your eyes and behind your nose. It can make an allergy attack feel like the sniffles.

If you have sinusitis, the chances are you may also have a pounding headache, pressure behind your eyes and cheeks, toothache, green or grey nasal mucus or postnasal drip (secretion of mucus from the cavities at the back of your nose). You may also lose your sense of smell and taste and have bad breath, along with chronic congestion. About half of all people with sinusitis have allergies, and the theory is that

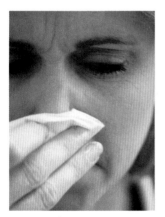

If you're prone to sinus infections ask your doctor to check you for allergies.

Can surgery help my sinusitis?

Chronic sinusitis affects 15 per cent of the UK population and often coexists with nasal polyps, which are estimated to affect one in 50 people. Both conditions reduce quality of life as symptoms include blocked nose, nasal discharge, facial pain and loss of smell and taste.

When medical treatment fails, or in cases of severe nasal obstruction, sinonasal surgery may be appropriate. To assess the effectiveness of such surgery, a national audit was set up with the Clinical Effectiveness Unit at the Royal College of Surgeons and ENT UK.

A survey of 3,128 patients who underwent sinonasal surgery in England and Wales during 2000 suggested that patients' symptoms improved following surgery, but deteriorated again slightly from three to 12 months. The majority of patients were satisfied with the results and, though many reported minor problems with bleeding after surgery, most returned to normal daily activities within two to three weeks. The rates of major complications were very low (0.26 per cent, with no long-term problems). Within a year of operation, around 8.6 per cent were awaiting or had already undergone further surgery for their sinonasal disease.

'One of the keys to preventing relapse of sinusitis,' comments Dr Chris Corrigan, senior lecturer in the Department of Respiratory Medicine & Allergy at Guy's Hospital, London, 'is to recognize and treat underlying allergic rhinitis.'

the allergies lead to the sinus infections. It works like this. Normally, mucus and liquids drain from the sinuses through tiny openings about the size of a tip of a pen. Swelling due to an allergy can block that drainage, resulting in a build-up of mucus and providing the conditions for bacteria or viruses to thrive.

If allergies are not treated, they can also lead to nasal polyps (pale, round outgrowths of the nasal lining) or swollen nasal turbinates (protruding tissues that line the inside of your nose). Sometimes surgery is needed to correct these problems. Untreated allergies can also cause dental and facial abnormalities, as described later, and can affect speech development in children.

In addition to the most common symptoms associated with allergic rhinitis – sneezing, runny nose and watery eyes – it often disturbs sleep, so people spend their days in a fog of fatigue. Consequently, their ability to think, study and process information is affected. They may also have difficulty remembering things, impaired hand-eye coordination and decreased capacity to make decisions. Some of these symptoms may be caused by over-the-counter allergy remedies and others by a lack of sleep.

If congestion blocks your ear canals, it can interfere with your hearing and affect learning and comprehension. Meanwhile, constantly blowing your nose and coughing can interrupt your concentration and ability to learn. But if you feel as if you're moving in slow motion and your brain has turned to cottonwool, don't worry. Once you have learned to control your allergies with our Breathe Easy Plan explained in part 3, you should regain your alertness.

Allergies can also affect your appearance. For instance, dark under-eye circles can make allergy sufferers look as if they've been out on the tiles for a string of late nights; these are actually caused by swollen blood vessels under the eyes. Also, because many people who suffer from allergies breathe through their mouths, they are more likely to develop a high, arched palate (roof of the mouth), an elevated upper lip and an overbite, which may require orthodontic work to correct. Then there's the nasal crease, a line across the lower part of the nose that forms from constantly rubbing it. Finally, allergy sufferers may look as if they are permanently tired, partly as a result of swollen adenoids, the lymph tissue that lines the back of the throat and extends behind the nose.

Other common symptoms are chronic coughing; wheezing or shortness of breath; conjunctivitis or red, swollen eyes; sore throat; frequent nosebleeds; postnasal drip; halitosis (bad breath); mouth ulcers; an itchy palate; stomach problems such as bloating, belching and heartburn; irritability and depression.

The trouble with allergies

When you think allergies, you usually think sneezing and wheezing. But allergies can affect your body in so many ways. Here are many of the possible affects, both short and long-term.

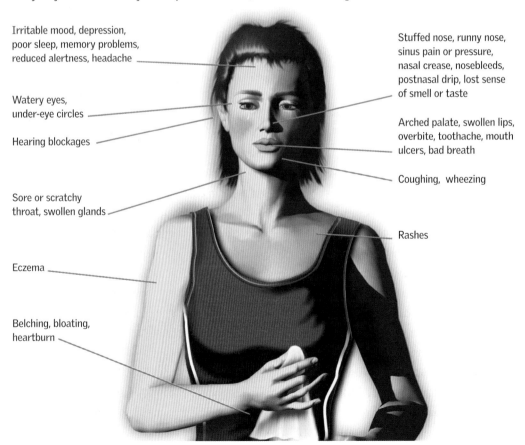

Irritable mood, depression, poor sleep, memory problems, reduced alertness, headache

Watery eyes, under-eye circles

Hearing blockages

Sore or scratchy throat, swollen glands

Eczema

Belching, bloating, heartburn

Stuffed nose, runny nose, sinus pain or pressure, nasal crease, nosebleeds, postnasal drip, lost sense of smell or taste

Arched palate, swollen lips, overbite, toothache, mouth ulcers, bad breath

Coughing, wheezing

Rashes

Allergy or irritation?

Just because your nose is running and you're sneezing, it doesn't mean that you have allergies. You could have a cold, sinusitis or a form of rhinitis that is not associated with allergies. *Rhinitis* is simply a medical term for the symptoms that result from nasal irritation, such as congestion or runniness. Although these symptoms can mimic allergic reactions they are not the result of the IgE immune response that occurs in allergies.

This is an important distinction. While your body may be irritated by any number of substances, an allergic response involves an immune system breakdown of a particular nature (described in detail in chapter 2). Some doctors believe that what many people consider to be allergies are often simply irritations caused by substances such as dust or smoke.

There are several different terms – sometimes overlapping – which medical experts use to describe rhinitis. If the condition lasts for less than six weeks, it is an acute attack, while persistent or recurring symptoms are called chronic. If symptoms usually appear only at one time of year, as in hay fever, the condition may be dubbed seasonal rhinitis, whereas symptoms that occur all year round are called perennial. Infectious rhinitis is caused by viruses or bacteria, such as when you have a cold, and can happen in anyone, whereas allergic rhinitis only occurs in people allergic to a particular substance, such as pollen or cat dander. Vasomotor rhinitis is a chronic form in which the membranes lining the nose are thickened and symptoms are provoked by factors such as a dry atmosphere, air pollution or medications.

Your nose normally produces mucus, which traps substances such as dust, pollen, pollution and germs. Mucus flows back from the front of your nose and drains down your throat. If there is too much mucus, it drains down the front of your nose, too, causing a runny nose. The more irritation, the more mucus your

What's your rhinitis type?

All allergic rhinitis is not created equal. Here are the three main types.

1 **Seasonal rhinitis** This is what we think of when we think of rhinitis – occurring at certain times of the year, primarily in the spring and autumn, when pollens (potent allergens) are at their peak. Although for you the timing of the allergy season depends on where you live, the climate and the season, that doesn't mean that moving will improve things. If you are prone to allergies, you'll probably simply become allergic to something else in your new environment.

2 **Perennial rhinitis** If you have perennial rhinitis, you have the dubious honour of being miserable all year round. It's likely that you are allergic to pet dander, dust mite and cockroach droppings, and mould – all allergy triggers that know no seasonality. You'll learn more about them later.

3 **Occupational rhinitis** Blame it on your job; that's what your doctor will do. Occupational rhinitis results from a sensitivity to something at work, be it a chemical, the plants in the lobby or the fibres in the carpet (but no, it's probably not the boss). If your symptoms occur only at work, improve or disappear at weekends and on holiday, or are shared by your colleagues, ask your doctor to consider that something at work is literally getting under your skin.

body produces in order to collect and dispose of the irritants. Rhinitis has many other causes, including temperature changes (your nose runs in cold weather), spicy food, certain medicines (including blood pressure drugs, birth control pills, aspirin and other drugs such as ibuprofen and naproxen), cigarette smoke, perfume, alcoholic drinks such as beer and wine, cleaning solutions and chlorine in swimming pools. Some people even become congested when sexually aroused.

Pinning the blame

You may be convinced that you are allergic to *something*. The question is, what? The only sure way to find out is with a skin or blood test, described in detail in chapter 6. Here we focus on the suspects responsible for allergic rhinitis. Bear in mind that you can be allergic to several of these triggers at the same time and that one allergy may disappear while another may come to take its place.

What's making my nose run?

You could be suffering from a cold. You could be encountering an irritant, such as smoke. Or you could possibly be having an allergic reaction. Here are questions to ask to find out whether your dripping nose is caused by nonallergic or allergic rhinitis.

1 Do you have a history of sneezing spells, itching of the nose and throat and a large amount of watery nasal discharge?   yes ☐   no ☐

2 Do you have a family history of allergies?   yes ☐   no ☐

3 Do your symptoms respond favourably to treatment with antihistamines?   yes ☐   no ☐

4 Do your symptoms get worse during certain times of the year, such as spring or autumn?   yes ☐   no ☐

5 Does exposure to animals such as cats or dogs cause nasal symptoms?   yes ☐   no ☐

Yes *answers to these questions are strongly suggestive of allergic rhinitis.*

1 Do you have fever and muscle or joint aches associated with your nasal symptoms?   yes ☐   no ☐

2 Do you have pain behind your eyes or above your upper teeth?   yes ☐   no ☐

3 Is your nasal drainage thick and/or discoloured (green or yellow)?   yes ☐   no ☐

4 Are any other members of your household ill at present?   yes ☐   no ☐

Yes *answers to these questions usually suggest infectious rhinitis.*

1 Are your nasal symptoms brought on by changes in temperature or humidity?   yes ☐   no ☐

2 Are you very sensitive to scents in the air, such as perfume and cologne?   yes ☐   no ☐

3 Do cigarette smoke, cooking odours and emotional stress cause nasal symptoms?   yes ☐   no ☐

4 Are antihistamines usually not helpful in alleviating symptoms?   yes ☐   no ☐

Yes *answers to these questions usually indicate vasomotor (non-allergic) rhinitis.*

Something in the air

Airborne allergens, ranging from pollen and dust to mould spores, pet dander and fibres, are the most common reason for rhinitis, with an estimated 12 million people in Britain allergic to these substances.

Let's start with pollen.

Even as many of us celebrate the end of winter and the glory of spring, millions of allergy sufferers head home, abandoning the golf course, giving up country walks and seriously considering investing in gas masks – all because the very same thing that is responsible for spring's beauty is also responsible for their misery. The culprit is pollen, the microscopic round or oval grains that plants use in lieu of sex to reproduce. Some use the grains to pollinate themselves, while others rely on insects, the wind or even your clothes to carry the tiny particles around so that they can fertilize other plants.

Generally speaking, it is not flowers that are to blame for your misery (although iris, geranium and clematis can produce hay fever symptoms). Rather, it is plants without showy flowers – trees, grasses and weeds. That's because, unlike flowering plants that depend on insects to collect and distribute their heavier pollen, these plants produce particularly small, light, dry pollen granules that are custom-made for wind transport. And they travel enormous distances. Scientists have found ragweed pollen – a principal cause of hay fever in the USA – 400 miles out at sea and two miles high in the air. That's why simply clearing the area around you of offending plants won't do any good. Plus, there is the sheer quantity of pollen: a single ragweed plant, for instance, can generate a million grains a day.

Pollen occurs everywhere, in every country on every continent (including Antarctica). Even living in a high-rise apartment building in the midst of a city is no protection. Scientists in northern Spain found that residents of tower blocks in the city of Valladolid actually had a *higher* risk of pollen allergies than people who lived in villages in the local countryside. In fact, wrote one of the scientists, 'Natural pollen sensitization appears to increase with the height of where the patient lived.'

The reason for this is that pollen rises as the air warms, then begins to fall as it cools in the evening. So if you suffer from pollen allergy and

allergy sufferers ask
Am I allergic to cigarettes?

The short answer is no. Nor can you be allergic to perfume. You can, however, have a *sensitivity* to such substances, which can make your eyes water and your nose run and have you sneezing – and if you have allergic rhinitis, you are more likely to have such sensitivities. In fact, if you've ever complained to a hotel that you're allergic to cigarette smoke and simply have to have a non-smoking room, it is not strictly true. It would be more accurate to say that you are 'greatly irritated' by smoke. But no self-respecting hotel would consider your demand an unreasonable request.

The usual suspects

Allergens come from lots of seemingly unrelated sources, as this rogue's gallery shows. But they do have something in common: they all are generated from living things. Your immune system is trained to attack viruses, bacteria and parasites, so it makes some sense that it might be hypersensitive to similar-size foreign proteins, organic chemicals and moulds.

Tree pollen

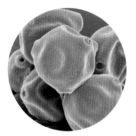

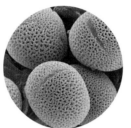

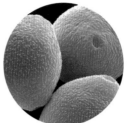

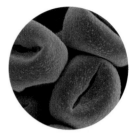

BIRCH Wide-spread tree releases pollen in large amounts in April in England and Wales, later in Scotland.

ASH Its pollen is mainly released in April, though sometimes during March in parts of England and Wales.

HAZEL Pollen from this tree, commonly found on the edge of woods, can be in the air as early as January.

OAK High oak pollen counts are often recorded from late April or May in the south, and early June in the north.

Grass pollen

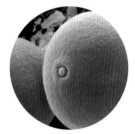

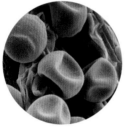

Cockroaches

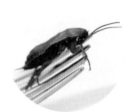

Pet dander

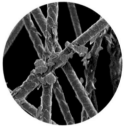

TIMOTHY GRASS One of many common grasses that trigger allergies. Others include rye, cocksfoot, meadow and fescue.

MEADOWGRASS One of the UK's most profusely pollinating flowering grasses. It is likely to cause problems in early spring.

The saliva, faeces, and bodies of these hardy urban bugs all generate allergens that can trigger attacks.

Cats and dogs constantly shed old skin cells, or dander, that carry all sorts of allergenic proteins.

Moulds

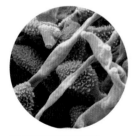

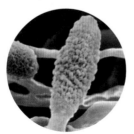

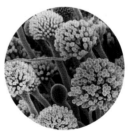

Dust mites

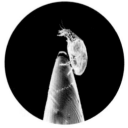

CLADOSPORIUM There are more than 30 types of moulds in this genus. They tend to flourish in water-damaged environments.

ALTERNARIA The unusually shaped mould tends to grow mainly on dead plants, particularly grasses and cereals.

ASPERGILLUS This grows on decaying vegetation, such as compost heaps and fallen leaves, and often in air-conditioning systems.

About half the size of a pen dot, these non-biting insects live for only three months. They love beds for the warmth and food.

live in a high-rise building, you should make sure that you keep your windows closed.

In the UK, during the spring, the main problem for hay fever sufferers is tree pollen. Although seasons vary slightly geographically and from year to year, alder and hazel can be in the air as early as January, followed by elm, willow and ash in March. Pollen from these affect only small numbers of hay fever sufferers but can trigger symptoms in people with allergies. Pollen from silver birch affects one in every four hay fever sufferers in the UK, and is followed by oak tree pollen, also a potent allergen. Other trees that have allergenic pollen include pine, poplar, beech, sweet chestnut, yew, juniper and walnut.

revealing **research**

Oral allergy syndrome

Some hay fever sufferers discover that they also develop oral allergies to specific fruits, vegetables and nuts. These people typically develop hay fever in early spring and then notice itching and swelling of the mouth and throat when they eat fresh fruit and vegetables.

This phenomenon is called the oral allergy, or pollen-food allergy, syndrome. Silver birch pollen allergy sufferers may develop oral allergies to apples, peaches, cherries, carrots, celery, hazelnuts, peanuts and walnuts. People who suffer from a grass pollen allergy develop oral allergies to tomatoes, melon and watermelon. Mugwort pollen allergy cross-reacts with apple, celery and carrot.

People who suffer from pollen-food allergy do not react to cooked or canned fruit and vegetables and the reaction almost always remains localized in the mouth and throat.

By far the most frequent cause of hay fever in the UK is grass pollen, which affects 95 per cent of hay fever sufferers. The grass pollen season generally lasts from late May until mid August, with a peak in June followed by a smaller peak in July. Weed pollens affect a small but significant number of sufferers from June to September peaking in August.

You may be allergic to several types of pollen. One clue to the cause of your allergy is when it occurs, so it is worth trying to identify local plants and trees and finding out when they flower. You can also check pollen forecasts at: **pollenuk.worc.ac.uk/** (National Pollen and Aerobiology Research Unit) or at **www.bbc.co.uk/weather**.

A pollen count is simply a measure of how much pollen is in the air. It represents the concentration of all the pollen in the air in a certain area at a specific time, expressed in grains of pollen per cubic metre of air sampled over a 24-hour period. Pollen counts are usually for grass, birch and nettles. During the pollen season plants release pollen early in the morning.

On a sunny day, as the temperature rises and more flowers open, pollens rise and tend to peak at 5-6pm in the countryside and an hour or two later in cities. On humid, windy days, pollen spreads further. If it rains, pollen may be cleared from the air and the levels will drop – although thunderstorms can actually spread pollen further. Bear in mind, however, that the pollen count reflects the *previous* 24 hours, not the coming day. Also note that while the amount of pollen makes a difference in the severity of your symptoms, the type is just as important. For instance, it takes just a little pollen from grasses, such as Timothy or rye grass, or trees (such as birch, oak and elm) to trigger allergies, but generally takes much larger quantities of pollens such as eucalyptus, which are heavier and don't disperse as easily.

But don't despair; later in this book we'll tell you how you can still enjoy the great outdoors despite your allergies.

Formidable fungi: moulds

Mould is now believed to be a potential health risk. More about its role in so-called sick building syndrome, is outlined later in the book. For now, we will focus on the role that common mould spores play in your allergies.

When allergies bloom

The pollen calendar below shows when the most common allergenic plants are in bloom in the UK. The timing will differ from south to north and also west to east and with height above sea level. The exact timing and severity of the pollen seasons vary from one year to the next depending on the weather and on biological factors. Note that flowers, with their oversize pollen grains, rarely cause allergies.

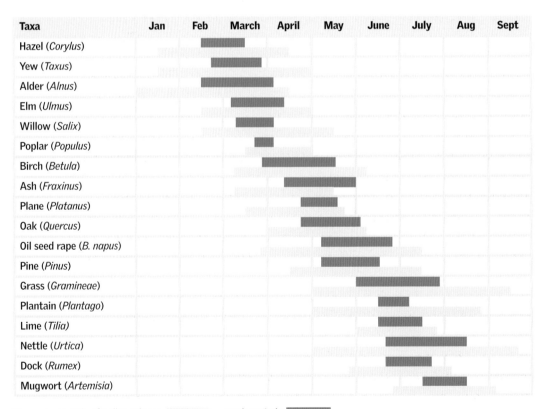

The main periods of pollen release   peak periods

Source: National Pollen Research Unit, University College Worcester

There are thousands of types of moulds and yeasts in the fungus family. Moulds are made of many cells that grow as branching threads called hyphae; yeasts are single cells that divide to form clusters. Although both can probably cause allergic reactions, in the UK only around 20 moulds have been identified as offenders.

If you're allergic to mould, your symptoms may worsen from spring to late autumn. Just as with plant pollens, there is a mould 'season', which peaks from July to late summer, but unfortunately, the first freeze doesn't put an end to the mould problem as it does with pollen. Moulds are tenacious little fungi that are able to grow at subfreezing temperatures. Even snow, while lowering the outdoor mould count dramatically by covering the fungi, doesn't kill mould spores. Come the spring, the moulds revive from their dormant state, thriving on the vegetation that has been killed by the winter cold. Small wonder that moulds are believed to be the oldest form of life on planet Earth.

In warm parts of the country, however, mould allergies can be perennial, or year-round, as can allergies triggered by indoor moulds. And mould is to be found everywhere, with thousands of mould species throughout the world, even in icy Antarctica. In fact, moulds outnumber pollens, possibly because it is easier for them to grow. They don't require much: just moisture, oxygen and a few other readily available environmental chemicals. And they can grow on anything, from rotting logs and fallen leaves to compost piles, grasses and weeds and on grains such as wheat, oats, barley and corn, not to mention your shower curtain. Anywhere there is any dampness in your house – in the base-ment, bathroom, refrigerator drip tray or even houseplants – there is likely to be mould.

It is not the mould itself that causes the allergic reaction, but its spores, which could be described as the mould's form of pollen. Each spore that germinates results in new mould growth, which in turn can produce millions of spores. These spores are so small that they easily evade the protective mechanisms of the nose and upper respiratory tract to reach the lungs. In some people, eating mould-containing foods, such as cheese, mushrooms and dried fruit, can also bring on allergic symptoms. But only a few types of mould are allergens. The primary source of allergy in the UK is Cladosporium, an

allergy **sufferers ask**

What about that yellow stuff on my car?

It's probably pine tree pollen. In spring and summer it blankets parts of the country with a layer of yellow dust, coating cars and pavements. Scotland has the highest count, in June. Elsewhere smaller amounts of the pollen are released earlier. But it's probably not the cause of your misery. The chemical composition of pine pollen appears to make it less allergenic than other types. Also, because it's heavy, it falls straight down and doesn't scatter, so it rarely reaches human noses.

A mould allergy on steroids: Aspergillus

Although allergic rhinitis caused by mould is fairly benign, there is a certain kind of mould that can cause a more severe respiratory reaction. Called Aspergillus, this form of mould, found throughout the environment, may lodge in your airways or in a distant part of your lung and grow until it forms a compact sphere known as a fungus ball.

Aspergillus mould can also lead to asthma or to allergic bronchopulmonary aspergillosis, a lung disease resembling severe inflammatory asthma. This condition, which occurs rarely in only a minority of people with asthma, is characterized by wheezing, low fever and coughing up of brown-flecked masses or mucus plugs. Corticosteroid drugs are frequently used to treat the reaction; immunotherapy (allergy injections) won't do much good.

airborne mould, found in summer on foods, uncleaned refrigerators, in poorly ventilated homes and low, damp areas. Other culprits include Alternaria, responsible for black spots on tomatoes and other foods, and Aspergillus, which thrives in soils, plant refuse and decaying vegetables and is associated with asthma and bronchitis (see box, left).

Penicillium the green-blue mould found on stale bread, fruit and nuts, is linked with indoor allergy. Present year-round, its concentrations reach a peak in winter and spring. There is no link, however, between a respiratory allergy to Penicillium and an allergy to the drug penicillin, which is made from mould. If you are not sure whether or not moulds are to blame for your allergy, think about your symptoms. Do they tend to occur most of the year, worsening in the summer, when you're near fields or after you have been gardening? It could be a mould allergy.

Mould spores are counted just like pollen, but the count is not as helpful. One reason is that the number and types of spores actually present in the mould count may change considerably within 24 hours, depending on the weather. Many common allergenic moulds are of the dry spore type, meaning that they release their spores during dry, windy weather. Other fungi require high humidity, fog or dew to release their spores.

Although rain washes many larger spores out of the air, it can also trigger the release of spores from moulds such as Didymella, which are sensitive to humidity. These spores thrive better in humid conditions and are thought to be one of the causes of so-called 'thunderstorm asthma'.

Dust mites and cockroaches

If you ever took a good look at what lives on the ostensibly clean surfaces of your home, it might make you sick. Billions of microscopic, eight-legged dust mites make their home in your bed, carpeting, curtains and furniture.

Their favourite food is flakes of your dead skin. And the dust you see floating in shafts of sunlight includes dead dust mites and their droppings. Dust mites love dark, warm, humid spaces such as upholstered furniture, mattresses, duvets, pillows, rugs, curtains and stuffed animals. Millions are probably making themselves comfortable in your pillows – which is why you may find that your allergies worsen when you're in bed or on the sofa. You're actually allergic not to dust mites but to their excrement. The same goes for cockroaches, another cause of allergic rhinitis, particularly in the USA. While dust mites are ubiquitous, cockroaches are most commonly found in crowded cities. But although minuscule mite and cockroach droppings, invisible to the naked eye, can wreak havoc with your immune system, help is at hand. We'll tell you more about how to stay one step ahead in chapter 8.

Animal dander

With over 14 million cats and dogs in the UK, plus 37 million small animals, there is no doubt that Britain lives up to its reputation as a nation of animal lovers. Statistics show that around 15 per cent of adults and more than 50 per cent of children are allergic to pets. Yet a growing body of research suggests that having a cat or dog in the house when you are very young may actually prevent the development of asthma or allergies, even if you are genetically disposed to them. Claudia Rock, a researcher at the University of Wisconsin-Madison, studied nearly 300 children who were at risk of developing allergies because of their family histories. Her study found that a year after birth, babies were no more sensitive to allergens if they had a cat or other animal in their home than if they didn't, and if they had a dog, their sensitivity significantly *decreased*. Exposure to dogs, the study found, increased levels of cytokines, chemicals that put the brakes on the body's reactions to allergens.

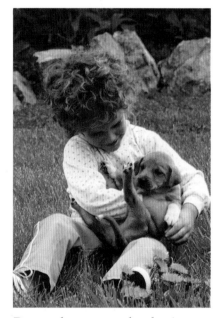

A recent German study produced similar findings. But household pets are still among the most common sources of allergy and some allergists won't begin treatment until a patient agrees to give up the family dog or cat. Plus, it can take as long as two years from the time you get a pet for the allergy to develop.

Research suggests that having a dog in the house when children are very young may actually help to protect them against asthma or allergies.

Don't blame your pet's fur or hair, and don't imagine that getting a hairless cat or a Chihuahua will solve the problem. It's not the fur that makes you sneeze but rather proteins that are secreted by oil glands in the animals' skin and shed in dander (scurf from the skin), as well as proteins in their saliva, which sticks to the fur when the animal licks itself. Another source of allergy-

What is dust?

Take one part mould, a few dust mites and their faecal matter, plus some animal hair and dander, then throw in minuscule bits of upholstery, lint and other fibres and mix well with particles of human skin, plants, food remnants and insect droppings.

That's dust, which we play a role in creating – but which also occurs when we're not around. You can go away on holiday, leaving your home immaculate with every surface shining, and when you return you'll still have some house dust. It took scientists years to work out the recipe and to realize that people are not allergic to dust itself, but only to some of its specific components.

causing proteins is animal urine. When the substance carrying the proteins dries, they are free to float into the air.

Cat dander is particularly ubiquitous. First, there's the basic lifestyle of cats. They lick themselves more, may be held more, spend more time all over the home close to humans, and may urinate and defecate in litter boxes in the house. Their dander also seems to hang in the air longer than dog dander – and it spreads faster.

Allow someone to bring a cat to stay at your home for the weekend, and within 30 minutes of the feline's entrance into your home, the air will be filled with allergy-causing proteins.

Some studies find that male cats that have not been spayed produce more allergy-causing proteins than female cats – another reason to have your kitten neutered. Another study found that dark-haired cats seem to cause more severe symptoms in their allergic owners than light-haired cats, though experts say in practice it makes little difference; both types can cause allergic reactions.

Pet allergies are not restricted to cats and dogs. Even small pets, such as guinea pigs, gerbils and birds, can cause allergic reactions, as can mice and rats. And getting rid of your pet won't magically clear your nose. Animal dander can remain on furniture, bedding, curtains and other surfaces for months after the pet is gone.

Even if you've never owned a pet you're still at risk, as animal proteins are stickier than glue. You can be exposed to pet proteins from the clothes of pet-loving colleagues at work or even the girl at the next table in the cafe. When researchers from Johns Hopkins University in Baltimore measured airborne concentrations of cat allergens in homes with and without feline occupants, they found low levels of cat allergens in the cat-free homes, 'as well as in every other building where it was sought, including newly built homes, shopping centres, doctors' surgeries and even hospitals'.

Despite the agony of allergies, some pet owners would rather live with the symptoms than give up their animals. Many people persist in keeping cats despite their allergy; in the USA about a third of the estimated 6 million people who are allergic to cats have cats at home – some even resort to immunotherapy (injections desensitivizing them to the pet dander allergen).

The eyes have it

The red, itchy eyes of allergies may be related to more than just your nose; you may have an eye allergy as well. According to a recent poll, up to 21 per cent of adults in the UK are affected by this allergy, only half of whom seek help for their symptoms. And don't imagine that you're immune because you don't have nasal allergies. A survey by the American College of Allergy, Asthma and Immunology in 2002 found that of the 82 per cent of people who reported itchy, watery eyes, only 37 per cent also had nasal allergies. Sufferers described their symptoms as 'feeling like they had sand in their eyes' and said that the symptoms interfered with their daily activities. Sometimes an allergic attack can be so intense that the surface of the eye swells, a condition called chemosis.

Eye allergies, or allergic conjunctivitis, accounting for 15 per cent of all eye problems, result from the same immune system malfunction that causes nasal allergies, this time affecting the mast cells in the eye (there are 50 million in each eye). The triggers are similar to those causing nasal allergies – pet dander, mould, pollen and dust mites – and the condition can be either seasonal or perennial. There are three rarer forms of allergic conjunctivitis that may affect your eyes:

▓ **Atopic keratoconjunctivitis (AKC)** This form is closely associated with the skin condition atopic dermatitis (you'll read more about skin-related allergies in chapter 14).

Of people with AKC, 95 per cent have atopic dermatitis and almost 90 per cent have asthma. It occurs most frequently in adolescence or early childhood. Symptoms include burning and tearing, along with corneal ulcers or cataracts; red, oozing lesions around the eye; mucus discharge; and sensitivity to light.

allergy **sufferers ask**

What is a sneeze?

It's as much a part of allergies as a stuffy nose, but what, exactly, *is* a sneeze? Well, it's an involuntary violent expulsion of air through your nose and mouth involving many upper-body muscles. The sequence is probably deeply implanted in your brain and spinal cord, which is one reason it's so difficult to suppress a sneeze once the irritation message is sent to the brain.

The sneeze occurs when the nervous system in your nose (which you probably didn't even know you had) is stimulated, causing a sudden contraction of dozens of muscles in your face, chest and abdomen. This contraction forces air out of your nose extremely fast, with the goal of expelling the irritation. How fast? It is estimated that a sneeze emerges as quickly as the fastest ball bowled by a professional cricket player – at about 160k/h (100mph). Sneezing comes in handy if you have a stuffed nose. The acceleration of air through the nose causes a drop in pressure, and this tends to draw excess mucus and other fluids from the sinuses, having the same effect as when you blow your nose.

And yes, sometimes looking at a light can trigger that just-on-the-edge sneeze into a violent explosion. Another bit of sneezing trivia: the US inventor Thomas Edison studied the sneeze, and in 1897, he created one of the first 'action' movies of the time by filming a series of still shots of a sneeze in sequence, then replaying them rapidly one after another.

■ **Vernal keratoconjunctivitis (VKC)** The condition tends to occur in spring, most often in boys under 10. If left untreated, it can result in scarring that could lead to vision loss. Symptoms include intense itching, sensitivity to sunlight, blurred vision and stringy or ropy mucus discharge.

■ **Giant papillary conjunctivitis** Inflammation of the conjunctiva lining the upper eyelid results from a combination of allergy and contact with a foreign body in the eye, often a contact lens and is associated with overuse of lenses. Symptoms include intense itching, burning and redness. Prevalence varies from 1 per cent of hard lens wearers to 1-5 per cent of people using soft lenses.

Treatment for common allergic conjunctivitis ranges from over-the-counter eye drops, such as tear substitutes and decongestants/antihistamines especially for the eyes, to prescription eye drops. The more serious forms of conjunctivitis require more aggressive approaches using prescription drugs. More about the specific treatments available is discussed in chapter 7.

Allergies through a lifetime

It has long been believed that people outgrow their allergies, or that if you had no allergies as a child, you won't get them as an adult. In fact, during the first year or two of life, children rarely develop allergic rhinitis. They're more prone to food allergies, particularly to milk and peanuts. This may be because very young children don't experience the outdoors. As they grow and have more exposure to both outside allergens (pollens and grasses) and indoor allergens (pet dander, dust mites and mould spores), the allergies begin. Conversely, as children grow older and their immune systems become better able to regulate the production of IgE, they may no longer react to certain food allergens.

Puberty provides another impetus for the development of allergies, with some adolescents pegging the start of their allergies to their spurt of reproductive hormones. And it is true that many people find that their allergies disappear as they grow older – a rare benefit of ageing. The reason, researchers suspect, is that people tend to produce less IgE as they age.

Putting it into perspective

Whether your symptoms are triggered by cat dander or pollen, mould or dust mites, the Breathe Easy Plan should help. The plan is introduced in part 3. If your only problem is allergic rhinitis, you may want to move on to those pages now, but if you suffer from asthma or food allergies, keep reading. The following two chapters are packed with information about these conditions.

Chapter **four**

All about asthma

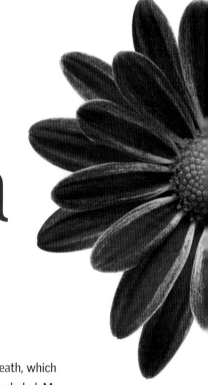

'Having an asthma attack requires a laborious intake and outtake of breath, which induces a maddening wheeze and whistle as each breath is drawn and exhaled. My lungs feel sticky, and it's as if the air is fighting its way to open the passages. As it opens those passages, there's often a release of mucus, which causes a constant need to cough or clear my throat. Sometimes it feels as if the air is sandpaper and is actually scraping against my lungs. Whether it's real or psychological, the attack is followed by an immediate feeling that I'm not getting enough oxygen and a bit of accompanying panic. At that point, the only thought in my head is to get to my inhaler, which immediately eases the breathing process.'

Dan Moore, *33, software developer, Manchester*

As Dan and other sufferers describe, having an asthma attack feels as if you're suffocating. That is why ancient Greek physicians used the word *asthma*, meaning 'gasping', to describe shortness of breath. Ironically, the problem is not only that you can't get enough air into your lungs; it's also that your lungs become so inflamed and congested that you can't get the air that's in them *out*.

Asthma is an ancient disease dating back to the 12th century, when Moses Maimonides, a renowned rabbi, philosopher and physician who practised in the royal courts of Egypt and Syria, wrote a treatise on the condition. Among his recommended treatments were: moderation in food, drink, sleep and sexual activity; avoiding polluted city environments; and, as a specific remedy, chicken soup. Not bad advice, given that inhalers and anti-inflammatory medications didn't exist at the time.

Some 800 years later, treatments are more sophisticated and yet the disease remains a conundrum. Today, identifying the cause (or causes) of asthma is as difficult as blowing up a balloon during an asthma attack. And because the causes are hard to pinpoint and the symptoms can be similar to those for other disorders, doctors quite frequently misdiagnosis the condition. They may advise patients that the problem is chronic bronchitis, pneumonia or hyperactive lungs. This misreading can delay the appropriate treatment.

The confusion stems from the disease itself. Unlike singular diseases such as chickenpox, asthma has many forms caused by different stimuli which all trigger a similar effect on the lungs.

Stated simply, asthma is a disease in which the airways of the lungs become hypersensitive to one or many irritants. When exposed to such irritants, the airways constrict, the lining of the bronchial tubes swells, and mucus production increases, making it hard for air to get into and out of the lungs. Repeated asthma attacks cause permanent scarring and compromise lung function over time. Fifty years ago, doctors thought asthma was a disease of the smooth

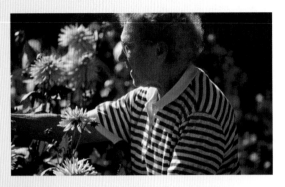

Are you over 65? Read this

You may have asthma and not know it. A study of 4,581 people age 65 and older, published in 1999 in the journal *Chest*, found that not only was asthma underdiagnosed in this group, it was also undertreated in the majority of those with the disease. This and other studies also found that asthma contributes to a decreased quality of life in elderly people, with those who have severe asthma reporting more negative feelings about life in general, describing their health as being poor, and having a greater degree of impairment during daily activities. Researchers in one study also found high levels of potential asthma triggers in the homes of the elderly people tested, from carpeting, older furnishings, high indoor relative humidity and mattresses that were not properly covered to block allergens. Sadly, the researchers noted, the poor quality of life many of the people reported meant that they were less likely to do the kind of housekeeping, such as vacuuming and dusting, that could reduce allergen levels in their homes, easing severe asthma.

The underlying message is: if you experience trouble breathing, chronic cough, wheezing or any other asthma symptoms, ask your doctor to evaluate you for asthma and prescribe proper treatment if you are asthmatic. Age is not a reason to ignore asthma.

muscles that wrap around the airways in a lung. A trigger would cause the muscles to go into spasms, narrowing the airways and thus limiting the flow of air. Such triggers included allergens, air pollution, exercise, cigarette smoke and cold air. Since these episodes waxed and waned over time – and disappeared after treatment – asthma was viewed as an intermittent illness that required minimal treatment between episodes. When it was discovered that steroid tablets and, later, steroid inhalers improved asthma, it was correctly deduced that asthma is an inflammatory disease and one that in recent decades has become more dangerous and far more prevalent. Doctors now know that it is also a chronic condition and that even without symptoms, the disease is still active. Some other new understanding about the disease includes:

Inflammation of the airways is a persistent feature of asthma – even between attacks – and plays a critical role in changing overall lung function. In other words, your asthma is changing the way your lungs work every minute of every day, even if you feel fine and are breathing well. That is why most people with asthma require medication daily, not only during an attack.

Complex reactions within the airways are a big part of an asthma attack These reactions are based in the immune system, meaning that they involve many of the cells that play a role in allergies: eosinophils, T lymphocytes, macrophages, neutrophils and basophils as well as mast cells and epithelial cells, which line the airways. It is these reactions that create the mucus and inflammation that further restrict breathing capacity.

Our improved understanding of asthma, however, still leaves us far from knowing what causes it. One of our greatest questions is: what exactly *is* the relationship between inflammation and asthma?

For instance, we know that asthma is always associated with inflammation of the airways and that the intensity of the inflammation determines the severity of the symptoms. We also know that there can be a spiralling effect in asthma: inflammation aggravates the hypersensitivity, which triggers more asthma attacks, which brings on more inflammation. No one knows what triggers this inflammatory response. But we do know that over time and without proper treatment, the inflammation can eventually change the physical appearance and function of your lungs, leading to the replacement of normal tissue with non-functioning scar tissue that no amount of treatment can reverse.

There are four main types of asthma. Each behaves somewhat differently, is triggered differently, and may respond to different treatments or interventions.

Allergic asthma (sometimes called extrinsic asthma) This is the most common form; if you suffer from asthma and allergies, you probably have allergic asthma. Attacks are triggered by allergens such as seasonal pollens or perennial allergens that you breathe into your system, including those caused by dust mites and animal dander. Allergic asthma often begins in childhood and stays with you for the remainder of your life.

▓ **Non-allergic asthma (sometimes referred to as intrinsic asthma)** This form of asthma is not associated with allergy and results from something 'intrinsic' within your body. It may be associated with chronic sinusitis and other features such as aspirin sensitivity. It generally develops later in life and very little is known about its causes. It is often more difficult to treat than allergic asthma.

▓ **Mixed asthma** Sometimes asthma is triggered by both allergies and non-allergic factors. For instance, your allergy to grass and tree pollen triggers your asthma, but you have symptoms even in winter, when there is no pollen.

▓ **Severe or 'brittle' asthma** If you have experienced this form of asthma, you know it. Attacks come on suddenly and very intensely but don't respond to the usual treatment. With this form, you often have so much trouble breathing that you become exhausted and collapse. You are also in significant danger of death; people with acute severe asthma can deteriorate very fast and die within the first 24 hours of an attack. One regional survey of fatal or near-fatal asthma attacks found that half occurred suddenly and unexpectedly, without any obvious predisposing factors. In the other half of attacks, psychosocial factors (such as stress), running in cold weather, overreliance on inhaled bronchodilators, and delays in seeking care were contributing causes.

Inside an asthma attack

'One of the easiest ways to describe how I feel when having an asthma attack is to imagine everything in slow motion. Each action requires the maximum effort – even speaking! I feel like I'm walking through treacle and my body aches. My breathing becomes laborious and I can hear the whistling in my chest start to begin. My immediate throughts are that I want clean fresh air into my lungs to help ease the pain and that I must try and relax to see my way through.'

Kate Hunter, 26, London

'My asthma attacks were originally associated with stress, either physical (school sports) or mental (getting important exam results). They start with a feeling of irritation in my throat, then an awareness that it is getting harder to breathe. After a while it feels like however much breath I draw in, I can't fill my lungs. Slow regular breathing helps but leaves me feeling short of oxygen. Asthma attacks were originally associated with stress, either physical (school sports) or mental (getting important exam results).

'They start with a feeling of irritation iin my throat, then an awareness that it is getting harder to breathe. After a while it feels like however much breath I draw in, I can't fill my lungs. Slow regular breathing helps but leaves me feeling short of oxygen.

'When I was younger, I would sometimes progress to the "wheezing" stage where the narrowing of the airways result in a characteristic noise when breathing in and out. These days I go for months or years without any attacks and, when they do come, they are usually mild.'

Bill Crum, *38, Norwich*

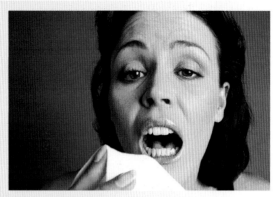

Warning signs of an asthma attack

Yours may differ, but signs generally include at least one of the following:

- Decline in blowing power
- Chronic cough, especially at night
- Difficult or rapid breathing
- A feeling of chest tightness or discomfort
- Mucus in your chest that you can't cough up
- Becoming out of breath more easily than usual
- Wheezing
- Fatigue
- Restlessness

An asthma 'attack' starts with a trigger, as does an allergy attack. It can be an allergen or something as seemingly innocuous as breathing in the first cold air of winter. The trigger irritates your airways. If you don't have asthma, you can simply cough and be done with it. If you do have it, this irritation results in the release of chemicals such as histamines and leukotrienes from the mast cells found in the lining of your airways.

This causes tightening of the muscles around your bronchial tubes, the small branches in the lung, which accounts for the tightness and pressure that asthma sufferers feel. The underlying inflammatory process inherent in asthma may also lead to bronchial spasms, in which the muscles around your bronchial tubes twitch, preventing air from entering or leaving the lungs and helping to explain the wheezing (as you struggle to get air in or out through clogged airways) and the feeling of choking or drowning many people with asthma describe.

Thanks to the inflammation that has been triggered, mucus and fluids quickly build up in your lungs. They overwhelm the cilia, the tiny hairlike projections on certain cells that keep the lungs clear by moving the fluids on.

The result so far: you try to cough to clear out the mucus, but at the same time, you are gasping for air. All of this is just phase one of an asthma attack. It doesn't end there. As this occurs, your immune system senses that something is

(continued on page 56)

Asthma in the UK

The charts below, largely based on research by Asthma UK, help to bring home the stark reality of asthma in Britain today. Prevalence continues to grow, while health services struggle to help people suffering from asthma to achieve a life free of symptoms.

Estimated annual cost of asthma in the UK

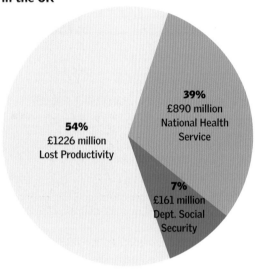

54%
£1226 million
Lost Productivity

39%
£890 million
National Health Service

7%
£161 million
Dept. Social Security

Asthma facts and figures

• Asthma is now three to four times higher in adults and six times higher in children than it was 25 years ago. More than 5 million people in the UK are receiving treatment and an estimated 8 million people in the UK have been diagnosed with asthma at some stage in their lives. But a 2005 survey suggests that the incidence of of asthma symptoms in children appears to be levelling off.

• The UK headed the asthma table in a survey carried out by the European Commission in 2003. It revealed that 13 per cent of people aged over 15 years experienced asthma at some time in their lives.

• Treating asthma costs the National Health Service almost £890 million a year.

How asthma affects quality of life

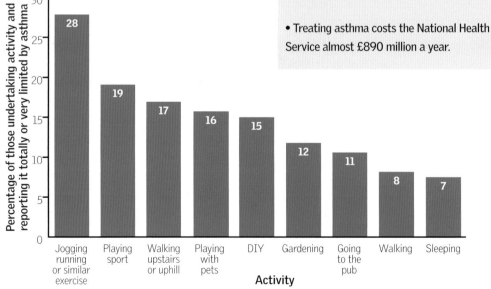

Percentage of those undertaking activity and reporting it totally or very limited by asthma

Activity	%
Jogging running or similar exercise	28
Playing sport	19
Walking upstairs or uphill	17
Playing with pets	16
DIY	15
Gardening	12
Going to the pub	11
Walking	8
Sleeping	7

Factors contributing to deaths from asthma

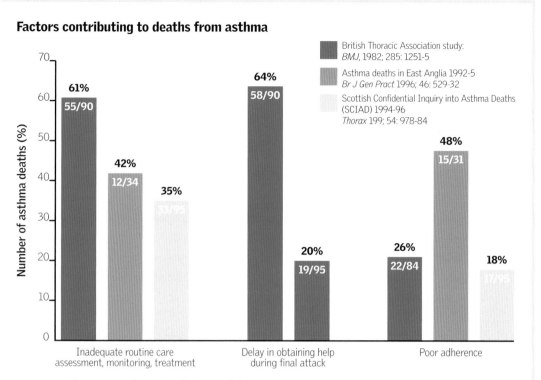

The graph reflects the findings of three reviews into asthma deaths between 1979-1996.

British Thoracic Association study:
BMJ, 1982; 285: 1251-5

Asthma deaths in East Anglia 1992-5
Br J Gen Pract 1996; 46: 529-32

Scottish Confidential Inquiry into Asthma Deaths
(SCIAD) 1994-96
Thorax 199; 54: 978-84

Deaths from asthma in the UK by age

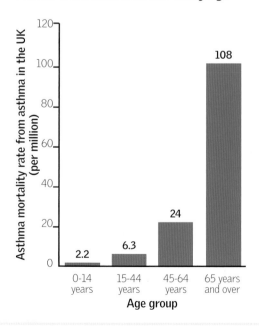

Mortality

• Some 1,500 people still die from asthma each year in the UK.

• Asthma mortality peaked in the 1960s and 1970s but has levelled off in recent years. Past reports suggest that better healthcare measures could have prevented many of these deaths; some improvements have been reported since the late 1970s.

• Although the majority of deaths are in the elderly, 25 children and more than 500 adults aged less than 65 years died as a result of asthma in 1999.

Source: Asthma UK

wrong and rushes in to try and fix things. Instead, this intervention only makes a bad situation worse. Various immune system cells release chemicals that activate the immune system's neutrophils and eosinophils. They then release chemicals that trigger inflammation. The result is the chronic inflammation that is characteristic of asthma.

These chemicals may also hamper how well the smooth muscles in your airways respond to signals from the nervous system to loosen their grip. What's more, they may prevent blood from picking up oxygen (starving your whole body of this vital element) and increase mucus secretion (clogging up the works even more).

Over a period of time, in some asthma sufferers these effects may result in permanent changes in the lungs, known as airway remodelling. This is due to leakage from tiny blood vessels, overgrowth of smooth muscle cells and the thickening of airway walls as scar tissue forms and other physical changes take place. The result can be irreversible alterations in the airways and permanent loss of lung function.

Constricted airways

An irritant lands in one of the bronchioles. For a person with healthy lungs, a cough moves it on or cilia sweep it away. But for a person with asthma, the irritant causes the release of histamines and other chemical responses that start the domino chain of an asthma attack.

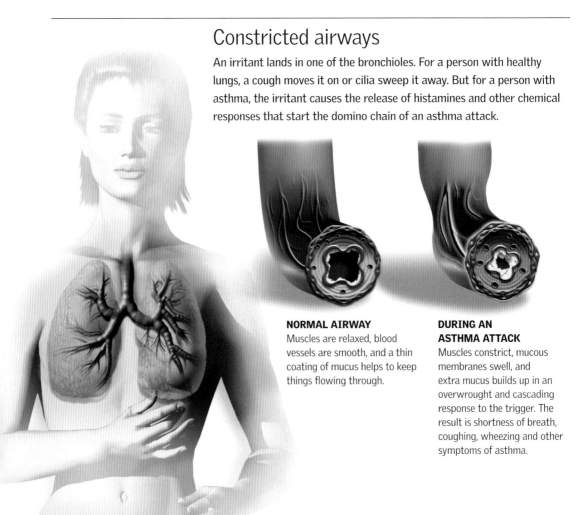

NORMAL AIRWAY
Muscles are relaxed, blood vessels are smooth, and a thin coating of mucus helps to keep things flowing through.

DURING AN ASTHMA ATTACK
Muscles constrict, mucous membranes swell, and extra mucus builds up in an overwrought and cascading response to the trigger. The result is shortness of breath, coughing, wheezing and other symptoms of asthma.

When asthma turns fatal

In the UK there are around 1,500 deaths annually due to asthma, 25 of which are children. Despite the soaring incidence of asthma, the number of deaths has levelled in recent years after peaking in the 1980s. Yet there is still no way to predict which people with asthma face an increased risk of death. (Death from asthma is usually related to respiratory arrest, when breathing stops suddenly, or pneumothorax, where air leakage causes the lungs to collapse.)

There are some clues, however, as to whether asthma may suddenly become severe and life-threatening. Researchers have found that many who died from the disease had histories of severe asthma, with some previously requiring breathing tubes. It is known that having a severe attack increases the risk of further severe attacks. It is also possible that people who have life-threatening episodes are unable to sense when their oxygen levels are dropping, thus delaying medical treatment.

Although some deaths are unexpected, more often there is evidence that those who've died ignored the progressive worsening of symptoms or failed to seek help soon enough or did not take their medications regularly. Too often, people may think they're doing fine and wean themselves off their daily medicines. This is very dangerous, and it can't be emphasized enough that asthma does *not* go away.

Common triggers of asthma attacks

Before getting into the details, you need to understand the difference between something that causes the disease called asthma and something that triggers an asthma attack. Most research has been conducted on what triggers attacks or makes symptoms worse in someone who already has asthma. The scientific investigation into the underlying cause of the disease itself is just catching up, so here we'll describe mainly the irritants that trigger an asthma attack or worsen symptoms. Keep in mind, though, that even when you're not having symptoms, the disease is still silently menacing your lungs.

The air we breathe

You don't need a book to tell you that most of us in the UK breathe some pretty dirty air. But did you know that breathing polluted urban air is almost as damaging to your health as living with someone who smokes cigarettes?

Admittedly, air quality has improved since the passage of the Clean Air Acts of 1956 and 1968. But although national and international legislation now address air pollution, much more could be done. The health of an estimated

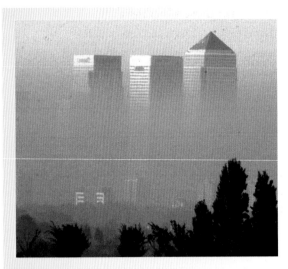

Air pollution in our cities

According to a report by the Chartered Society of Physiotherapy published in 2005 air pollution caused by nitrogen dioxide from traffic fumes far exceeds government targets in many of our cities. The report shows that the air around London's Marylebone Road had more than twice the level the government believes to be safe. The top ten locations, with their nitrogen dioxide cigarette equivalent in 24 hours, are:

1	Oxford	61.4
2	Bath	46.8
3	Glasgow – Kerbside	44.7
4	London's Marylebone Road	30.0
5	London's King's Road	29.6
6	Exeter	27.7
7	London's Hammersmith Broadway	27.3
8	Bristol City Centre	27.1
9	Sheffield – Tinsley	27.1
10	Brent	26.7

one in five people in the UK is at risk from air pollution, and during the 2003 heatwave up to 800 premature deaths are thought to have been attributable to poor air quality. The Department of Health estimates that air pollution accounts for several thousand deaths a year and up to 20,000 hospital admissions, as well as several thousand instances of illness, distress and discomfort. Health experts agree that there is a consistent, though modest, link between exposure to traffic fumes and asthma prevalence in children.

While research continues into air pollution as a possible cause of asthma, Asthma UK's medical officer warns that over 80 per cent of people with asthma find that air pollution aggravates their symptoms. This is of particular concern during the summer months when ground level ozone increases. According to Asthma UK, 66 per cent of people with asthma say that traffic fumes trigger their symptoms; and 42 per cent say that they try to avoid walking or shopping in congested areas so as to avoid exhaust fumes.

Specific air-related asthma triggers include:the following:

■ **Ozone** A respiratory irritant, ozone forms when sunlight acts on vehicle exhaust fumes and industrial pollution. High levels of ozone, which typically occur on hot summer days, are to people with asthma what a burning cigarette is to a drought-stricken forest. That's why many cities issue ozone alerts when levels are high, warning people with respiratory conditions such as asthma to stay inside. In fact, scientists suspect that high ozone levels may be one reason for our current asthma epidemic: a 2002 US study found that children who played a lot of outdoor team sports in areas of high ozone concentration were up to three times more likely to develop asthma than those who didn't participate in such sports. The study offered the first evidence that ground-level ozone could be a 'causative factor' in the development of childhood asthma rather than one that merely aggravates it. Asthma UK advises sufferers to avoid exercising outdoors when pollution levels are high, especially in the afternoon.

Particulate matter First, there are the fine solids in the air, such as dirt, soil dust, pollens, moulds, ashes and soot. Then there are the aerosols that form in the atmosphere from the by-products of combustion: volatile organic compounds (VOCs), sulphur dioxide and nitrogen oxides. Particulate pollution comes from diverse sources such as factory and utility smokestacks, vehicle exhaust, wood burning, mining, construction and agriculture.

When it comes to asthma and other respiratory illnesses, the main concern centres on fine particles – less than 2.5 microns in diameter. (For comparison, a human hair is about 75 microns in diameter.) You can easily inhale them into your lungs, where they may be absorbed into the bloodstream or remain embedded in your body's cells for long periods of time. One US study found a 17 per cent increase in the risk of death from asthma and other respiratory conditions in areas with higher concentrations of small particles.

Indoor air pollution Surprisingly, the air we breathe inside our homes, offices and other buildings often has more pollutants than the air we breathe outside. These air pollutants may come from combustion sources such as gas stoves, fireplaces and cigarettes, plus treated woods, paints, furnishings, carpets and fabrics. Sprays, pesticides, window cleaning products and even laundry detergents produce more pollutants. That's in addition to known indoor allergens such as animal dander, cockroaches, dust mites, moulds and fungi.

A 2002 study in *Environmental Health Perspectives*, conducted by Dutch researchers, concluded that more than half a million children under the age of six with asthma would not have the disease if risk factors such as pet dander, moulds, cigarette smoke and gas cookers were removed from their homes.

revealing **research**

Possible causes of asthma

Looking for the cause of asthma is like searching for the proverbial needle in a haystack. The possibilities are endless, and each month brings another theory.

For instance, a Swedish study suggests that women exposed to high levels of pollen in the last trimester of pregnancy are more likely to have children with asthma, possibly because the antibodies the mother produces in response to the pollen may cross to the foetus and make allergies and asthma more likely. Another study examining children's two upper baby teeth – which provide a good picture of nutrition in the womb – suggests that babies who do not receive enough of the minerals iron and selenium while in the womb may have a higher risk of wheezing in early childhood and possibly of developing asthma later on.

With our growing understanding of the genetic underpinnings of disease, researchers are also isolating numerous genes associated with asthma, and have found nearly 300 linkages so far.

Irritants

Irritants are exactly that: external conditions or substances such as smoke that are irritating to almost everyone. For a person without asthma, an irritant might evoke a cough; for a person with hypersensitive lungs, it could trigger the muscle spasms and inflammation that launch an asthma attack. Common irritants include cigarette smoke, cold air, perfume and paint fumes.

Then there's the chlorine in swimming pools. Researchers found that the high concentrations of chlorine in the air above swimming pools can irritate the lining of the lungs, making it easier for pollen, dander and other allergens or irritants to trigger an asthma attack. Ironically, people with asthma are often urged to exercise in indoor swimming pools, since the warm, humid air is believed to be beneficial for the lungs. If you are a swimmer and you have asthma, talk to your doctor about the relative risks and benefits.

The weather

Even the weather can exacerbate your asthma. For years, doctors in casualty wards throughout the world knew that thunderstorms brought in a rush of patients with asthma attacks. In 2003, their anecdotal observations were scientifically validated after researchers at the University of Ottawa Health

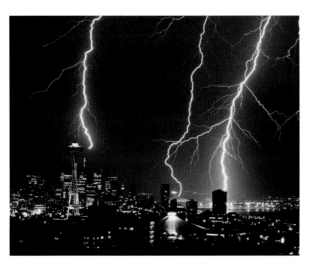

Research suggests that the rise in asthma attacks during thunderstorms may be related to the creation of ozone, an increase in airborne fungal spores, or changes in barometric pressure.

Research Institute in Canada examined four years of records from the Children's Hospital of Eastern Ontario that correlated asthma attacks with information on weather patterns, airborne allergens and pollution collected at a nearby airport. They found that asthma-related hospital visits jumped 15 per cent during thunderstorms, from an average of 8.6 visits on clear days to 10 on stormy days. Researchers suspect that the rise is related to an increase in airborne fungal spores, which nearly double during thunderstorms. In fact, when levels of these spores were high – storm or not – asthma-related hospital visits increased.

Another reason may be the creation during thunderstorms of ozone, which, as mentioned earlier, is a well-known asthma trigger. Some studies also suggest that changes in barometric pressure may affect asthma. In the UK, the coincidence of heavy storms and particularly high pollen counts in June 2005 saw a six-fold increase in hospital admissions for asthma. According to Dr Jean Emberlin, Director of the National Pollen Research Unit (NPRU) at Worcester University, pollen counts had been at record levels for the time of year in many areas, and at their highest ever in some sites.

Cold, dry air is another weather-related asthma trigger, particularly for those with exercise-induced asthma, while wind increases asthma flare-ups because it sends more pollen and mould spores into the air, where they can be breathed in by an allergic person and trigger an asthma attack.

Emotional anxiety and stress

In the mid-1900s, some doctors thought that asthma was purely psychosomatic (caused by emotional conflicts). Today, there is clear evidence to disprove this. For instance, lung transplants from donors with asthma have resulted in recipients developing asthma, showing that it occurs at the cellular level.

Yet there is no doubt that stress and emotional anxiety can trigger asthma symptoms; and research suggests that they may even contribute to the initial development of the disease. Parents with depression or anxiety disorders are more likely to have children with asthma and other allergy-based conditions, according to a 2005 study at New York's University of Columbia. In a survey of 9,000 parent and child pairs of which 554 were non-biological parents, it was found that biological parents with major depression were 67 per cent more likely to have a child with asthma or another allergy-based condition than those in good mental health, with an increased risk of 46 per cent for parents who had anxiety disorders. By contrast, adoptive parents with depression did not show higher levels of asthma in their children. The findings provide more evidence that common genes may contribute to the development of both asthma and anxiety disorders. Martin Dockrell of Asthma UK commented: 'Manifestly, anxiety and asthma reinforce each other, but this study suggests that they may also share a common cause. The correlation does not imply causation,' he added. 'It would be wrong to say simply that a parent's anxiety causes a child's asthma, or that a parent's asthma causes a child's anxiety.'

A small UK study suggests that stressful life events more than quadruple the risk of children suffering asthma attacks. A research team from University College, London studied 60 children, aged between six and 13 years, who had suffered from asthma for at least three years. All the children were asked to keep diaries for 18 months recording their symptoms, attacks and their peak flow measurements – an indicator of airway function. The team also recorded any instances of negative life events during regular interviews with the parents. During the study, 361 episodes of rapidly worsening asthma symptoms were recorded and 124 negative life events, such as deaths, parents' separations, house moves and illnesses in the family. Results showed that children were almost five times more likely to suffer a sudden worsening of asthma symptoms within 48 hours of experiencing a stressful life event than if such situations had not occurred.

The connection between stress and asthma varies. One explanation has to do with the complex effects of stress on the immune system, which dampen its ability to control inflammation (a key problem in asthma). Also, people who are under a lot of stress are less likely to take the kind of preventive steps that can reduce asthma symptoms. And then there's the shallow, tight breathing you tend to do when you're stressed. If you hyperventilate, you may think you are having an asthma attack when you're actually just breathing too fast.

Other illnesses

Often, asthma exists in conjunction with other illnesses, most commonly gastro-oesophageal reflux disease (GORD), acute or chronic sinusitis and other infections such as the common cold. Here's what you need to know.

Gastro-oesophageal reflux disease

Figures from Core, the national charity fighting gut and liver disease, show that as many as 60 per cent of people with asthma have GORD, a chronic form of heartburn, compared with between 20 and 30 per cent of the general population. GORD occurs when the oesophageal sphincter, which normally keeps food and acid in your stomach, repeatedly fails to close sufficiently tightly, allowing stomach acid to flow back, or reflux, into the oesophagus and create a burning sensation.

Heartburn is just one symptom of GORD, however; others include cough, chronic sore throat, bad breath and laryngitis. The condition may also be symptomless, when it is known as silent reflux. But if you have asthma and GORD, and GORD is undiagnosed or untreated, it may lead to serious repercussions for your asthma.

The link between the two is still being debated, but doctors suspect that changes in chest pressure that occur during asthma help to relax the oesophageal sphincter. The effects work the other way, too. Acid in the oesophagus can irritate the lungs, by being breathed, or aspirated, into them or by stimulating the bronchial nerves into spasms. To make things even more complicated, some studies also show that theophylline, a medication sometimes used to treat asthma, may worsen GORD symptoms.

The potential environmental and dietary changes you can make to alleviate GORD as an asthma trigger are discussed in more detail in later chapters. For the moment, however, if you often have heartburn (particularly when you lie down), have increased asthma symptoms after meals, and have respiratory symptoms such as frequent coughing and hoarseness, you might ask your doctor if you should be evaluated and treated for GORD. One review of 12 studies found that treating reflux improved asthma symptoms in 69 per cent of the 326 patients enrolled in the studies. Another study found that children who have both GORD and asthma could reduce their use of asthma medication by half if they were effectively treated for reflux. The link remains controversial but a Cochrane review suggests that it is worth investigating and treating GORD in asthmatics.

Sinusitis and allergic rhinitis

Is your nose constantly running? Does it feel as if someone has shovelled concrete behind your eyes? You probably have sinusitis (inflammation of the sinuses) and/or allergic rhinitis. Both are guaranteed to aggravate the symptoms of anyone with asthma. During a sinus infection, mucus draining into the nose, throat and lungs can cause asthma symptoms, while the inflammatory response triggered by an allergen (and causing allergy symptoms) spills over to the lungs, making asthma symptoms worse. However, you can have asthma without having allergies. That's why an asthma diagnosis shouldn't necessarily make you give up your cat; the pet needs to go only if you are allergic to its dander.

Infections

Infection with the rhinovirus, which causes the common cold as well as other respiratory illnesses, can cause wheezing, often sending an asthma sufferer into a fully-fledged attack. Other infectious agents linked to asthma symptoms include respiratory syncytial virus (RSV), *Chlamydia pneumoniae* and *Mycoplasma pneumoniae*. In fact, asthma patients who are infected with mycoplasma have six times more mast cells in their lung tissue than uninfected asthma patients, meaning that they have a much greater risk of inflammation.

Some researchers suspect that many asthma attacks attributed to colds could instead be the fault of this bacterial infection. In some cases, a course of antibiotics may make a huge difference in your ability to control your asthma symptoms.

Your job

During the early 1700s, the Italian physician Bernardino Ramazzini studied bakers exposed to wheat and rye flour, mill workers exposed to grain dust, and farmers sensitive to animal dander and described a link between their asthma and their occupations. All had what today would be called work-related or occupational asthma.

Occupational asthma is the most frequently reported occupational respiratory disease in Britain. According to the British Occupational Health Research Foundation, each year some 3,500 people develop new asthma at work because of the substances to which they are exposed while doing their jobs (occupational asthma). In addition, 750,000 employees find that exposure to allergens and irritants at work aggravate their existing asthma (work-related asthma). Together these cause the loss of more than 12.7 million working days

Is your job stealing your breath?

The following list illustrates the wide range of occupations and agents that are associated with occupational asthma.

Occupation	Allergic to...
Bakers, farmers, flour mill workers and grain elevator workers	flour and grain dust
Research laboratory workers, silk-processing workers, pest control workers	insects; rat and mouse urine proteins
Prawn and fish processors	seafood and other marine organisms
Laboratory workers and animal handlers	animal dander
Detergent producers, food industry workers and blood-processing lab workers	various enzymes
Carpet manufacturing workers, pharmaceutical industry workers, latex glove manufacturing workers and health-care workers	latex and gums
Plastic, rubber or foam manufacturing workers; spray painters; foam insulation installers	diisocyanates such as toluene, diphenylmethane, and hexamethylene
Solderers and electronics industry workers	abietic acid (in rosin, used in soldering fluxes)
Cosmetics, plastics and other industrial workers	castor bean dust from castor oil
Refinery workers	metals such as chromium, platinum and nickel
Textile workers	dyes
Plastic and epoxy resin workers	anhydrides, such as trimellitic and phthalic anhydride
Adhesive handlers	acrylates
Health care workers	glutaraldehyde and formaldehyde
Pharmaceutical industry workers	certain pharmaceuticals

each year. An estimated 9 to 15 per cent of asthma cases in adults of working age are caused by occupational factors, such as wood dust, paints, flour, animals, latex, hair dyes and nickel – substances that are commonly present in many workplaces.

Under the Health and Safety at Work Act, employers are obliged by law to take certain measures to protect employees and others from exposure to substances harmful to health. The Health and Safety Executive (HSE) publish clear advice on how to prevent occupational asthma and employ medical inspectors to advise employers and ensure compliance with the law. In some workplaces, such as shops, offices or hotels, the local council's environmental health office can provide the same service. For further advice on oocupational asthma visit **www.hse.gov.uk/asthma/causes.htm** or telephone the HSE Infoline, 0541 545500 or write to the HSE Information Centre, Broad Lane, Sheffield S3 7HQ.

Medications

Each time you go to the doctor, you are asked if you have any allergies to medications. You probably don't even think about aspirin. But if you have severe asthma and/or nasal polyps, you may have a form of asthma known as aspirin-sensitive asthma, in which the very common pain-killing drug actually makes your asthma symptoms worse.

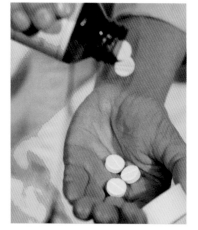

About one in five adults with asthma have attacks triggered by sensitivities to aspirin and other similar drugs.

Overall, 21 per cent of adults with asthma have attacks triggered by sensitivities to aspirin and other similar drugs, known as nonsteroidal anti-inflammatory drugs (NSAIDs). These include ibuprofen (Nurofen, Brufen), naproxen (Naprosyn, Synflex), diclofenac (Voltarol, Diclomax, Motifene) and several others. The older you are, the more likely you are to experience this reaction, and it can be quite serious. Studies show that anywhere from 3 per cent of patients with asthma seen in a private allergy practice to 39 per cent of adults with asthma admitted to an asthma-referral hospital had severe and even fatal asthma attacks after taking aspirin or NSAIDs.

Aspirin and the like are believed to affect sensitive individuals because of their effects on an enzyme called COX-1, which plays a role in producing chemicals that help your lungs to work properly. By preventing the COX-1 enzyme from doing its job, NSAIDs also prevent production of these critical chemicals.

Other medicines known to worsen asthma symptoms include beta-blockers often used to treat high blood pressure, such as propranolol (Inderal), and eye drops prescribed for glaucoma, such as timolol maleate (Timoptol).

Chemicals

This category includes chemicals to which you may have a sensitivity rather than an allergy. Among them are sulphites, often used to preserve foods and beverages, including tuna, salad-bar food, processed potatoes, prawns, dried apples and raisins, lemon juice, grape juice, beer and wine. Some foods containing sulphites may carry warning labels but if you're not sure that a food is safe, avoid it. You may want to check labels for tartrazine, a dye found in many foods and medicines, including cough syrups and liquid cold and flu remedies.

Asthma and women

The overall incidence of asthma is rising, and the rate of increase is notably higher among women than men. In women aged 16 to 44 asthma is more common than any other long-term condition including back pain. Between the 1980s and 1990s asthma levels rose 114 per cent in males and 165 per cent in females. Some of that increase may be due to improved diagnosis, but some is probably related to gender differences.

The turning point appears to be puberty. 'What happens in early childhood is that asthma tends to be two to three times more common in boys,' says Stephen Holgate, Professor of Immunopharmacology (the study of the use of drugs to treat allergies) at the University of Southampton.

That appears to happen until the age of 13 to 14, when the girls catch up. Some children seem to 'outgrow' their asthma but what happens with true asthma is that the symptoms might wane with time but the bronchial inflammation is still there causing excessive sensitivity of the airways.

Professor Holgate admits that the whole question of asthma distribution between the sexes is not clear-cut. 'It's one of those phenomena that might be staring us in the face but we can't see it because we haven't been asking the right questions. There's a dearth of research into the severe end of asthma and how cases are allocated in different groups.'

Although experts cannot explain the gender discrepancy in the incidence of asthma, they have theories. Hormones are thought to play a role and up to 40 per cent of women with asthma find that their symptoms worsen just before and during menstruation. This is probably due to the effects of progesterone, levels of which rise sharply and then drop abruptly towards the end of the menstrual cycle, just before menstruation. Scientists don't yet know exactly how progesterone affects asthma, but the hormone does play a role in inflammation. There is also some evidence to suggest that oral contraceptives, which contain oestrogen, progesterone, or both together, can aggravate asthma symptoms. The hormonal link is supported by a recent study in Norway, which found that

Why does my asthma get worse at night?

Do you often wake up in the middle of the night coughing? Do most of your asthma attacks occur at night? You may have sleep, or nocturnal, asthma, which affects about 70 to 80 per cent of people with asthma. (A persistent nocturnal cough, especially in children, should prompt suspicion of asthma if not already diagnosed).

Symptoms often include shortness of breath and wheezing at night, and may help to explain why 80 per cent of severe asthma attacks occur between midnight and 8am.

Unless you have GORD (described on page 62), your symptoms are probably not related to lying down but rather to the time of day. Asthma, like many diseases, follows the clock or, as they say in medical circles, has its own chronobiology. The study of chronobiology focuses on biological processes that have time-related rhythms.

Basically, it seems that your lungs work better at certain times of the day, regardless of whether or not you have asthma. They are at peak efficiency at around 4pm and much less efficient at around 4am. If you have normal lungs, you don't notice these changes in efficiency, but if you have asthma, your lung function can change as much as 50 per cent throughout the day.

Researchers disagree on whether nocturnal asthma represents a worsening of asthma or whether it is a separate form, like exercise-induced asthma. They do know the symptoms are related not to lying down but to the time of day or night when you sleep, so even if you work nights and sleep during the day, you can still experience sleep asthma. They have also found that the chronobiology of asthma, and hence the propensity for nocturnal symptoms, worsens with age. There are several theories about the cause, but no single answer. Changes in hormones related to sleep and circadian rhythms, which may affect the relaxation of smooth muscles (as in the lungs), and inflammation may play a role.

If you have nocturnal asthma more than once a week, it's a sign that your asthma is not being treated properly. Drugs to treat nocturnal asthma include theophylline and salmeterol (Serevent). You'll learn more about these drugs in chapter 7.

women with irregular periods are more likely to have asthma and allergies. In a study of 6,000 women, those aged 26 to 42 who had erratic periods were 54 per cent more likely to have diagnosed asthma than those with a regular menstrual cycle and almost one-third more likely to experience hay fever.

A woman's weight also contributes to her risk of asthma, with a 1999 study published in *Archives of Internal Medicine* finding that women who gained weight after the age of 18 were at increased risk of developing asthma. The study, part of the long-term, ongoing Nurses' Health Study in the USA, tracking the health of nearly 86,000 women, found that the higher a woman's body mass index (BMI), the greater her risk of asthma. The risk was almost three times greater for women whose BMI was 30 or more than for those whose BMI was less than 20. (A healthy BMI is between 19 and 25.)

Asthma may also worsen or improve during pregnancy. In general, a third of pregnant women with asthma tend to improve, a third find that their symptoms worsen, and a third stay the same, with all returning to their pre-pregnancy

Can I outgrow asthma?

The idea that children can outgrow asthma stems from the fact that wheezing in infancy is often caused by viral infections which may be misdiagnosed as asthma.

As they grow older, children may stop wheezing when those infections strike, suggesting that they have 'outgrown' their asthma. If a child is indeed asthmatic, symptoms may also abate but bronchial inflammation will remain and symptoms could recur.

asthma status once they deliver. Although no one really knows why these changes occur, factors such as increased stress, infections, increased production of inflammatory chemicals known as prostaglandins, and increased resistance to the steroids often used to treat asthma are all reasons why an expectant mother's asthma may get worse. Of course, that doesn't explain why asthma improves in some pregnant women. Women with asthma can have safe and normal pregnancies provided that they keep their asthma under control. This is crucial because asthma attacks cause a decrease in blood oxygen levels, which can affect the amount of oxygen that the baby receives. There is also a certain amount of evidence to suggest that poorly controlled asthma may affect the size of the baby. For that reason, doctors may decide to prescribe medications to pregnant women. Generally speaking, they tend to favour inhaled medications because with these less of the drug reaches the baby. Also, medications that have been used for several years by the mother are less likely to carry risks for the baby. The same medications are also generally safe to use while breastfeeding. We'll talk more about the use of medication during pregnancy in chapter 7.

Living with asthma

Study after study confirms that with the proper treatment – both medical and environmental – you can live a normal life with asthma, avoiding the lung-scarring and life-threatening repercussions of this chronic disease. Yet too few people with asthma receive proper treatment or comply with treatment advice. According to Asthma UK, one in every three asthmatics admitted to hospital in Scotland receives no information about follow-up treatment. Furthermore, three out of four asthma-related hospital admissions could be avoided if proper information and support was given by care workers.

Here's where the Breathe Easy Plan comes in. The book not only shows you how to get the right diagnosis but also explains about treatment options so that you can work with your doctor to ensure you are receiving the right treatment. You'll learn how to use medications properly; and how to evaluate your life so that you can change those things that could be making your asthma worse – except, perhaps, the weather.

Chapter five

All about
food
allergies

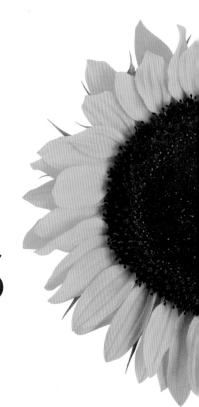

Remember the days when peanuts were considered to be
perfectly normal party fare, without the hint of a health threat? Today, most
parents and schools are well aware that they could trigger a lethal allergic
reaction in susceptible people.

An increasing number of children in the UK are allergic to peanuts, and
peanut allergy, the most common food allergy to cause fatal or near-fatal
reactions, has more than doubled over the past 10 years and now affects one
in 70 children.

It is not known exactly how many people in the UK have a food allergy. As
many as one in five people believe they are intolerant to one or more foods, yet
tests show that only about 1 to 2 per cent of adults and 4 per cent of children in
the UK has a true food allergy – about 1 million people. More than one child in
100 is believed to suffer severe allergic reactions to peanuts, other types of nut
or both. A small but significant number are affected by other foods.

Food allergies, whether to peanuts, other nuts, shellfish, dairy products or
egg whites, are serious. They are the leading cause of anaphylaxis, the life-
threatening reaction that causes difficulty breathing, swelling in the mouth and
throat, a sudden drop in blood pressure and in some cases loss of consciousness.

Hospital admissions for allergies have increased sharply. In 1990, 1,960 people were admitted to hospital because of allergic reactions. By 2001, that figure had more than trebled to 6,752. Hospital admissions for allergic swellings and anaphylaxis were up 70 per cent, while food allergies went up fivefold, or 500 per cent. Each year there are between six and ten reported deaths due to food induced anaphylaxis.

That is why people with severe food allergies carry a strong antidote with them at all times. The drug is a synthetic version of the naturally occurring hormone adrenaline (epinephrine), which counteracts anaphylaxis. It comes in the form of a pen (Epi-Pen or Anapen).

There is also increasing evidence that food allergies may be a risk factor for severe asthma in children, with one study finding that 56 per cent of children with serious asthma also had food allergies, compared with just 10.5 per cent of those with mild asthma. The results suggest that life-threatening asthma attacks may be triggered by food allergies in susceptible patients with asthma.

The rising prevalence of food allergies cannot be due solely to increased consumption; in oriental countries, for example, nut allergies are rare despite high levels of nut consumption. Scientists suggest that reasons for the rise in peanut allergies may include exposure to allergens earlier in life as a result of early weaning, the use of nut ingredients in baby oils and products to ease sore nipples in breast feeding, or the increased allergenicity of roasted nuts.

Unlike allergic rhinitis or asthma, there is no effective treatment for food allergies. All you can do is avoid the food in question, which takes a Herculean effort these days. Food allergens can be so pervasive that some people have had serious reactions simply because they walked through a fish market or kissed someone who had recently eaten seafood. For some, even inhaling the fumes from frying or steaming foods to which they're allergic can trigger a reaction.

Food allergies defined

If you have a food allergy, blame your parents: it's an inherited predisposition. In other words, if your family has a history of allergies, you are much more likely than, say, the child of allergy-free parents to develop a food allergy. The development of a food allergy begins with one simple step: exposure to the food. If you never touch or eat a peanut, you'll never develop a peanut allergy. Even that first peanut butter cracker may be innocuous, but as you digest it, it triggers your immune system to produce IgE antibodies that will be activated the next time you eat the food. Actually, it's not the food that triggers the reaction but rather proteins within the food that cooking, stomach acids or digestive enzymes don't break down. These proteins are absorbed through the gastrointestinal lining into your bloodstream then travel through your body.

From there, the process is familiar: the proteins interact with the IgE molecules on the surface of mast cells, triggering the cells to release

Watch what you eat: common culprit foods

Theoretically, any food containing protein can contribute to a food allergy. In reality, the following seven foods account for the vast majority of the food allergies in the UK.

1 **Peanuts** These are the leading cause of severe allergic reactions to food, including food-related anaphylaxis.

2 **Seafood** If you have a seafood allergy, the chances are you react to shellfish, generally prawns, crayfish, lobster or crab. Some people, however, are also allergic to both fresh and salt-water fish. Once you have a seafood allergy, you will probably have it for life.

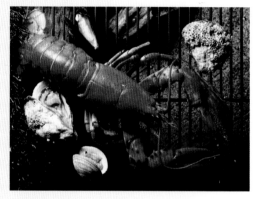

3 **Tree nuts** Almonds, Brazil nuts, cashews, hazelnuts and walnuts are included in this category.

4 **Eggs** The whites in particular cause reactions. More children than adults have an allergy to eggs, and children with atopic dermatitis (dry, scaly, itchy skin) have an increased risk of an allergic response to eggs.

5 **Cow's milk** The principal culprits are the proteins in milk, such as lactoglobulin, lactalbumin, casein and whey. Milk allergies almost always begin in the first year of life, soon after cow's milk or cow's-milk-based formula is introduced to a child's diet. Between 2 and 7 per cent of infants under one year old suffer from cow's milk allergy, making it the most common food allergy of childhood.

6 **Soya** The prevalence of soya-based formulas and baby foods today is leading to an increase in soya allergies among babies, with gastrointestinal symptoms most common.

7 **Wheat** Don't confuse a wheat allergy with gluten sensitivity. Gluten is the component of wheat, barley, rye and other grains that provides the 'glue' holding the grain together. It is associated with a disease called gluten-sensitive enteropathy, or coeliac disease, caused by an abnormal response to gluten. A wheat allergy, on the other hand, means that you are allergic to certain proteins in wheat. If you eliminate wheat from your diet and your symptoms disappear, you have a wheat allergy; if the problem persists even after you substitute other grains, the chances are your symptoms are related to gluten. Of course, an allergy test is generally the best way to find out what's plaguing you.

inflammatory chemicals such as histamine. *Where* those chemicals are released determines your reaction. For instance, the mast cells on your skin are most likely to be affected by food allergies, leading to hives or atopic dermatitis (eczema), a skin condition characterized by itchy, scaly red skin. If mast cells in your ears, nose and throat are activated, your mouth may itch, and you may have trouble breathing or swallowing. If they are activated in your gastrointestinal tract, you may have abdominal pain, diarrhoea or vomiting. If it happens in your lungs, you could have an asthma attack.

A food reaction can vary from mild tingling in the mouth to full-blown anaphylaxis with collapse. The reaction can start almost instantly as the food touches your mouth, or may develop more slowly over the next hour or so. This sequence is known as IgE-mediated food allergy, for the obvious reason that IgE antibodies are integral to the reaction.

You can also have a *non*-IgE-mediated food reaction. This occurs when a food triggers the production of T cells, which in turn call in other substances that activate your immune response, including inflammation. Most non-IgE-mediated food reactions result in gastrointestinal symptoms, such as gas, and are not life-threatening.

A third possibility is a combination of IgE-mediated allergy and non-IgE-mediated food sensitivity. For instance, you could have a bona fide allergy to milk and at the same time be lactose intolerant, meaning that you lack the enzyme that enables you to digest the milk sugar lactose.

If you are allergic to one food, you are more likely to be allergic to others. For instance, if you have a history of allergic reactions to prawns, you're likely to be allergic to crab, lobster and crayfish as well. Doctors call this cross-reactivity. Furthermore, people who have a birch-pollen allergy may also react to hazelnuts, apples, carrots and celery. And if you're allergic to latex, watch out for bananas.

Some people suffer from exercise-induced food allergy. In this form, if you eat a certain food and exercise soon afterwards a reaction is triggered. As you work out and your body temperature rises, you begin to itch, become light-headed, and soon have allergy symptoms such as hives or even anaphylaxis. The cure is simple: don't eat for a couple of hours before exercising.

Food allergy or food intolerance?

Each time you drink a glass of milk or eat an ice-cream cone, you feel bloated, with gas, stomach pain and diarrhoea. Does this mean that you are allergic to milk? Probably not. Usually only young children are allergic to milk and other dairy products; you are probably lactose intolerant. If you lack the enzyme lactase, your body can't digest lactose, a sugar found in dairy products. Lactose intolerance affects 5 per cent of the population, but among Black and Asian communities, where milk is not traditionally consumed as part of the typical adult diet, it is far more prevalent, developing in 80 to 90 per cent of people.

In this area, self-diagnoses tend to be faulty. Although only between 1 and 2 per cent of adults in the UK have food allergies, as many as 20 to 30 per cent *think* they do. Although the allergy rate among children is higher, a far greater percentage of children are misdiagnosed as having food allergy. And you should be careful not to eliminate too many foods from the diet, such as milk and wheat, as this can lead to nutritional deficiencies causing significant problems.

Instead of an allergy, what many children have is a food intolerance – an abnormal response to a food that is not an allergic reaction. It differs from an allergy in that it doesn't involve the body's immune system but rather an inability to digest the food.

It's understandable that people might think that they have food allergies, since the symptoms mimic those of reactions to infectious agents and other substances, as well as digestive problems. For instance:

■ **Micro-organisms** Foods contaminated with micro-organisms, such as bacteria, and their products, such as toxins, can trigger symptoms that mimic an allergic food reaction. In reality, the problem is food poisoning.

■ **Histamines** Some natural substances, such as histamines, can occur in foods and stimulate a reaction similar to an allergic reaction. For example, histamine can reach high levels in cheese, some wines and certain kinds of fish, particularly tuna and mackerel. In fish, histamine is believed to stem from bacterial contamination, particularly in fish that has not been refrigerated properly. If you eat a food with a high level of histamine, you may experience histamine toxicity, a reaction that strongly resembles an allergic reaction to food.

■ **Food additives** Compounds used to preserve, colour or flavour foods are often linked with adverse reactions that can be mistaken for food allergy. These include: sulphur dioxide and sulphites (E220-28), found in soft drinks, sausages, burgers and dried fruit; and benzoic acid and benzoates (E210-19),

Preventing food allergies

The majority of studies suggest that exclusively breastfeeding babies for their first four to six months helps to reduce their risk of allergies, particularly to milk or soya. If you or your partner have a history of atopy and you breastfeed, Allergy UK recommends that you try to avoid nuts, including peanuts, and have a normal, healthy mixed diet unless your baby has had an obvious allergic reaction to a specific food you have eaten. Allergy UK also has a factsheet, available on request, which explains how to wean to reduce the risk of your child developing food allergies.

common in soft drinks and naturally occurring in fruit and honey; both can trigger asthma in susceptible people. Tartrazine (E102), a yellow dye widely used in soft drinks, sweets and sauces, can cause nettle rash (urticaria), dermatitis, asthma or rhinitis.

■ **Gluten** Some people are gluten intolerant, a condition associated with a disease called gluten-sensitive enteropathy, or coeliac disease. It is caused by an abnormal immune response to gluten, a component of wheat and some other grains. A blood test that looks for anti-gliadin antibodies can diagnose this problem.

■ **Psychological factors, or food aversion** Certain foods may be associated with bad memories. Say, for instance, that when you were young, your parents took you regularly to a local Chinese restaurant. You hated the food: spare ribs, egg fu yung and wonton soup, and had a miserable time yelling and screaming in protest. Today, when you eat those dishes, you have what seems to be an allergic reaction. Since the foods remind you of those awful experiences, they may trigger a physical reaction to the psychological distress.

■ **Diseases** Some diseases that share symptoms with food allergies (such as vomiting, diarrhoea, cramping or abdominal pain that becomes worse when you eat) include ulcers, colitis and cancers of the gastrointestinal tract.

The challenges of avoiding foods

You may be wondering, what's the problem? If you're allergic to peanuts, simply avoid peanuts and foods that contain them. Allergic to shellfish? Don't order the prawn dishes on the menu.

But it's not that easy, particularly given our increasing dependence on prepackaged and processed foods. Up to 50 per cent of people who are allergic to peanuts experience an accidental peanut ingestion every four years, even if they are exceedingly careful. It is also possible that a juice drink boxed on a packaging line that is also used for milk products could receive enough milk protein contamination to trigger an allergic reaction. The same is true of tofu desserts packaged in ice cream plants. Maureen Jenkins, an allergy nurse consultant in Sussex and an adviser to Allergy UK, notes that a banana slice lying against a slice of kiwi may contain enough kiwi protein to provoke an allergic response and even crisps in a bowl previously containing nuts may prompt an allergic response in a nut-allergic person.

Simply working out what's *in* certain foods is a major challenge. Terminology and the inclusion of less than obvious ingredients complicates matters. For instance, it can be particularly hard to avoid eggs. Did you know that most commercially processed cooked pastas (including those used in prepared foods such as soup) contain eggs or are processed on equipment shared with pastas that contain eggs. Or that eggs may be used to create the foam or milk topping on specialty coffee drinks and are put in some cocktails? Or that flu vaccines are grown on egg embryos and may contain small bits of egg protein?

Many medications contain food proteins. And if you're allergic to fish, watch out for Worcestershire sauce and Caesar salad dressing; they both contain anchovies.

Then there's milk. Just because the label says a product is dairy-free, that doesn't mean it's milk-free. Current labelling guidelines allow the use of the term *dairy-free* even for foods that contain milk by-products.

As noted, milk and soya proteins are often added to increase protein content or enhance flavour to a wide variety of foods. Likewise, spices (such as garlic and coriander) and seed derivatives (such as mustard and sesame seeds) are included for flavouring in many prepared foods. Peanut and nut products are added to flavour and thicken sauces (such as spaghetti sauce, gravy and barbecue sauce) and baked goods. And eggs and milk may be added to boost the nutrients in other food products.

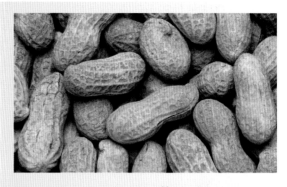

More on peanut allergies

There are plenty of beliefs in circulation about peanut allergies. One widely held belief is that peanut allergies are always life-long. Until recently this was thought to be true. However, a growing body of recent evidence suggests that some children may, in fact, outgrow peanut allergies.

Another belief is that merely inhaling the odour of peanuts or sitting next to someone who is eating a peanut butter sandwich can trigger a reaction. There is some evidence to support this. Although inhaling allergens is a very rare source of reactions, it can and does occur in susceptible people. As a precaution, many airlines have now stopped serving roasted peanuts with drinks during flights because the dust could trigger allergy attacks in passengers.

Manufacturers are improving labelling but you have to find out a lot about the content of foods yourself. For example, some people who react adversely to peanuts also react to unrefined or gourmet peanut oil. Peanut oil is sometimes called groundnut or arachis oil, and many manufacturers often label foods as containing 'vegetable oil', which may well contain peanut oil. Possible contamination is usually addressed by 'may contain nuts' labelling.

But it appears that UK consumers are generally becoming more aware of food labelling. In its 2004 survey of consumer attitudes, the Food Standards Agency found that 78 per cent of consumers claim to check food labels, 31 per cent always, 26 per cent usually and 21 per cent occasionally. Three in five people found information on food labelling easy to understand, though one in five found some labels 'fairly difficult' to understand, and one in 20 found them 'very difficult'.

While confidence in the accuracy of food labelling appears to have slightly increased, more than half of the consumers interviewed for the survey were concerned about the accuracy of health claims made for various products, although the majority (58 per cent) were 'fairly' rather than 'very'concerned.

Supermarkets are also becoming more 'allergy-friendly'. Most major supermarkets now have lists of foods that are 'free from' (nuts, egg, milk, gluten and other culprit foods). These are available on request so it is worth telephoning the customer services department of your local store for more information.

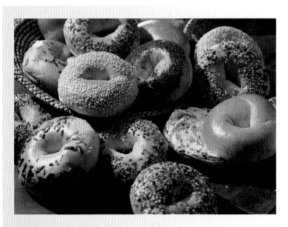

Other food culprits

The vast majority of food allergies are triggered by one of the seven foods listed on page 71. Yet there are other potential culprits. Seeds, for one. These include sesame seeds, sunflower seeds and poppy seeds. The problem is much bigger than you'd think. Just consider your local bakery, where seeded rolls and bagels – including poppy seeds and sesame seeds – sit side by side, or think of sesame-seeded hamburger buns at a fast food restaurant. In addition, sesame and poppy are considered to be spices by some food manufacturers, so they don't have to be listed as separate ingredients on labels.

The good news? The oils from cottonseed and sunflower seeds are usually highly refined, meaning they are free of proteins, so they are unlikely to cause a problem for anyone allergic to various seeds.

Diagnosing food allergies

Diagnosis of food allergies is sometimes very straightforward. If clearly allergic symptoms like urticaria or anaphylaxis occurred immediately after eating a single suspect food such as a nut or a prawn, your doctor may ask a few questions and then proceed straight to a skin or blood test to confirm diagnosis.

In other cases, the link between a food and a reaction is not as obvious, for example, if symptoms were less specific (like headache or diarrhoea), occurred some time after eating, or were prompted by a food with many ingredients, such as a curry or pie. And food sensitivities, as distinct from true allergies, can be much harder to pin down. In these cases your doctor will probably take a detailed medical history of your symptoms: such as when they occur, how long they last, what treatments have worked, with what food they might be associated, how much you ate before the reaction began, how the food was prepared, and what other foods you were eating at the same time as the one you may suspect made you ill. You will also probably be asked to keep a food diary like the one below, in which you make a note of everything you put into your mouth. Such steps may enable your doctor to reach a diagnosis with no further testing; in this case, he or she will probably put you on an elimination diet, in which you eliminate the suspect food for a week or two and see if the symptoms disappear. Again, the food diary will come in handy in tracking whether this works. If your symptoms disappear when you eliminate the food, then reappear when you eat it again, it's almost certain that the food is causing the symptoms.

To confirm a food allergy, your doctor may carry out medical tests that measure the allergic response. These include:

Skin prick test The skin test lancet is dipped into the suspect fresh food, then scratched or pricked into the skin on your forearm or back. Any swelling or redness, called a wheal, indicates a local allergic reaction, meaning you have IgE on your skin's mast cells specific to the food being tested.

RAST blood test If you have severe reactions to the suspect food that lead to anaphylaxis, or if you develop severe skin rashes or hives, your doctor will probably suggest a blood test such as the RAST test to measure the presence of

Keeping a food diary

The best way to find out if you have a food sensitivity is to keep a food diary for at least two weeks. It seems tedious, but it's what your doctor will tell you to do, too. Keep track of everything you put in your mouth, including chewing gum, as well as processed and other prepared foods. If you have a bad reaction, go back and add greater detail about the ingredients of your most recent meal. This written record should provide the data you need to identify the culprit. You can set up your chart like this one.

Date	Time	Food	Symptoms	Time elapsed between eating the food and start of the symptoms

Cookbooks and recipes

Looking for a recipe for chocolate cake that doesn't include eggs or milk? How about tips for shopping, substituting foods, and cooking when you or a family member has food allergies?

There are plenty of cookbooks to help you. Those below are all recommended by Allergy UK on their website www.allergyuk.org/info_booklist.html and are available from bookshops or from Amazon.co.uk You'll find more at www.dontgonuts.co.uk/books.htm

- *The Allergy Free Cookbook* by Michelle Barridale-Johnson (Thorsons, £6.99)
- *The New Allergy Diet* by Dr J.O. Hunter (Vermillion, £8.99)
- *Recipes for Health: Easy Wheat, Milk and Egg-Free Cooking* by Rita Greer (Thorsons, £6.99)
- *The Sensitive Gourmet: Imaginative Cooking Without Wheat, Gluten or Dairy* by Antoinette Savill (HarperCollins, £17.99)
- *Allergy Free Cooking for Kids* by Antoinette Savill (Thorsons, £12.99)

The internet also has some excellent sites if you are looking for recipes for someone with a food allergy or food intolerance. Simply type 'special diet cookery' or 'special diet recipes' (or anything similar) into your search engine and see what comes up.

food-specific IgE in your blood. It takes about a week to get results.

While an immediate allergic reaction to food, backed up by a positive skin prick or RAST test is usually sufficient to diagnose IgE-mediated food allergy, skin tests cannot be used to predict allergic reactions to foods; many patients who test positive to particular foods do not react when they actually eat them. Occasionally a skin test is misleading if the wrong food was tested.

Double-blind food challenge
This involves placing various suspect and non-suspect foods in individual opaque capsules. You swallow a capsule, and the doctor waits to see if you have a reaction, then you continue the process until you've taken all the capsules. The study is considered 'blinded' because neither you nor the doctor know what food the capsules contain until the test is finished. (Alternatively, the suspect food may be disguised in other foods.) Someone with a history of severe reactions can't be tested this way, and, because the test takes time, it's fairly expensive. Studies show that fewer than half of all people who suspect that they have a food allergy test positive in a double-blind food challenge.

Treatment for food allergies

Currently, there is no treatment – in terms of medication – for food allergies. There is hope on the horizon, however, in the form of an experimental drug that locks on to circulating IgE, thus preventing it from locking on to the mast cells. The IgE is rendered harmless before it can 'hit' any targets. In a study published in 2003 in the *New England Journal of Medicine*, researchers reported that the injectable drug kept people who were allergic to peanuts from having serious reactions. You'll learn more about this drug in chapter 7.

There is some evidence that traditional Chinese medicines may have anti-allergenic properties, which may be useful for treating peanut allergy. When researchers from Mount Sinai School of Medicine and Johns Hopkins University investigated the effects of a Chinese herbal formula, FAHF-1, on mice that were bred to have severe peanut allergies, they discovered that the compound completely blocked anaphylactic symptoms and significantly reduced peanut-specific IgE levels after two weeks of treatment.

Researchers are also making progress in the development of a vaccine for peanut allergies, with several groups reporting the production of a vaccine against allergy-causing proteins that proved 'very effective' in mice with peanut allergies. A vaccine for peanut allergies has also been tested on dogs. It is hoped that human trials will begin within the next few years.

As if that weren't enough, other researchers are trying to genetically alter foods such as peanuts and soybeans to remove the allergy-causing proteins. Someday, the thinking goes, people with food allergies may be able to eat whatever they want – without having to read complicated food labels.

Skin-food alert!

If you or members of your family have adverse reactions to specific foods you are probably scrupulous about checking food labels in food stores and supermarkets. But do you check the labels on skin care products?

Many soaps, cosmetics and so-called 'personal care' products contain food ingredients to which some people may have a sensitivity. Under recent EU legislation, any preparation that is applied to the skin, eyes, mouth, hair or nails must carry a list of ingredients to enable consumers to identify products that might be harmful to them. The only problem is that ingredients are listed using their Latin names, which may not be instantly recognizable. An example is 'arachis oil', which is the International Nomenclature of Cosmetic Ingredients (INCI) name for peanut oil.

The solution is for you to have a list with the Latin names of ingredients you may wish to avoid, and to refer to it whenever buying such products. A list of Latin (INCI) names is available from the Cosmetic Toiletry and Perfumery Association on their website www.ctpa.org.uk/home.asp

Below are some common food ingredients with their INCI names as they appear on the packaging of skin care products.

• Avocado	Persea gratissim
• Bitter almond	Prunus amara
• Brazil nut	Bertholletia excelsa
• Coconut	Cocos nucifera
• Cod liver oil	Gadi iecur
• Egg	Ovum
• Hazel nut	Corylus rostrata/americana/ avellana
• Melon	Cucumis melo
• Milk	Lac
• Mixed fish oil	Piscum iecur
• Pea	Pisum sativum
• Peanut oil	Arachis oil
• Sesame	Sesamum indicum
• Soy	Glycine soja
• Sweet almond or almond oil	Prunus dulcis
• Walnut	Juglans regia/nigra

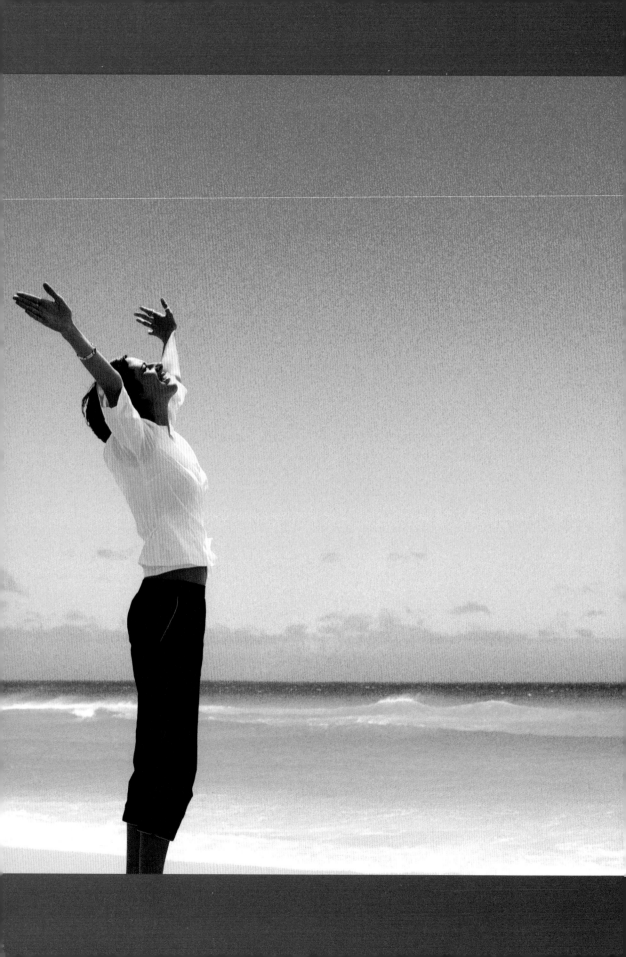

PART TWO

The solutions

You CAN control your allergies and
asthma. No matter what the
severity or cause of your condition,
researchers have developed
outstanding medications to end the
attacks and prevent new ones
from occurring. Equally important,
there are many things in your
power to improve your situation.

Chapter **six**

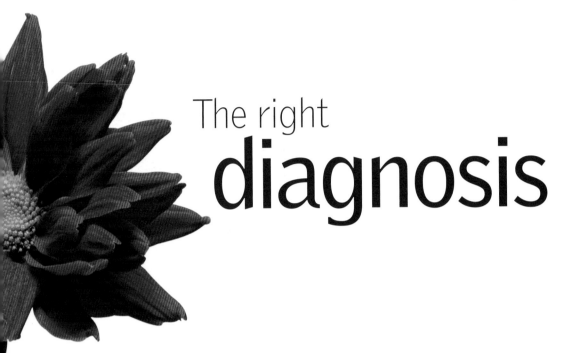

The right
diagnosis

So you're tired of spending every spring and summer wheezing, with your eyes red and your nose clogged. It's time to get a proper diagnosis and get those allergies taken care of.

You may think that this is quite unnecessary. After all, you have just identified your problem. Next, you'll be thinking that you don't need a doctor and that all you need to do is pop to the chemist's and stock up on antihistamines.

If that is the case, you could fall into one of the biggest traps in the allergy/asthma world: thinking that you can self-diagnose and, by extension, self-treat your symptoms.

First, as discussed earlier, allergies and asthma are extremely good at masquerading as other ailments and vice versa. In one 2002 survey conducted by the The American College of Allergy, Asthma and Immunology, 41 per cent of those with allergies thought they had colds or viral infections when they first began having allergy symptoms.

But even doctors and health care workers don't always reach a correct diagnosis. A recent survey of members of Allergy UK showed that only half of asthma patients reporting symptoms of allergic rhinitis have been diagnosed as suffering from both conditions. Sometimes asthma patients are not aware that they have hay fever and believe that they are suffering from a persistent cold. Only about two out of three (69 per cent) patients are aware that asthma and allergic rhinitis are associated.

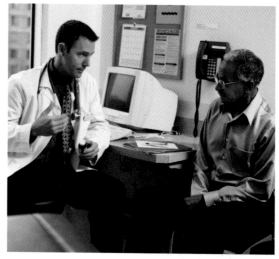

A report by the Respiratory Alliance in 2003 identified a shortfall in NHS services for people with allergies and respiratory disease. For example, although rhinitis is recognized as a risk factor in the development of asthma, and treatment of rhinitis can help to alleviate asthma symptoms, it is often missed by health professionals or not treated properly. This is in line with Asthma UK surveys which found that only half of people with asthma had been told what to do in the event of an attack.

A recent Asthma UK audit found that even when asthma is diagnosed, many people do not receive adequate information and advice. The organisation's reports show that only half of asthma sufferers feel they have a full discussion with their doctor or nurse about the best medication for them; only 3 per cent of patients have a personal written action plan agreed with their health professional; and one-third of patients with severe asthma had not been seen by a health professional for more than a year for a treatment review.

Yet even despite any such shortcomings in healthcare services, you should always seek a professional diagnosis. Here's how to go about it.

If your symptoms trouble you, a proper medical diagnosis is advisable as early allergy symptoms can be easily confused with colds and viruses.

Choosing a doctor

If you have recently moved house and are not already registered with a local NHS doctor, ask for a list of GPs in your area. Lists are available from NHS Direct, the local library or your local Health Authority. It is also a good idea to ask neighbours, friends and the local pharmacist to recommend a good GP.

Then you should pay a visit to the surgery – you can tell a great deal about a medical practice from even a short visit. Are the receptionists welcoming and efficient? Is the waiting room clean and not too crowded? Are there magazines or newspapers to read and toys for children to play with? What leaflets and posters are on display? Confidence in your doctor is all-important, so you should choose a doctor you feel you can talk to, who doesn't make you feel rushed, who takes your symptoms seriously, answers your questions and explains things in language that you can understand. It is worth remembering that you can't insist that a particular GP accepts you as a patient, and an NHS doctor is not obliged to provide a reason for turning you down.

Most medical care for asthma is provided within primary care, by a GP or an asthma nurse, often in dedicated clinics. Ask whether your practice has a GP or nurse who is a member of the General Practice in Airways Group (GPIAG): if so, you are likely to receive better care. Severe cases of asthma are referred to respiratory physicians: few people get to see an allergist or clinical immunologist.

At present there are only a few specialist allergy clinics in the UK. These are mainly located in London and the south-east of England, and allergy services tend to be poor elsewhere in the country. Out-patient waiting times for referral to these centres vary from three months to two years. One key reason for this is the relative shortage of qualified experts in this field. In the UK there is only one full-time consultant allergist per 2.1 million people, compared with a rate of one consultant per 90,000–100,000 people for mainstream specialities such as cardiology or gastroenterology.

You will need to see your GP for an initial diagnosis and may then be referred to an allergy or asthma specialist if any of the following apply.

- Your GP has difficulties diagnosing your condition.
- Your symptoms continue despite the treatment prescribed.

Cold or allergy?

So you think you have an allergy. But can you be sure? Although an estimated 18 million people in the UK suffer from allergies, other conditions – such as colds – are very good at mimicking them. Before you make an appointment with your doctor, take a few minutes to answer the following questions.

1 Do your symptoms, including sneezing, congestion, runny nose, watery eyes, fatigue, and headaches, occur simultaneously?   yes ☐   no ☐

2 Is the duration of your symptoms variable – for instance, sometimes a month or more and sometimes just a couple of days or even hours?   yes ☐   no ☐

3 Is the mucus discharge from your nose clear?   yes ☐   no ☐

4 Do you sneeze frequently, particularly two or three times in a row?   yes ☐   no ☐

5 Do your symptoms occur more often between spring and autumn?   yes ☐   no ☐

6 Are your nasal symptoms unaccompanied by aches and chills?   yes ☐   no ☐

SCORING *3 to 5* yes *answers:* It's quite likely that your symptoms are related to allergies. See your health care provider for further testing. *3 to 5* no *answers:* You probably have a cold or other respiratory ailment. Wait a few days, and if it doesn't clear up on its own, see your health-care provider.

You need specialist allergy testing or immunotherapy (allergy injections).

You have other conditions that make your allergies or asthma symptoms worse, such as polyps, gastro-oesophageal reflux, chronic bronchitis or emphysema.

The best way to find a specialist is to start with recommendations from your doctor, or from friends or relatives. If that is not satisfactory, you may want to search for your nearest clinic on the website of the British Society for Allergy and Clinical Immunology at: **www.bsaci.org/clinics/UK**

Preparing for the first visit

Your initial evaluation session will go more smoothly if you take time preparing for it before going to your doctor's surgery. To help you to do this properly, we have produced the personal assessment project below. It is worth while trying to do this, both for your own benefit and that of your doctor, who will then be in a much better position to make a fast, correct diagnosis. Here are the elements of your home assignment:

1 Track your allergy/asthma symptoms, using the log provided overleaf.
2 Gather salient health history facts, using the health history form provided (for your benefit and that of your GP, who should have these on record).
3 Finally, when it is closer to the time for your appointment, you should try to prepare your answers to the 10 questions that your doctor is likely to ask (see box on page 89).

Make copies of these forms as required, and remember that it is in your best interest to be thorough and honest in all your answers.

allergy & asthma **sufferers ask**
Are our needs being met?

The prevalence, severity and complexity of allergy in the population is rising rapidly yet there are major inadequacies in the current provision of allergy services in the UK. Those working in primary care often lack the training, expertise and incentives to deliver allergy services. Furthermore, a 2003 report by the Royal College of Physicians found only six full-time centres (concentrated mainly in the south-east) staffed by consultant allergists with expertise in all types of allergic problems.

Among its proposals for an improved NHS allergy service over the coming decade, the report proposed creating more consultant posts and funded training posts in allergy, and setting up regional, appropriately staffed, specialist allergy centres evenly distributed throughout the country. Acknowledging that primary care must ultimately provide the front line care for allergy care, it proposed including clinical allergy training on the undergraduate medical curriculum and improved training of GPs and practice nurses.

A 2004 House of Commons Health Committee report on the provision of allergy services strongly endorsed the proposals, urging the Department of Health to respond with a strategy document to show that it takes seriously the growing problem of allergy and to provide a catalyst for change.

Form one

Symptom tracking log

Each time symptoms occur, use this log. Rank each symptom on a scale from 1 to 10, with 1 being barely noticeable and 10 interfering with your ability to function.

Date and circumstances*	Missed school or work	Decreased exercise tolerance	Tight chest/short of breath	Waking up at night	Sneezing	Postnasal drip	Nasal congestion	Itchy nose	Runny eyes	Headache	Wheezing	Cough

*Note whether you were around pets, at work or working in the garden; sudden changes in the weather; the foods you ate and medications you took; whether you were exercising; and so on.

Form two

Your health history

NAME _____

DATE OF BIRTH _____   SEX   male ☐   female ☐

OCCUPATION _____

MARITAL STATUS   single ☐   married ☐   widowed ☐   divorced ☐

CURRENT MEDICINES

Prescription_____

_____

Non-prescription (list all you take regularly, including antacids, pain relievers and healing supplements)

_____

_____

CURRENT/CHRONIC MEDICAL CONDITIONS _____

_____

PAST MEDICAL PROBLEMS (include year they occurred) _____

_____

SURGERY (include year it occurred) _____

_____

ALLERGIES   yes ☐   no ☐

To which of the following are you allergic (be specific)?

Insects _____

Plants _____

Medications _____

Foods _____

Other _____

TOBACCO USE   yes ☐   no ☐   Current use (type/amount) _____

Started (year or age) _____ Stopped (year or age) _____

ALCOHOL USE   yes ☐   no ☐

Estimated number of drinks (beer, wine, spirits) per day/week _____

Are you or others you know concerned about your use of alcohol?   yes ☐   no ☐

SUPPLEMENT USE

Daily vitamin: yes ☐   no ☐   Occasional vitamins: yes ☐   no ☐

List vitamins taken _____

DIET /EXERCISE

My current diet is: very healthy ☐   healthy ☐   variable ☐   unhealthy ☐

Concerns: _____

My current exercise/activity level is: very high ☐   high ☐   moderate ☐   low ☐

Concerns: _____

My current weight is: much too high ☐   somewhat high ☐   acceptable ☐   too low ☐

Concerns: _____

I have previously used a diet or other programmme to gain/lose weight: yes ☐   no ☐

I have previously used medicines or supplements to gain/lose weight: yes ☐   no ☐

FAMILY MEDICAL HISTORY

No knowledge of family medical history ☐

Race/ethnicity (optional) _____

Relative	Age	Health status	If deceased, cause/age at death
Father			
Mother			
Siblings			
Children			
Other			

Please tick all conditions that apply to members of your family (brother, sister, father, mother, aunt, uncle, grandparent) below and note the relationship or additional concerns.

☐ Alcohol/substance abuse _____

☐ Arthritis _____

☐ Asthma/allergies _____

☐ Bleeding/clotting disorder _____

☐ Breast disease (benign) _____

☐ Breast disease (cancer) _____

☐ Chronic lung disease _____

☐ Diabetes _____

☐ Headaches _____

☐ Heart disease _____

☐ High blood pressure _____

☐ High cholesterol _____

☐ Mental illness _____

☐ Seizures/epilepsy _____

☐ Stroke _____

☐ Thyroid disorder _____

☐ Ulcers _____

☐ Other (specify) _____

_____

_____

Mission: diagnosis

Although doctors use several tests for allergies and asthma, they are mainly used to confirm a diagnosis and provide more detailed information. The most important part of any diagnosis is the physical examination and medical history, so it's vitally important that you are completely honest with your doctor during your initial examination, answering every question as fully as possible. For instance, if you suspect that you are allergic to cats, hiding the fact that you have a kitten at home won't do you any good. Also tell your doctor *why* you think you have a certain allergy. Be specific; it's not enough to say you think you have allergies; describe your symptoms in some detail and refer to your symptom tracking log so that you can provide your doctor with a proper overview of your condition.

During the physical examination, depending on your presenting symptoms, your doctor may focus on your eyes, ears, nose and throat, looking for such signs as the boggy, pale grey-blue lining of the nose characteristic of allergies; any nasal polyps or sinus infection; dark circles under your eyes; redness of your throat; and postnasal drip. Your doctor may also want to listen to your chest and/or check your skin condition.

Diagnosing allergies

Many GPs can diagnose allergic rhinitis simply on the basis of your medical history. That is sufficient for run-of-the-mill allergies, but if yours are significantly interfering with your life or are not easily controlled with standard medications, you may need to undergo blood tests or be referred to a specialist for more sophisticated testing. The aim would be to pinpoint the exact cause so that a more targeted treatment plan can be developed for your specific problem. You can then try to find ways to avoid the allergens. You are also more likely to require allergy testing if you have allergic asthma (asthma that is triggered by allergens).

The two main types of allergy tests are skin tests and blood tests.

Questions your doctor may ask

1 When did your symptoms begin?

2 What makes them better or worse?

3 When do they typically appear?

4 Have you ever been diagnosed with allergies or asthma?

5 Do you wheeze or cough a lot, particularly at night?

6 Do you ever have difficulty breathing?

7 Are you oversensitive to heat, cold or temperature changes?

8 Do your symptoms persist when you go away from home on holiday? Do they get worse?

9 Do you have any relatives with current asthma or allergies?

10 Do you have relatives who have or had a history of allergies?

1 Skin tests

Gold-standard, immediate-type hypersensitivity (IgE) skin tests are typically used to test for a skin reaction to airborne allergens, foods, insect stings and penicillin. A positive skin test implies that the problem is due to IgE antibodies to a particular allergen. Skin tests can also help to diagnose some drug hypersensitivities and food allergies (but your doctor may not do a skin test if you have had a very bad reaction to a food or drug – a blood test is safer.) Skin tests for food are best done with the fresh product – your doctor may ask you to bring these with you to the clinic. Although early skin tests used a 'scratch' technique, in which the allergen was applied to the skin and the skin was scratched, this has been largely replaced by the more accurate prick/puncture test (see page 91).

Before having any tests, talk to your doctor about which, if any, medicines you should stop taking. Generally, you will need to stop all antihistamines for three to five days and sometimes more, depending on the drug, since they may affect the test's accuracy. You may also need temporarily to stop taking any other drugs with antihistamine properties, including those for schizophrenia, such as chlorpromazine (Largactil); the anti-nausea medication prochlorperazine (Stemetil); and tricyclic antidepressants, such as amitriptyline (Triptafen) and doxepin (Sinequan). In addition, your doctor may advise you to stop taking beta-blockers for the day of your tests. These drugs, such as propranolol (Inderal) and atenolol (Tenormin), block the actions of adrenaline, an emergency medicine used if you have a severe allergy attack. If you are taking long-term or high doses of oral corticosteroids, skin prick tests tend to be less sensitive and you may be asked to have a blood test as well.

Given all of this, it is easy to see why it is so important to take a list of all your medications to your first appointment. It is essential that you consult your doctor before you stop taking any drugs.

Conditions that mimic asthma

One reason why it is so important to get the correct diagnosis if you suspect that you may have asthma is that several conditions – some of them quite serious – mimic it.

- **Coronary disease** can produce asthma-like constriction of the chest.
- **Early congestive heart failure** – with shortness of breath and even wheezing – can mimic asthma; it was formerly called cardiac asthma and was treated with aminophylline, still occasionally used to treat asthma.
- **Recurrent blood clots** in your lungs (pulmonary emboli) produce shortness of breath and in some cases even some wheezing.
- **Airway and chest tumours** may cause wheezing and coughing.
- **Immunologic lung diseases**, such as pulmonary vasculitis, have asthma-like features.
- **Vocal cord spasms** have symptoms similar to asthma. In one study, when 56 patients diagnosed with asthma were treated with vocal retraining by speech pathologists, more than 90 per cent improved.
- Other conditions that mimic asthma include **hyperventilation**, or panic disorder, acute **infectious bronchitis** and adult mild **cystic fibrosis**.

Your doctor will perform a 'negative control' test using a saline solution before testing for specific allergens. You shouldn't have any reaction to this test; if you do, you are oversensitive, making accurate readings of other skin tests much more difficult. The doctor should also conduct a 'positive control' test, injecting histamine under your skin, which causes an allergic reaction. It should produce a bump; if not, you are under-reactive, which also makes evaluating future skin tests difficult. This test is also used for comparison with allergen skin testing to find out how severely you react to an allergen.

Sensitive vs. specific

If you were a fly on the wall, listening to allergists discussing you or any other patient, you might hear them talking about a test's sensitivity or specificity. Allergists are also likely to use these terms when discussing your tests with you.

Here's what they mean:

The more *sensitive* a test is, the more likely it is to identify all people who have the allergy. However, it may also include a fair number of 'false positives', which are positive readings for someone who really doesn't have the allergy.

The more *specific* the test, the more guaranteed that a positive test is accurate. However, because of its tougher criteria, a highly specific test is likely to miss some people who have the disease.

Skin prick (percutaneous) tests These tests are the most convenient, least expensive, and most specific screening method for detecting IgE antibodies, and they tend to be the best for determining the causes of allergic rhinitis. They are usually performed on your upper back or forearm. Using a diluted solution of various airborne allergens common in your geographical area, the doctor or other medical professional places a drop on your skin, then either punctures or pricks the skin with a special tool, allowing the allergen to come in contact with deeper layers of skin.

Intradermal tests These are generally performed only if a skin prick test is negative for IgE antibodies but symptoms strongly suggest an allergic mechanism. It involves using extremely fine needles to inject the diluted allergen just below the skin surface on your upper arm or forearm. It's not as painful as it sounds; the needles are so fine that you may feel only a slight burning sensation. These tests are more appropriate for people with low skin-test sensitivity, but they should be performed only *after* a negative prick/puncture test because they carry a slightly higher risk of reaction.

About 15 minutes after performing a skin test, the doctor 'reads' the resulting wheal, a small, raised, reddened area like a mosquito bite, and the amount of redness on your arm, measuring the wheal and comparing it with the positive control test performed earlier. A wheal that is at least 3mm larger than any wheal that appeared after the control test implies the presence of allergen-specific IgE. The larger the prick/puncture skin test reaction, the more likely that it's clinically significant. But a positive skin test does not necessarily mean the allergen tested is the one causing your symptoms; it only implies that you have an IgE response to it.

Many people have positive skin prick tests to allergens, including grass pollen and food allergens, but never develop any symptoms, so these tests can't be used to predict allergic reactions but only to confirm or refute the cause of suspected allergic reactions..

Expect to spend about an hour or more in your doctor's surgery undergoing skin testing. In some instances, you may require up to 30 skin prick tests, possibly followed by some intradermal tests to identify what is causing your allergic rhinitis. Don't be alarmed if you see redness, hardness or swelling at the site of the test 1 to 2 hours or more after the application of the allergen; this is the delayed allergic reaction we've talked about, which is normal and generally disappears within one to two days.

Patch skin test Also called delayed-type hypersensitivity skin test, this test (usually performed by dermatologists, rather than allergists) is used to see if you have a skin sensitivity, called contact dermatitis, to substances such as rubber, medications, fragrances, hair dyes, metals and resins. The diluted allergen is put on your upper back, and the site is covered with tape, which is left on for at least 48 hours. Then the patch is removed, and the site is checked for a reaction. The patch is replaced, and the site is checked again at 72 and/or 96 hours (or earlier if a reaction occurs).

Question these tests

The tests below are not regarded by conventional medical practitioners to be relevant, standardized or repeatable, and are considered to have no place in the diagnosis of true allergy.

- **Leukocytoxic or cytotoxic test**, a blood test to evaluate the effects of allergens on white blood cells

- **Neutralization-provocation**, in which diluted allergens are injected under the skin to elicit a response, then a weaker or stronger dilution is injected to relieve the symptoms

- **Electrodermal diagnosis or Vega testing**, which measures the electrical resistance between two points on the skin in a 'circuit' which may contain a phial of allergen solution.

- **Applied kinesiology**, in which the practitioner presses down on your arms after you have eaten or held an allergen, or had it injected

- **'Reaginic' pulse test**, or auricular cardiac reflex method, in which your pulse rate is measured after you have been exposed to a potential allergen

- **Chemical analysis** of hair or body tissues

2 Blood tests

Radio-allergosorbent testing, or RAST, was the first blood test developed for allergen testing, in the mid-1960s. Since then the UniCap RAST test, used almost universally in hospitals, and several others including 'dipstick' RAST blood tests have been approved in the UK.

The test is carried out on a small sample of blood, at your GP's surgery or at a hospital. It is usually taken from a vein in the arm, using a fine needle and a small syringe, causing minimal discomfort. RAST tests are particularly useful when the patient has a risk of an anaphylactic (shock) reaction, so skin prick testing would be considered unsuitable; when extensive eczema makes skin prick testing impractical; when antihistamine medication cannot be stopped because of the severity of the symptoms; and when unusual and rare allergens are suspected. Blood tests may also be the preferred method of identifying cases of food allergies.

Compared with skin tests, RAST tests have lower sensitivity and a limited range of allergens that can be detected. It takes longer (up to 14 days) to get RAST test results, which may be inconclusive.

A new test for monitoring asthma

In May 2003, the US Food and Drug Administration (FDA) approved a first-of-its-kind, non-invasive test to measure the concentration of nitric oxide (NO) in exhaled human breath, using a device called the NIOX Nitric Oxide Test System. Nitric oxide levels are higher in the breath of people with asthma because of the inflammation of their airways. Thus, measuring levels of nitric oxide is a good way to test whether your anti-inflammatory medications are working.

At present the device is used primarily for research, and by a few respiratory specialists in the UK. It should make its way into doctors' surgeries before too long as it becomes simpler to use and the price drops.

Diagnosing asthma

It wasn't until the early 1800s that an asthmatic French doctor, René Laënnec, designed the first crude stethoscope (a rolled-up piece of paper) to listen to a patient's heart and lungs, and not until the 1830s that microscopes allowed doctors to examine patients' lung tissue and secretions. But perhaps the most important diagnostic discovery for respiratory illnesses such as asthma was made in 1850, when a British surgeon, John Hutchinson, developed the spirometer – the instrument that measures the amount of air entering and leaving the lungs – for his research into respiratory physiology.

Nowadays, electronic digitized spirometers, along with peak flow meters, are essential tools for any allergy/asthma specialist. They are used to monitor the speed and strength of your breathing as well as your lung capacity.

These machines are only tools, however, best used to confirm a diagnosis or track your progress. Most of the work your doctor will do in determining the diagnosis involves talking to you, examining you and taking a detailed medical history as described earlier. However, tests can be useful.

If you have allergic asthma, that is caused entirely or even in part by allergies, you will probably undergo skin testing as described earlier in this chapter. In addition, there are a few other tests that your specialist will want to conduct, not only to help diagnose your asthma but also to monitor how well you are controlling it once you have both agreed on an appropriate course of treatment.

Using a peak flow meter

The following steps describe precisely how you should use this breath-measuring device at home.

1 Be sure the device reads zero or is at base level.
2 Stand up.
3 Breathe in as deeply as possible.
4 Put your mouth around the meter and close your lips around the mouthpiece.
5 Blow out as hard and fast as possible in 1 to 2 seconds.
6 Don't cough, spit or let your tongue block the mouthpiece.
7 Write down the value you get.
8 Repeat the process twice more and record the highest of the three numbers in your chart.

A new pocket-sized 'Piko' electronic peak flow meter is now available on prescription in the UK. The device logs peak flow levels, along with the time they were taken, which can then be downloaded to a computer for tracking, making it easier for people with asthma to monitor their symptoms and so help to reduce the incidence of asthma attacks. It could encourage people to take readings more regularly and remove margins for error, according to health professionals.

1 Pulmonary function tests

These tests measure the degree of obstruction in your lungs and involve blowing into a machine that measures your exhaled breath. There are three main types.

Spirometers Using a spirometer is fairly easy. Hold the tube in your mouth, inhale as much air as you can, then exhale forcefully until your lungs are empty. The spirometry measurements provide clues to the health of your lungs in the same way that blood pressure and blood cholesterol numbers indicate the health of your cardiovascular system. The results are described in terms of:

Forced expiratory volume (in 1 second), or FEV1. This is the amount of air you can force out of your lungs in the first second after you begin exhaling, or your lung velocity. You should be able to get the majority of air out of your lungs in the first second; you want the result to be 80 per cent or better. The lower the number, the narrower your airways, particularly the small airways (bronchioles).

Forced vital capacity, or FVC. This is the total amount of air you breathe out after a full inhalation, or your lung capacity. Any remaining air is known as residual volume. As we discussed earlier, people with asthma have a more difficult time exhaling than inhaling. The FVC should be normal in most people with asthma unless the disease is very severe. You want a result of 90 per cent or better; any lower means that either you haven't tried hard enough to blow or you have extra air trapped in your airways, suggesting severe asthma.

Challenge test (bronchoprovocation) This test is used if spirometry indicates normal or near-normal lung function, but it still seems that asthma is causing your symptoms. First, the doctor gives you a baseline spirometry test, then you inhale a drug (usually methacholine or histamine), which constricts the airways in asthmatics, but not non-asthmatics. The spirometry test is repeated. If your airways constrict, the doctor will give you an airway-opening drug. If you are sensitive to methacholine (indicated by a drop of at least 20 per cent in your spirometry test) and respond to an airway-opening drug (indicated by an improvement in your spirometry test), you probably have asthma. However, the test is not always 100 per cent accurate. You could have a marginally positive test result and not have asthma; for instance, sometimes people with allergic rhinitis have sensitive airways, resulting in a positive test, but that doesn't mean they have clinical asthma. It is sometimes positive in other lung disorders such as chronic obstructive pulmonary disease caused by smoking.

Peak flow meter This test is to asthma what a thermometer is to fever and a finger prick is to diabetes: it helps you to monitor your asthma at home, determining whether or not your medications are working effectively. The peak flow meter is a small, hand-held device that you breathe into. It measures the rate at which you can force air out of your lungs, called your peak expiratory flow rate (PEFR). It is not good at measuring small-airway obstruction; it indicates only obstruction in the large airways.

During the test, you breathe in as deeply as you can and then blow into the device as hard and fast as possible. If your asthma symptoms are about to worsen, your peak flow readings will drop. Such drops are a clue that you probably need to increase your medication. Ideally, you don't want your peak flow readings to vary more than 15 per cent from the previous reading.

Although your doctor will use the peak flow meter test in order to assess the severity of your asthma, you should view it as an early warning system, alerting you to the possibility of major problems.

2 Other tests
In addition to pulmonary function tests, your doctor may perform other tests, more to rule out other problems than to actually confirm an asthma diagnosis. These include:

Chest X-ray An X-ray to view the inside of your lungs helps to rule out other possible causes of your symptoms, including bronchitis, pneumonia and lung cancer.

Sinus X-ray or CT scan This test uses X-rays to see if you have nasal polyps (growths in your sinuses) or sinusitis (inflammation or swelling of your sinuses due to infection), both of which may make it more difficult to treat and control asthma.

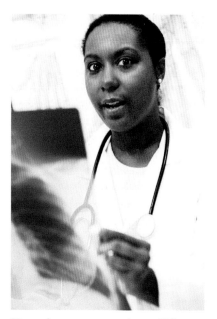

Your doctor may order a CT scan or chest X-rays to rule out other possible causes of your symptoms.

Sputum evaluation It may not sound appealing but this test evaluates the mucus you bring up from your lungs, looking for eosinophils, the white blood cells that increase during asthma attacks and are triggered by allergies.

Complete or full blood count (CBC or FBC) Here, the doctor is looking for elevated levels of white blood cells that could indicate an infection such as bronchitis or pneumonia; high levels of eosinophils also suggest an allergic component to your asthma.

The next steps

By now, you should have found a suitable doctor, received a diagnosis of allergies or asthma (or both) and find yourself clutching a handful of prescriptions. The complex world of drugs is explored in detail in the next chapter.

Chapter **seven**

The right
medications

A large part of the Breathe Easy Plan involves lifestyle changes: changing your environment, your diet and even the supplements you take to minimize asthma and allergic reactions. Equally important to the programme and to your health is taking the right prescription and over-the-counter (OTC) medicines – and taking them correctly. Some people with asthma and allergies may not appreciate the importance of this. Even those who are careful about the way they take their medicines may discover that they are taking the wrong medication or are taking it at the wrong times, in the wrong manner or in the wrong doses. Because this may be dangerous and also because some £659 million a year is spent on prescription drugs and £117 million on dispensing for asthma alone in the UK , it is important to get it right.

Today, there is a wealth of options available for allergy and asthma treatment, both OTC and prescription. This chapter provides an overview of each major category of medications for allergic rhinitis and those for asthma. In some instances, a medication may be used for both.

Before considering the detail, it is important to emphasize a major caveat. *Don't start or stop taking any medication without first talking to your doctor.* The advice given here is just that – advice. It is not prescriptive and its principal aim is to arm you with enough knowledge and information to have an educated, informative discussion with your doctor or specialist about your particular allergy or asthma.

It is also critical that you tell your doctor about *all* medications you're taking, including OTC drugs, vitamin and mineral supplements and herbs, and about any medical conditions you have other than allergies or asthma. Many drugs recommended for asthma in particular can be dangerous if you have heart disease, diabetes or liver disease. And if you are looking for medication for your child, be sure to ask if the drug is approved for use by children. Specific drugs for children are discussed later in the book.

What follows is an overview of the medications available.

Medicines for allergies

People who have allergies today have one advantage. The past decade has seen an enormous increase in the numbers and types of allergy medications. At the same time, many drugs have been improved. Yet the choice of medications, whether over-the-counter or prescription, can seem bewildering.

In 2004, some £75.7 million was spent on OTC remedies for hay fever alone, and around 10 per cent of the annual GP prescription budget is spent on treatments for allergies, partly because allergy sufferers often require more than

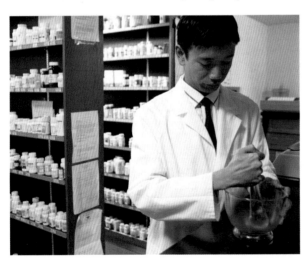

one drug. Many people with hay fever find that oral antihistamines don't act fast enough. As a result, they end up switching medications or using additional treatments.

Individual doctors may treat symptoms in different ways. But there are now clear guidelines from the British Society for Allergy and Clinical Immunology (BSACI) to help primary care physicians – our GPs – to manage hay fever and allergic rhinitis (see page 100). The

If you have allergies today, consider yourself lucky, because drugs are much improved. Still, you can't expect miracles.

guidelines explain clearly how different drugs should be prescribed according to the severity of the disorder.

The important thing is that when you have explained your symptoms, your doctor works *with* you, taking your health and all your concerns into consideration, in order to develop a treatment plan tailored to your needs.

Antihistamines

- **NON-PRESCRIPTION (sedating)** Allerief, Boots Allergy Relief Antihistamine Tablets, Calimal Piriton Allergy (all contain chlorphenamine)
- **NON-PRESCRIPTION (non-sedating)** Benadryl Allergy Relief (acrivastine), AllerTek, Benadryl One A Day, Piriteze Allergy, Zirtek Allergy, Zirtek Allergy Relief (all contain cetirizine), Boots Hayfever and Allergy Relief All Day, Boots Hayfever and Allergy Relief Fast Melting Tablets, Clarityn Allergy (all contain loratadine)
- **PRESCRIPTION (sedating)** Dimotane (brompheniramine), Chlorphenamine, Piriton (chlorphenamine), Tavegil (clemastine), Periactin (cyproheptadine), Phenergan (promethazine)
- **PRESCRIPTION (non-sedating)** acrivastine, cetirizine, Neoclarityn (desloratadine), Telfast (fexofenadine), Xyzal (levocetirizine), Loratadine, Mizollen (mizolastine)

As the name implies, antihistamines counter the effects of histamine, the inflammatory chemical released by your body's mast cells during an allergic reaction. Histamine is to blame for the sneezing, nasal swelling and drainage, and itchy eyes, throat and nose that are the hallmarks of allergic rhinitis. Today, you are likely to hear antihistamines referred to in two ways: their level of sedation (sedating or non-sedating) and their duration (short or long-acting).

Sedating cough medicines

It is not generally known that many cough medicines on sale to the public contain sedating antihistamines. They include the following: Benylin Chesty Coughs original, Benylin Children's Night Coughs, Benylin with Codeine, Benylin Cough and Congestion, Benylin Dry Cough, Benylin Four Flu, Benylin Night Tablets, Boots Night Time Cough Syrup 1 Year Plus, Multi-action Actifed Dry Coughs, Multi-action Actifed Syrup, Multi-action Actified Chesty Coughs, Night Nurse, Robitussin Night-Time, Sudafed Plus, Tixycolds, Tixylix Cough and Cold, Tixylix Night-Time, Tixyplus Active Relief for Colds and Flu, Vicks Medinite.

First-generation, sedating antihistamines

Oral antihistamines, which come as pills, tablets and syrups, have long been considered a first-line defence against the misery of allergies, with their use dating back to the 1940s. They work well, but there is one major problem: some OTC antihistamines have such a strong sedative effect that you can feel quite wiped out. That is because their active ingredients cross the blood/brain barrier, affecting your central nervous system.

Most sedating antihistamines are now sold principally in cough medicines rather than specifically as allergy relief preparations. Some include diphenhydramine, the same active ingredient as that used in most OTC sleeping pills. No wonder, then, that some people say they are less effective at work on days when they take such cough medicines.

Furthermore, studies suggest that even those who say such medications don't make them drowsy may have impaired reaction time, visual-motor coordination, memory and learning capacity, as well as poorer performance on arithmetic exercises and driving tests.

In the USA, one study showed that the standard 50mg dose of a sedating antihistamine drug impaired driving ability (as measured in a driving simulator) as much or more than alcohol, making the subjects legally drunk. Most worrying was the fact that those tested had no sense of impairment after taking the medicine. They thought they were driving competently even though they were severely impaired. Also, children who take diphenhydramine score significantly lower on tests of learning ability than those who receive similar amounts of non-sedating antihistamines.

So it is hardly surprising that you may be considered officially unfit to drive if you are taking a sedating antihistamine. For instance, pilots are not permitted to fly if they have taken such a drug within 24 hours of a scheduled flight.

In the UK, chlorphenamine is the biggest selling OTC sedating anti-histamine sold, under the brand names Boots Allergy Relief Antihistamine Tablets, Allerief and Calimal. The effects of these sedating antihistamines don't last long, so you need to take a dose about every 4 hours. They do play a role in the treatment of allergies but newer, less-sedating options are now available on prescription, and few doctors now recommend using sedating anti-histamines to treat allergy.

They remain quite popular because they work relatively fast, providing quick relief. They are also inexpensive and many brands are available at any chemist or supermarket pharmacy. But be sure to read the instructions carefully. These

---

The hay fever treatment guide

The British Society for Allergy and Clinical Immunology (BSACI) provides primary care physicians with guidelines for helping patients to manage hay fever and allergic rhinitis. They are summarized below.

- **Always** Avoid exposure to pollens as far as possible, and other irritants such as smoke, aerosols, dust.

- **For minor symptoms that do not interfere with work/school/sleep** A daily non-sedating antihistamine (these can be taken as required in very mild cases, but regular treatment works best).

- **For anything more than minor symptoms** Add a daily topical nasal corticosteroid (these *must* be taken regularly, preferably starting a few weeks in advance of the anticipated start of symptoms).

- **If copious watering of the nose is a particular problem** Add a daily topical nasal anticholinergic.

- **For very severe symptoms or in anticipation of major events such as exams** Add a short course (3-10 days) of an oral corticosteroid.

The GP should also consider referral to an allergy specialist for allergy diagnosis, specialist advice and treatment such as immunotherapy.

are most effective if taken half an hour before you think you might encounter an allergen, such as before visiting a house with cats. For chronic allergies, timed-release antihistamines that work for up to 12 hours may be most suitable.

Keep taking antihistamines as directed until you feel better. Sometimes the medication needs to build up in your bloodstream to provide maximum relief. If you find that an antihistamine that was working well is suddenly no longer effective, seek advice from your doctor; you may require a different or stronger drug.

Second-generation, non-sedating antihistamines

The advent of the newer (so-called 'second generation'), non-sedating anti-histamines such as acrivastine, fexofenadine, cetirizine, levocetirizine, loratadine, desloratadine and mizolastine brought relief – and a clear head – to allergy sufferers. The active ingredients in these medications have very little effect on the central nervous system because they are composed of larger molecules that cannot get past the blood/brain barrier. So they don't make you tired, irritable or confused. That is why these drugs are recommended as the most appropriate initial treatment for allergic rhinitis.

While all these drugs work in a similar way, individuals may find that one is more effective for them than another. So you may try several before finding the one that works best for you; then you must use it regularly for maximum relief.

Antihistamine nasal spray

Two antihistamine nasal sprays are licensed in the UK, azelastine (Rhinolast) and levocabastine (Livostin). Available only on prescription, these work quickly and can be used as required, though, like antihistamine tablets, they are better used regularly. Although effective on the nose they do not relieve sneezing and itching elsewhere, as do anti-histamine tablets, and they don't work if the nose is already blocked, for example, by nasal polyps.

Antihistamine nasal sprays have two main advantages. They provide targeted therapy, unlike oral anti-histamines, which must first travel through the digestive system and bloodstream. And they are approved for treating both allergic and non-allergic rhinitis, because they also help to clear congestion (which oral antihistamines can't touch).

Antihistamine warnings

It is known that sedating antihistamines can have a powerful effect on your brain and body, so be sure to heed the product warnings. When you are taking a sedating antihistamine:

- Avoid driving.
- Don't use any motorized equipment.
- Don't drink alcohol.
- Don't take any form of sedative or tranquillizer.
- Watch for side effects such as dryness of the mouth, nose and eyes.

Antihistamine eye drops

For severe eye symptoms caused by hay fever, there are also antihistamine eye drops available. These include Optilast (azelastine), Emadine (emedastine), Relestat (epinastine), Zaditen (ketotifen), Livostin Direct (levocabastine), Alomide (lodoxamide), Opatanol (olopatadine). They may be useful in addition to regular antihistamine tablets. Optilast is available over the counter, as is Otrivine-Antistin, an antihistamine (antazoline) combined with a local decongestant (xylometazoline); Otrivine-Antistin must *not* be used if you have glaucoma.

Decongestants

- **NON-PRESCRIPTION TABLETS (decongestant only)** Boots Decongestant Tablets, CAM, Contac Non Drowsy 12 Hour Relief, Galsud, Non-Drowsy Sudafed Decongestant Tablets, Non-Drowsy Sudafed 12 Hour Relief
- **NON-PRESCRIPTION NASAL SPRAYS/ DROPS** Afrazine, Dristan, Sudafed nasal spray, Vicks Sinex (all contain oxymetazoline), Non-Drowsy Sudafed Decongestant Nasal Spray, Otradrops, Otraspray, Otrivine, Tixycolds Nasal Spray (all contain xylometazoline), Fenox (phenylephrine)
- **PRESCRIPTION NASAL DROPS** Ephedrine

Soothing allergic conjunctivitis

As part 1 explained, your eyes contain thousands of mast cells, which means they are prime targets for allergies. If you suffer from eye allergies, most commonly known as allergic conjunctivitis, several forms of eyedrops can provide relief, including these.

Tear substitutes There are more than 50 different artificial tear preparations available over the counter these days. They temporarily flush out allergens and moisten your eyes. Most contain preservatives, which is no problem if you use them less than three times a day. If you use them more often, choose a brand without preservatives, which will be more expensive but safer for your eyes in the long run. For extra soothing power, put the eyedrops into the refrigerator before use.

Decongestants and antihistamines You can get over-the-counter eyedrop decongestants that constrict blood vessels in your eyes, thereby reducing redness, and antihistamines, which help with itching. A word of warning. Don't use decongestant drops if you have glaucoma, and don't use them for more than two or three consecutive days; like nasal decongestants, they can actually cause congestion if overused.

Prescription medications If you can't find an over-the-counter preparation that works for you, talk to your doctor about prescription eyedrops. There are prescription antihistamine drops, mast cell stabilizers and nonsteroidal anti-inflammatory drops that help with itching, and corticosteroids for chronic and severe eye allergy symptoms. Some carry a risk of side effects, however. Also, most need to be used twice a day, and some may be recommended for use for only a limited time.

In addition to hitting at the source of your allergy symptoms – histamine – you also want to unclog your nose. That's where decongestants come in. They work by restricting the blood supply to the nose and sinuses, thus reducing swelling, excess secretions and congestion.

Decongestants are found in a wide range of medicines not sold specifically for allergies, and are often combined with antihistamines (such as Benylin, Dimotane, Robitussin, Sudafed or Tixylix), or with an expectorant (such as Meltus, Boots Cough and Decongestant Syrup, Sudafed Expectorant or Robitussin Chesty Cough with Congestion) or with painkillers and cough suppressants to relieve cold and flu symptoms (such as Advil Cold and Sinus, Beechams Powders Capsules with Decongestant or Benylin Four Flu. Decongestant tablets should be used with caution or avoided by people with heart disease, hypertension, diabetes or glaucoma, as well as pregnant women, men with prostate problems, and those taking medication, such as anti-depressants, for behavioural or emotional problems. OTC decongestant nose drops and sprays tend to be ineffective and may have side effects; long-term use can damage the nasal lining.

Insider information Men with prostate enlargement may have urinary problems while taking decongestants.

Steroids

- **PRESCRIPTION (nasal)** Beconase (beclometasone), Betnesol and Vista-Methasone (betamethasone), Rhinocort Aqua (budesonide), Dexa-Rhinospray Duo (dexamethasone with ephedrine, a decongestant), Syntaris (flunisolide), Flixonase (fluticasone), Nasonex (mometasone), Nasacort (triamcinolone)
- **NON-PRESCRIPTION (nasal sprays)** Beclogen, Beconase Allergy, Beconase Hayfever, Boots Hayfever Relief, Care Hayfever Relief, Nasobec Hayfever, Pollenase Hayfever, Tesco Hayfever Relief, Vivabec (all beclometasone); budesonide, Flixonase (fluticasone), Nasacort (triamcinolone)

As allergies and asthma are first and foremost inflammatory diseases, the world of medicine's best anti-inflammatories – corticosteroids, so-called glucocorticoids or steroids – are the most important class of drugs for treating all but the mildest cases.

Several nasal steroids, some available over the counter, are approved for seasonal and perennial rhinitis. They work by driving out mast cells and other inflammatory cells from the nose, so that there is no histamine release

Insider information To reduce the risk of nasal bleeding when using nasal corticosteroids, aim the spray towards your ear and away from the septum, the wall of cartilage that divides the nose. This works best if you hold the inhaler in one hand and spray the medicine into the opposite nostril; that way, the inhaler is turned slightly to the outside, so there is less irritation of the septum and less potential for bleeding.

Hay fever treatment: over-the-counter or prescription?

Anyone who suffers from hay fever knows that it's not always possible to avoid pollen or mould allergens completely. Hay fever symptoms develop rapidly – within half an hour in 35 per cent of cases and less than 2 hours in 70 per cent – and it is often much quicker and more convenient to obtain over-the-counter (OTC) medicines than to wait for a GP appointment.

For severe symptoms, those that persist despite OTC treatments or if you are unsure of your diagnosis, you should consult your doctor. It is also advisable to see your GP if there is a particular problem, such as the need to avoid hay fever symptoms during exam time.

Many hay fever treatments, both sedating and non-sedating, are available OTC and a pharmacist can give you advice. In general, avoid sedating antihistamines; if you do take them, do so at night when drowsiness doesn't matter (and may even be helpful) but be warned: you are still likely to feel woozy in the morning. Research shows that a sedating antihistamine and its by-products can linger in the body the next morning, decreasing alertness. If you are driving or operating any machinery, take care to use a non-sedating agent. Remember, for all but the mildest hay fever you will benefit from a regular nasal steroid. Several are available OTC and you should try to start them early and make sure you take them regularly.

You may be concerned about prescription charges but buying drugs OTC may not be cheaper; your GP can often prescribe several months' treatment for a single prescription fee.

when pollen (or any other allergen) is inhaled. Nasal steroids work better than antihistamines on nasal blockage (which is the main reason that hay fever sufferers cannot smell or taste and lose a good night's sleep). They also reduce the size of nasal polyps.

There are two key things that consultants advise you should remember about steroid nose sprays: they produce no immediate relief and work only if taken daily whether you have symptoms or not, preferably starting several weeks before you know the symptoms are going to start.

These are *not* medicines that you take 'as required', rushing down to the chemist's to stock up when symptoms are terrible. They must be used regularly in addition to antihistamines for all but the mildest hayfever. Some sprays can be used for children as young as six years old. They are safe for long-term use.

Anticholinergic nasal spray

• **PRESCRIPTION** Rinatec (ipratropium bromide 0.03%)

Ipratropium bromide belongs to the tongue-twisting class of drugs known as anticholinergic agents. They block the effects of acetylcholine, a neuro-transmitter that stimulates mucus production, which makes them effective in combating runny noses. Available only in a prescription spray (Rinatec), ipratropium bromide 0.03% is approved for non-allergic and allergic rhinitis and 0.05% is for relief of runny nose due to the common cold.

Cromoglicate sodium spray

• **PRESCRIPTION (nasal spray)** brand names Rynacrom (4%), Vividrin (2%)

Rather than treating the symptoms of an allergic attack, this nasal spray, available only on prescription, stops attacks before they start by preventing the release of chemicals such as histamine from mast cells, thus serving as an anti-inflammatory agent. It has few side effects when used as directed, and it significantly helps some people with allergies. Cromoglicate sodium is most effective if started two to four weeks before you are exposed to allergens.

But it may be up to three weeks before you experience the full benefit and it doesn't work for everyone. Another drawback is that you have to use the spray up to four times a day. The nasal spray is sometimes used in children but, for anything other than mild allergy, topical nasal steroids are preferable.

Cromoglicate and nedocromil (a related drug) are also effective for eye allergies but their effect is quite short-lived so, like the nasal spray, they must be used quite frequently. Prescription-only eye drops include Sodium Cromoglicate (generic), Hay-Crom Aqueous, Opticrom Aqueous and Vividrin. OTC eye drops include Boots Hayfever Relief, Clariteyes, Optrex Allergy and Vivicrom. Anti-histamine eye drops are more long lasting and you may find them more effective.

Saline nasal spray

Salt water can relieve stuffiness and congestion. Buy this over the counter at pharmacies (Ocean, Ayr or Dristan Saline Spray) or make your own by adding ½ teaspoon of salt and a pinch of bicarbonate of soda to a cup of lukewarm water. Then use a bulb syringe like the ones used to clear an infant's nose to spray the solution into your nose a few times. Follow with a good, hard blow.

Emergency medications

• **PRESCRIPTION (injected)** Adrenaline, EpiPen, EpiPen Junior, Anapen, Anapen Junior
• **PRESCRIPTION (nebulized)** Ventolin (salbutamol)

Anyone with severe allergies knows the benefits of adrenaline, administered via injection in the event of a severe allergy attack or anaphylaxis. If you are severely allergic, particularly to insect stings and certain foods, you should carry

A life-saving bracelet

If you have severe allergies you should always carry an emergency treatment kit with you in case of an anaphylactic reaction. In addition, since you may be unable to communicate during an attack, it's worth considering wearing a MedicAlert bracelet or necklet. The charity MedicAlert provides a life-saving system for people with allergies and hidden medical conditions, supported by a 24-hour emergency telephone service. Your bracelet is engraved with your main medical condition(s) and vital details, a personal ID number and a 24-hour emergency telephone number which accepts reverse charge calls that can access your details from anywhere in the world in more than 100 languages.

adrenaline with you at all times as part of your emergency treatment kit. That kit should also include a list of medications you are currently taking and any that your doctor recommends in the event of an anaphylactic reaction, a list of your symptoms during anaphylaxis, a written treatment plan from your doctor, and your doctor's name and contact details. You might also consider wearing a MedicAlert or Medi-Tag bracelet in case you are unable to communicate during an attack. Asthmatics are particularly vulnerable to severe attacks during anaphylaxis. For this reason, your doctor may ask you to keep a salbutamol inhaler in your emergency kit – this can be used repeatedly if you become tight-chested in an anphylactic reaction. If you have a nebulizer, you can use nebulized salbutamol but this is not necessary in every case.

Immunotherapy: long-term allergy treatment

The idea of having an injection once or twice a week for six months or more probably holds little appeal. But what if that could enable you to enjoy spring days with no fear of allergy attacks? Suddenly, opting for a course of simple injections doesn't seem so bad, does it?

Treatment with allergy injections, or immunotherapy, was pioneered at St Mary's Hospital, London, in 1911. It is the only treatment for allergies that reduces symptoms over the long term rather than simply treating them for a few hours.

Immunotherapy works similarly to a vaccine, albeit one that is given many times over a long period. Each successive injection contains a tiny bit more of the substance to which you are allergic. Eventually, your body becomes desensitized to the allergen, decreasing the IgE reaction to it by blocking IgE antibodies and minimizing their action. Thus, when you encounter the allergen in the future, you have a reduced or very minor response to it and fewer symptoms.

There is evidence that it works. Experts analysing 24 studies involving more than 900 people with asthma who also had documented allergies found that allergy injections effectively treated allergic asthma in 71 per cent of them,

How do I know if immunotherapy is right for me?

Allergy injections are generally considered for people with perennial and seasonal allergies to airborne allergens, such as pollens, pet dander, dust mites and mould, or to insect stings; those whose symptoms are not well controlled with medication; those who want to avoid long-term use of medication; and those who are willing to make the long-term commitment to treatment. The British Society for Allergy & Clinical Immunology (BSACI) offers the following guide-lines for immunotherapy:

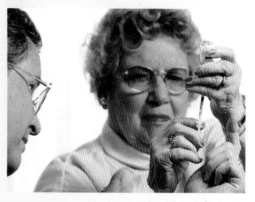

- It should be prescribed only by an allergist, immunologist, or other physician trained in the therapy.
- It should be given only in facilities equipped to treat anaphylaxis.
- You need to be healthy prior to every injection. If you are ill, especially with asthma or respiratory difficulties, you should not receive immunotherapy until your condition improves.
- Tell your doctor about any medications you are taking. Beta-blockers, for instance, block the effect of adrenaline, which may be needed to treat a severe reaction to an allergy injection.
- You should wait at the allergy centre for at least an hour after an injection, or longer if you are at high risk of a reaction.

You are probably not a suitable candidate for immunotherapy if you:
- Have an extreme response to skin tests. This may predict a dangerous allergic reaction to the injections.
- Have uncontrolled or severe asthma or lung disease.
- Are taking certain medications, such as beta-blockers.

And if you have been having immunotherapy treatment for 12 to 18 months without seeing any improvement, you should probably stop.

---

resulting in fewer symptoms, less lung inflammation and a reduced need for medications. Overall, other studies found that immunotherapy can reduce the sneezing and wheezing of allergic rhinitis by 80 per cent and the need for allergy medications by 88 per cent.

Some research also suggests that immunotherapy may prevent the development of new allergies and asthma in children who have allergic rhinitis. And a study presented at the annual meeting of the American Academy of Allergy, Asthma and Immunology in 2000 found that allergen immunotherapy for three years significantly improved patients' overall quality of life even as it reduced the need for doctor's visits.

Yet while immunotherapy has been enthusiastically adopted as the treatment of choice for allergic rhinitis and asthma in the USA and parts of Europe, it is not used to treat asthma in the UK. In 1986 the practice of immunotherapy was virtually halted here after the *British Medical Journal* published a Committee on the Safety of Medicines (CSM) report citing 26 anaphylactic deaths over a 30-year period. The deaths arose mainly from inappropriate use of the procedure to treat uncontrolled asthma.

Two decades on from the report's publication, immunotherapy is still not recommended by the British Society for Allergy & Clinical Immunology and the British Thoracic Society for treating asthma in the UK, because there is insufficient evidence to suggest that it is any more effective than standard anti-asthma treatments, and fatal reactions can occur in patients whose asthma is not properly controlled. Nor is immunotherapy useful in treating non-allergic rhinitis, atopic dermatitis, chronic urticaria or food hypersensitivity. But it is widely and successfully used in the UK to treat patients with severe hay fever or allergy to allergens such as pet dander or house dust mites that do not respond to the standard treatment with topical nasal steroids and antihistamines. It is also recommended for the treatment of bee and wasp venom allergy.

Yet immunotherapy is not always appropriate for people with such allergies. In the first place, many people have an aversion to injections. The therapy is also fairly intensive and takes much more time than swallowing a pill. A normal course of immunotherapy would comprise one injection a week for the first 8-12 weeks, and then further injections every 4-6 weeks for a total of three years depending on the nature of the particular allergen.

Immunotherapy is performed at present at only a few specialized allergy centres in the UK, located mainly in the south-east of England, and must be supervised by an experienced consultant allergist. To allow for treatment of any adverse effects, patients normally have to remain in the clinic for at least 60 minutes after

An alternative to needles: SLIT immunotherapy

The biggest drawback of immunotherapy is the needle. By the time you finish immunotherapy you may have received well over 100 injections. That is why a growing number of doctors in Europe have turned to sublingual immunotherapy (SLIT).

SLIT involves placing drops of the allergen solution under your tongue for a minute or two before swallowing. The treatment remains controversial, however, with opponents insisting that the delicate allergens cannot survive the rigours of the digestive tract long enough to have any significant effect on the immune system. Yet a growing body of research shows that SLIT may have a role in immunotherapy. Of 18 double-blind, placebo-controlled clinical trials in the past 15 years, 16 confirmed the effectiveness of SLIT in reducing allergy symptoms triggered by grass pollen, house dust mites or birch pollen. Other studies found that drops were as effective as injections, and safer, and that patients preferred them. In November 2003 the World Health Organization supported the use of SLIT, in particular for those patients who don't take their medications, refuse injections and/or have systemic reactions to injection immunotherapy. A 2005 Cochrane Review concluded that SLIT is a safe treatment for allergic rhinitis that significantly reduces symptoms and medication requirements. The treatment is still undergoing evaluation in the UK.

the injection. After completing the course, symptoms will remain controlled for several years. If they do return after that, you may need another course of treatment. Two types of adverse reactions may occur with immunotherapy.

Local reactions You may develop some swelling at the injection site. If so, try an oral antihistamine and apply ice packs. Let your doctor know so that the dose can be adjusted next time.

Systemic reactions This type of reaction is much less common. It can be mild, marked by sneezing, nasal congestion or hives. In these mild cases, the symptoms respond rapidly to medications such as antihistamines. Sometimes, however, more serious systemic reactions, such as anaphylaxis, occur. Typically, if you have a reaction, it will occur within 20-60 minutes of the allergy injection, which is why you need to remain in the allergist's clinic afterwards. However, reactions can occur even later, so remain alert to any symptoms.

A recent report from the Mayo Clinic on 79,593 immunotherapy injections over a 10-year period showed the incidence of adverse reactions was less than 0.2 of 1 per cent. Most were mild and responded to immediate medical treatment. There were no fatalities during the study.

Medicines for asthma

The goal in treating asthma is to use the smallest amount of medication necessary to achieve two goals: keeping the airways in your lungs open, both during attacks and over the long term, and reducing the ongoing inflammation that is the cornerstone of the disease.

The anti-inflammatory drugs that doctors typically prescribe for asthma are inhaled corticosteroids and leukotriene modifiers. To keep your airways open, they often prescribe short and long-acting bronchodilators known as beta2-agonists. These are discussed later.

How your doctor chooses to treat your asthma depends on the severity of your disease. In the UK asthma is treated according to the British Thoracic Society's guidelines, which specify the following 'steps' of therapy.

Step 1 Prescribe a short-acting beta2-agonist for when attacks occur. If patients need one or more doses in a day of short-acting beta2-agonist to control symptoms, go to Step 2.

Step 2 Prescribe a daily low dosage of an inhaled corticosteroid as well as a short-acting beta2-agonist as required.

Step 3 If symptoms are still not controlled, add in a daily inhaled long-acting beta2-agonist. A further option is to add in a leukotriene modifier and/or theophylline or aminophylline. These produce less predictable benefits for asthmatics than a regular long-acting beta2-agonist, and their use should be justified by documented improvement in symptoms or lung function.

■ **Step 4** If patients are still symptomatic after taking a low or moderate dose of inhaled steroid and regular long-acting beta2-agonist, it may be necessary to increase the dosage of inhaled steroid and add in extra drugs including leukotriene modifiers and/or theophylline as above.

■ **Step 5** If patients continue to have troublesome symptoms despite maximal dosages of inhaled steroid, a regular long-acting beta2-agonist and one or more extra drugs, a regular dose of oral steroid tablets may be necessary.

For steps 1-3, it is a realistic aim to abolish symptoms completely. This is often practical provided that the patient is shown clearly how to use the medicine, and most particularly the inhaler device which is used to deliver it. Once symptoms are under control, the goal is to gradually reduce the amount of medication to the lowest possible level necessary to control your asthma. Some patients with severe asthma never achieve perfect control, and here the aim is to balance the amount of medication (and any troublesome side effects) with the quality of life achieved.

Corticosteroids

- **PRESCRIPTION (inhaled)** Aero Bec, Asmabec Clickhaler, Beclazone Easi-Breathe, Becodisks, Becotide, Qvar (beclometasone), Pulmicort (budesonide), Flixotide (fluticasone), Asmanex (mometasone), Alvesco (ciclesonide)
- **PRESCRIPTION (nebulized)** Pulmicort Respules (budesonide)
- **PRESCRIPTION (systemic)** prednisolone (oral), hydrocortisone (injected)

Steroids are broad spectrum anti-inflammatory medicines (meaning they have a wide range of action on all the components of an inflammatory process), and so are useful in anything more than very mild cases of allergy and asthma. For asthma, the following types of steroidal medicines are used.

Inhaled

These drugs must be used regularly for all degrees of asthma other than very mild. It may take a month of daily doses before you notice any differences in your symptoms and derive the drugs' full benefits. Eventually, you may be able to reduce your dose as studies have shown that for people with mild asthma, the amount taken daily can be reduced in time without compromising the drugs' effectiveness. Inhaled corticosteroids are typically prescribed in either a metered-dose inhaler (MDI), a dry-powder inhaler, or a compressor-driven nebulizer.

Systemic

Unusually, your doctor may prescribe oral prednisolone to treat your asthma, in the short term (up to 7 days) for reversal of a sudden, severe attack, or in the longer (sometimes indefinite) term if you continue to have severe symptoms. Short-term treatment with steroids is harmless (if not used too often) and is the *only* treatment likely to reverse an acute, severe attack. The injectable equivalent of prednisolone, hydrocortisone, may be used for this purpose in hospital. Used long term, side effects could include cataracts, glaucoma, osteoporosis and diabetes – conditions for which patients must be monitored.

allergy & asthma **sufferers ask**

How dangerous are inhaled and nasal steroids?

Steroids have a bad name because they can cause significant side effects, including osteo-porosis and cataracts. The steroid nasal sprays and inhaled corticosteroids used to treat allergies and asthma, however, have far fewer side effects because they affect only a small part of your body (your respiratory system), unless they are used excessively. While they are safer than oral steroids, they do carry some slight risks and may have some side effects. That's why your doctor will put you on the lowest possible dose to treat your symptoms and control your asthma. The potential side effects may include:

Headaches and nosebleeds These are rare but should be reported to your doctor immediately.

Impaired growth The major concern for children is whether inhaled steroids adversely affect growth. There is little or no evidence that they reduce overall height at adulthood (whereas there is evidence that severe childhood asthma reduces growth). More research is required.

Eye diseases One possible side effect of inhaled steroids is glaucoma, a known side effect of oral steroids. In addition, some ophthalmologists have observed higher pressure in the eyes (a risk factor for glaucoma) in some people who use nasal steroid sprays. Some studies also suggest a higher risk of cataracts

in patients over 40 who use steroids, although no increased risk has been found in younger patients. Regardless, if you are using any form of steroids, be sure to see an ophthalmologist annually for a complete eye exam.

Nasal injury Steroid sprays may injure the nasal septum (the cartilage that separates the nasal passages) if the spray is directed onto it and can lead to septal perforation (a hole in the septum). This complication is very rare.

Decreased bone density There is better news here. While oral steroids can have a negative effect on bone density, a large study published in the January 2003 issue of the *Journal of Allergy and Clinical Immunology* found that inhaled steroids did not reduce bone mineral density in postmenopausal women with asthma, the group at highest risk for such a side effect.

Oral yeast infections Topical corticosteroids may lead to an overgrowth of yeast in the mouth and throat, so you should rinse your mouth and gargle after each inhalation. Be sure to spit out the water. The new inhaled steroid ciclesonide, which is activated in the lungs but not the mouth may be useful for this problem.

Other possible side effects Other rare, short-term effects may include euphoria, depression, water retention, increased appetite, hyperactivity and weight gain.

Delivering the medicine to your lungs

Most asthma medications need to be inhaled directly into the lungs. Luckily, people with asthma have far more options today than the cigarettes, pipes and other rudimentary devices that asthma sufferers used until the early 20th century. Here are the options and how to use them properly to ensure that you get the maximum amount of medication.

Nebulizer therapy

A nebulizer is a device used to deliver liquid medicines to the lungs. It is composed of an air compressor (which turns the liquid into a mist), tubing and a container for the medication. The force of the compressor helps you to receive the medicine without having to take a deep breath, so they are particularly beneficial for infants and small children. (They use a mask that fits snugly around the nose and mouth instead of a mouthpiece.)

Nebulizers are most often used in a GP's surgery, casualty ward or hospital. Their use is discouraged at home. Nebulizers are useful for delivering beta2-antagonists, such as salbutamol, in an emergency. However, if your (or your child's) asthma is frequently out of control, you may have one at home. To use it properly:

1 Put the liquid medication in the nebulizer cup.
2 Attach the nebulizer unit to the compressor with the tubing, making sure all connections are tight. Check the mouthpiece for foreign objects.
3 Place the mouthpiece in your mouth and close your lips around it to make a seal (or fit the mask snugly over your nose and mouth), then turn on the compressor.
4 Breathe in and out as you normally would (don't take any extra breaths). With each fifth breath, hold the medicine in your lungs for 5 to 10 seconds, then exhale. Continue until all the medicine is gone.

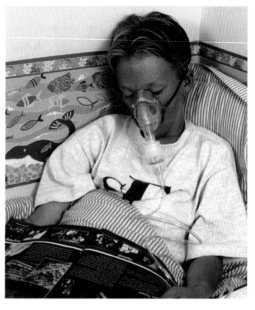

Metered-dose inhalers (MDI)

The term *metered dose* means the medication inside the pressurized canister is released in a single, measured, controlled dose every time you use the inhaler. You must shake the canister vigorously so that the ingredients mix properly and you get the right amount of medication with each dose. When using this form of inhaler, it is very important to properly time your breathing with the release of the medication; otherwise, the medicine may end up in your mouth instead of your lungs.

(For people who have particular trouble with this, breath-activated inhalers, such as Clickhaler and Easi-Breathe are available; the Novolizer inhaler is also useful for such patients. Otherwise the user of a 'spacer' ,see opposite, will solve the problem.)

To use the MDI inhaler properly:

1 Shake the inhaler.

2 Breathe out slowly and completely for 3 to 5 seconds.

3 Put the mouthpiece in your mouth. Press the top of the metal canister down firmly once and breathe in deeply through your mouth until your lungs are full. (You must start to inhale 1 second before you press down on the canister and release the medication.)

4 Lower the inhaler, press your lips together, and hold your breath while counting slowly to 10. This allows the medication to spread throughout your lungs.

5 Breathe out slowly.

6 Wait the prescribed length of time, then repeat as necessary.

Holding chambers and spacers

These devices can help with the delivery of metered-dose inhaled medication to the airways and are particularly recommended for anti-inflammatory medication. To use them:

1 Insert the inhaler mouthpiece or canister into the holding chamber according to the manufacturer's directions.

2 Shake well.

3 Exhale slowly and completely. Put the mouthpiece of the holding chamber into your mouth.

4 Slowly inhale medication for about 5 seconds.

5 Hold your breath for 10 seconds, then exhale slowly.

6 If you are prescribed two puffs, wait the recommended amount of time, shake, activate the inhaler and repeat the previous steps.

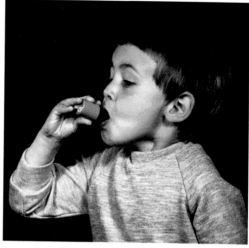

Dry-powder inhalers

These inhalers come in different shapes and sizes and are set to deliver bronchodilators as well as anti-inflammatory medications. They are easy to use and very effective. Because the particles of medication are so small, they can easily reach the tiniest airways. And, unlike metered-dose inhalers, you are less likely to taste or feel the medication when using it. You also don't need a spacer with dry-powder inhalers. Make sure that you follow the manufacturer's directions because various brands may differ slightly. In general, though:

1 Prime your inhaler following the manufacturer's instructions, then load the prescribed dose.

2 Breathe out slowly and completely for 3 to 5 seconds.

3 Put your mouth on the mouthpiece, then inhale deeply and forcefully.

4 Hold your breath for 10 seconds, then exhale slowly.

5 Repeat until you have taken the prescribed number of doses.

Bronchodilators

- **PRESCRIPTION (short-acting inhaled beta2-agonists)** Airomir, Asmasal Clickhaler, Salamol Easi-Breathe, Ventodisks, Ventolin (salbutamol), Bricanyl (terbutaline), Bambec (bambuterol)
- **PRESCRIPTION (short-acting nebulized beta2-agonists)** Ventolin Nebules (salbutamol), Bricanyl Respules or Respirator Solution (terbutaline).
- **PRESCRIPTION (long-acting inhaled beta2-agonists)** Serevent Accuhaler, Serevent Evohaler, Serevent Diskhaler (salmeterol), Foradil, Oxis Turbohaler (formoterol).

Bronchodilator medications open (and keep open) the large and small airways in your lungs. The short-acting type (known as rescue medications) are used when your symptoms are worsening or you're having an asthma attack; the long-acting type are used daily to prevent your asthma from getting worse.

These medications have very little effect on inflammation, though, so they won't provide the long-term relief you need for this chronic condition. And they may not work as well if you're taking other drugs, specifically beta-blockers, often prescribed for high blood pressure and heart conditions. Tell your doctor about all medications you are taking. If you have diabetes, heart disease, high blood pressure, an enlarged prostate, hyperthyroidism, or a history of seizures, ask your doctor if broncho-dilators are right for you. They are very safe but can cause side effects, particularly if overused, such as tremor, nausea, anxiety and a fast heart rate.

Short-acting beta2-agonists

Beta2-agonists relax and open constricted airways during an asthma attack. They are inhaled (via a nebulizer or other delivery system) and work for 3 to 6 hours. While they relieve the symptoms of acute attacks, they do not control the

revealing **research**

Hormones may improve lung function and asthma

A study published in the March 2003 issue of the journal *Annals of Allergy, Asthma & Immunology* found that progesterone and oestrogen may improve lung function and asthma across women's life spans.

It seems that the hormones play a role in strengthening respiratory muscles and increasing the relaxation of bronchial smooth muscle, reducing airway constriction. They also have some anti-inflammatory properties. That may partly explain why some women have increased asthma episodes and are hospitalized more often for asthma during their premenstrual and menstrual phases, when these hormone levels are low. It also possibly explains why some women have improved lung function and a decrease in asthma problems when they take oral contraceptives and hormone replacement therapy.

If you are susceptible to the effects of hormonal cycles, for example, if you suffer from premenstrual syndrome (PMS), tell your doctor. He or she may be able to adjust your asthma treatment to help you to avoid the worst attacks, which might also suggest how your asthma could be controlled during pregnancy.

underlying inflammation. If your asthma symptoms continue to worsen while taking these drugs, talk to your doctor about the possible need for anti-inflammatory agents.

Long-acting Beta2-agonists

Long-acting beta2-agonists such as salmeterol (Serevent) and formoterol (Foradil, Oxis) are taken regularly to help to prevent asthma attacks.

Generally these drugs are taken regularly twice daily, along with a regular inhaled steroid for patients at Step 3 or higher of the asthma treatment guidelines (see page 109) Combinations of drugs (Seretide contains fluticasone and salmeterol, Symbicort contains budesonide and formoterol) are also available for this purpose. The standard dosage of salmeterol produces the maximum bronchodilator effect, whereas taking additional dosages of formoterol can produce some additional relaxation of the airways. For this reason formoterol and the combination with budesonide (Symbicort) are licensed for extra 'as required' use in addition to regular use for treating asthma.

Long-acting beta2-agonists are designed to be taken regularly, twice daily, since they last for about 12 hours. Despite the fact that they have no anti-inflammatory effect on their own, they do reduce the need for inhaled steroids which is why the two are often prescribed together. Occasionally, intermittent doses of long-acting beta2-agonists may be prescribed, for example, for exercise-induced asthma.

revealing **research**

Considering genetics along with prescriptions

One of the most widely prescribed drugs for asthma is salbutamol, sold in various proprietory preparations, of which the most common is Ventolin. But it is not equally effective in all people with asthma. It turns out that your genetic makeup may determine how well salbutamol and quite possibly other asthma medications work.

In a study published in September 2000 in the journal *Proceedings of the National Academy of Sciences*, researchers determined the genetic fingerprints of 121 asthma patients. The patients later underwent spirometry, a test to measure their lung function, before inhaling salbutamol and were tested again 30 minutes later. Those with a certain genetic code for the beta-2 receptor responded best. Those with a different type responded worst.

While it's unlikely that your doctor will start doing genetic tests before writing a prescription, if you find that salbutamol is not working for you, you should talk to your doctor about other treatment options.

Theophylline

• **PRESCRIPTION** available under several brand names including Nuelin SA, Slo-Phyllin, Uniphyllin Continus and Phyllocontin Continus.

These days theophylline is rarely used to treat asthma, even though it was once one of the primary asthma drugs. It works by relaxing the muscles around the

Monitoring asthma drugs

Just because you have collected your prescription medications and are using them as instructed by your doctor doesn't mean you can stop thinking about your drug treatment. Now it's up to you to monitor how your regimen is working so that you can fine-tune your medications whenever necessary.

For those with asthma, one of the most important tools for monitoring the condition is a peak flow meter, described in chapter 6 (see page 95).

You should use it daily, tracking the results on a chart like the one opposite. You should always be trying to match or beat your 'personal best' – in this case, the highest peak flow number you can reach over a two to three-week period when your asthma is under control.

Your doctor will help you to determine this goal (in children, it will increase as they grow). Once you have a personal best, aim to maintain a peak flow reading within 80 per cent of that number. The following three zones tell you how well you are doing at controlling your asthma.

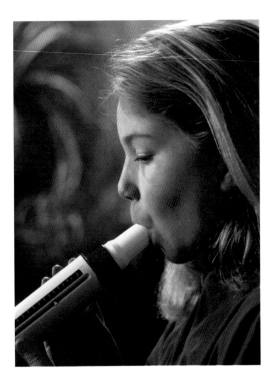

• **Green zone** Peak expiratory flow rate (PEFR) 80 to 100 per cent of personal best. You are relatively symptom-free and can continue your current asthma-management programmme.

• **Yellow zone** PEFR 50 to 80 per cent of personal best. Your asthma is getting worse. You need a temporary increase in your asthma medication, and, if you're on chronic medications, you may need to increase your maintenance therapy. Consult your doctor for some fine-tuning.

• **Red zone** PEFR below 50 per cent of personal best – the danger zone. Use your bronchodilator to open your airways. If your peak flow readings don't return to at least the yellow zone after using your bronchodilator, consult your doctor.

airways and stimulating breathing. One study reported that it may also have anti-inflammatory qualities even in low doses. But it can be dangerous. The main concern about theophylline is that it could build up to toxic levels in your blood. This risk increases if you have liver problems, such as hepatitis, or are taking drugs, such as erythromycin and systemic antifungal medications, that can interfere with your liver's ability to break down theophylline.

Chronic smokers absorb the drug much more quickly than non-smokers, so they require higher doses. Theophylline also interacts with other drugs for a variety of medical conditions, including, ironically, asthma. Theophylline

My asthma symptom and peak flow diary

1 Start-of-the-week readings

My personal best peak flow reading is _____   Last week, my best reading was _____

2 Daily readings

	MON		TUES		WED		THU		FRI		SAT		SUN	
	A.M.	P.M.	A.M.	P.M.	A.M.	P.M.	A.M.	P.M.	A.M.	P.M.	A.M.	P.M.	A.M.	P.M.
My peak flow reading was: Enter the number from your meter														
My peak flow ranking was: more than 80% of personal best														
50%–80% of personal best														
less than 50% of personal best														
The severity of my symptoms was: None														
Mild*														
Moderate**														
Serious***														
I used a medicine for my symptoms: (Yes/no)														
My activities were curtailed: (Yes/no)														

3 End-of-the-week readings

This week's best reading was _____   The general peak flow direction was (↑ ↓ ↔) _____

4 Notes _____

_____

_____

_____

_____

*only during physical activity; **also at rest, affecting sleep or activity level; ***serious while at rest, affecting ability to breathe or talk

should never be used as a rescue medication if you have an asthma attack, and it should not be taken by people with peptic ulcers.

If you are elderly or have heart or liver disease, hypertension, seizure disorders, gastro-oesophageal reflux or congestive heart failure, you should use extreme caution in taking this drug, and should probably talk to your doctor about alternatives.

That said, some asthmatics get their greatest relief with theophylline. If their blood levels are closely monitored while they are taking the drug, they may do well on it.

Asthma and allergy medications during pregnancy

Pregnant women often think that as soon as the stick turns pink, they have to come off all medications – prescription and OTC – lest taking them harm the developing baby. While that may be true of certain drugs, there are also numerous medications considered to be completely safe if taken during pregnancy. Furthermore, unilaterally abandoning your medication without consulting a doctor could put both mother and foetus at risk. Here are some guidelines regarding treatments for asthma and allergy.

Asthma symptoms may tend to worsen or improve in pregnancy, but whatever happens it is important to keep the disease very closely under control, particularly when labour approaches.

All UK physicians are agreed that asthma should be treated in exactly the same way in pregnancy as it is out of pregnancy, except perhaps that leukotriene modifiers would not normally be initiated in pregnancy because there is little experience to support their safe use in this context (although they would probably not have a harmful effect).

All other drugs, particularly inhaled bronchodilators and steroids, are considered risk-free in pregnancy and should be continued as usual. Nasal steroids are safe taken in pregnancy.

• **Short-acting bronchodilators** These generally pose no risk to expectant mothers. Terbutaline (Bricanyl) is particularly safe to take during pregnancy since it is often used intravenously to halt premature labour.

• **Inhaled budesonide** A Swedish study that evaluated 99 per cent of the births in Sweden from 1995 to 1998 found that mothers who took budesonide had babies that were born on time and at normal weights and lengths, with no increase in stillbirths or multiple births.

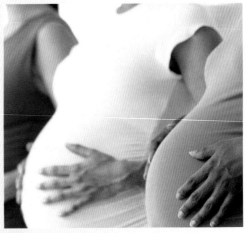

• **Decongestants** Although pregnant women have used the decongestant pseudoephedrine (Sudafed) for years, reports suggest a slight increase in abdominal wall defects in newborns, so it is advisable to avoid oral decongestants during the first trimester. One of the best treatments of all for congestion may be simple irrigation – washing out your nose with a saltwater solution.

• **Antihistamines** While there is no evidence that any antihistamine is harmful in pregnancy, at present most manufacturers err on the side of caution and advise that cetirizine, desloratadine, hydroxyzine, loratadine, mizolastine and terfenadine should be avoided. This leaves the more traditional, or sedating, antihistamines such as chlorphenamine, which are regarded as safe but also make you drowsy. For hay fever, nasal steroids used regularly are quite safe, as are sodium cromoglicate eye drops (Opticrom).

• **Immunotherapy (allergy injections)** You can continue immunotherapy treatment at a constant dose during pregnancy, but you should not start injections for the first time while pregnant because the initial injections are most likely to cause allergic reactions which are best avoided at this time.

Leukotriene modifiers

• **PRESCRIPTION** Accolate (zafirlukast), Singulair (montelukast)

Leukotrienes are among the molecules that mast cells, eosinophils and macrophages release when they encounter asthma triggers. They are partly to blame for the increased mucus production, airway constriction and inflammation of asthma and for the runny and stuffy nose of allergies.

They are particularly useful for preventing exercise-induced asthma and asthma triggered by allergens and aspirin. They also have some broncho-dilating effects, opening up airways within 2 hours of taking them.

Leukotriene inhibitors are not considered a substitute for regular anti-inflammatory inhaled steroid medication and so are only used in patients who already take inhaled steroids and usually a regular long-acting beta2-agonist as well.

Not all patients show any useful response to these drugs, so response must be monitored initially. There are few side effects. Leukotriene modifiers have also recently been licensed for treating allergic rhinitis.

Anticholinergics

• **Prescription (inhaled)** Ipratropium bromide aerosol, dry powder inhaler, nebulizer solution, Atrovent Aerohaler and nebulizer solution, Respontin nebulizer solution (ipratropium bromide), Spiriva HandiHaler (tiotropium bromide)

Anticholinergic medicines such as ipratropium reduce mucus production and cough, and also relax the airways, although not as quickly as beta2-agonists. They are sometimes useful for asthmatics with particularly troublesome cough or mucus production but are not used routinely. The longer acting drug tiotropium is used in patients with chronic bronchitis.

Sodium cromoglicate

• **PRESCRIPTION (inhaled:** Sodium cromoglicate, Cromogen Easi-Breathe, Intal aerosol, Spincaps and nebulizer solution

Sodium cromoglicate is a weak anti-inflammatory agent and can reduce allergen and exercise-induced asthma. Its actions are, however, inferior to inhaled steroids and it is now rarely used.

Anti-IgE drugs: new hope for the future

November 2005 may prove to be one of the most exciting times in the treatment of allergies and asthma. That was when the UK government approved omalizumab (Xolair), the first in a new class of drugs for the treatment of allergic asthma. Eventually, this class of drugs – called anti-IgE drugs – is expected to revolutionize the treatment of allergies.

Xolair is a genetically engineered drug called a monoclonal antibody. It works by stopping an allergic reaction before it starts by blocking the IgE antibody that causes the reaction. Everything else in our allergy arsenal treats only the allergy symptoms or blocks reaction to specific allergens.

Xolair – already approved in the USA – came about as a result of the discovery in 1998 of the precise shape of the receptor molecule that triggers the allergic response in your immune system. These receptors, called high-affinity immunoglobulin-E receptors, sit on the surface of mast cells and serve as 'docking stations' for IgE.

Once scientists found the docking stations, the race was on to work out how to prevent IgE from getting to them in the first place. If the IgE antibodies couldn't 'park' on mast cells, they couldn't trigger the cells' release of histamine and other inflammatory chemicals. So, put very simply, the molecules that make up Xolair grab IgE antibodies and keep them from ever reaching the mast cells.

Xolair has been licensed in the UK for moderate to severe allergic asthma for youngsters aged 12 and older whose disease has not responded well to other treatments. It is given by subcutaneous (under-the-skin) injection once or twice a month. Its use can really change your life. People taking Xolair are often able to live very normally for the first time ever, being able to visit a friend with a pet, for instance, or sleep with the windows open in spring and summer – the kinds of things those of us without allergic asthma take for granted.

Many people are also able to significantly reduce their use of other medications. For instance, in studies of Xolair in adults and children, some of those taking the drug were able to cut back on or even stop using inhaled corticosteroids. Eventually, Xolair will probably be approved to treat allergic asthma in children as well.

One problem with Xolair is the cost. It is likely to be very high compared to existing treatments – around £8,500 per patient per year. This is because it requires a very sophisticated manufacturing method. Also, it is given by injection once every two to four weeks, a regimen

Medicines of the future

Pharmaceutical researchers are anxious to discover the next allergy and asthma treatment. Research into other anti-IgE medications continues, but scientists are also exploring the following potential treatments.

Immunotherapy and vaccines

■ Researchers are studying so-called rush immunotherapy. Patients achieve the full maintenance dose with several injections a day over a period of three to five days instead of the three to six months it normally takes.

■ Researchers plan to begin clinical human trials of a vaccine against peanut allergies in 2006. Studies in mice have found that the vaccine, made from

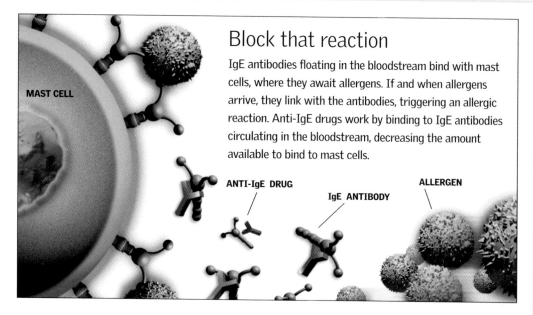

Block that reaction

IgE antibodies floating in the bloodstream bind with mast cells, where they await allergens. If and when allergens arrive, they link with the antibodies, triggering an allergic reaction. Anti-IgE drugs work by binding to IgE antibodies circulating in the bloodstream, decreasing the amount available to bind to mast cells.

MAST CELL

ANTI-IgE DRUG

IgE ANTIBODY

ALLERGEN

that may have to be maintained indefinitely. Studies find that once Xolair is stopped, IgE levels gradually return over several months to where they were before the drug was started.

Ideally, as more drugs in this class are approved and are used more widely, the price should come down. Additionally, there is some thought that a short course of Xolair treatment for those with allergic rhinitis who have not developed asthma may prevent asthma from developing at all. Anti-IgE medications may also prove effective for people who don't follow their daily medication regimens very rigorously, and possibly for those who have atopic dermatitis that is difficult to manage, allergies to foods that are hard to avoid, and latex allergies. Studies using another anti-IgE formulation on people with peanut allergies found that it significantly reduced their reactions to peanut proteins.

So it is worth keeping an eye out for further news about Xolair and other anti-IgE medications in the future. These revolutionary new drugs may very well change the way you and your doctor treat your asthma and allergies.

bacteria genetically engineered to produce modified peanut proteins that are then killed with heat treatment, blocks reactions in mice with peanut allergies.

In early 2003, a Danish pharmaceutical company began conducting clinical trials of a gel-cap, tablet-based immunotherapy for allergies.

Anti-inflammatories

A new class of anti-inflammatory compounds currently under investigation works to inhibit phosphodiesterase-4, a chemical involved in the inflammatory reaction. These drugs are related to theophylline, but have far fewer side effects. Among the drugs that were in late-stage clinical trials in late 2003 was a compound called roflumilast, which is also being investigated for future use in treating chronic obstructive pulmonary disease.

Asthma medications and dental health

Antihistamines and possibly corticosteroids may dry out your mouth to such an extent that it puts your teeth at risk. That's because you need a steady saliva flow to wash away sticky food particles, which adhere to your teeth, become a breeding ground for bacteria, and lead to cavities and gum disease.

The solution is obvious: you should drink plenty of water to keep your mouth moist. It is also advisable to brush and floss your teeth more frequently than usual, since water is less effective than saliva at keeping your mouth clean.

Inhaled corticosteroids

Ciclesonide (Alvesco) is newly available in the UK for asthma therapy. The drug is not activated until it comes into contact with the surface of airways in the lungs, thus minimizing its effects on the throat or the rest of your system.

Nasal sprays

Olopatadine, a prescription eyedrop for allergic conjunctivitis, may soon be licensed in the USA as a non-steroidal nasal spray; its current brand name is Patanase.

Immunomodulators

These drugs, originally used to prevent organ transplant rejection, work to suppress the immune system. Applied to the skin, immunomodulators tacrolimus (Protopic) and Elidel (pimecrolimus) have already been approved to treat atopic dermatitis (eczema), an allergic skin condition. An inhaled form of tacrolimus is now being tested for asthma. It would be ideal for those who don't respond to or don't want to take steroids but still need an anti-inflammatory.

Novel compounds

Heterocyclic thiourea (HCT) compounds This new class of drugs works to prevent the release of leukotrienes from mast cells. Work on them is still quite preliminary, however, and it will probably be 10 years or more before drugs in this class are available.

GE2 molecule This genetically engineered molecule, called a fusion protein, works to prevent mast cells and basophils from releasing histamine. It binds to two receptor molecules on mast cells. One acts as a kind of accelerator pedal, starting the allergic response, and the other as a brake, stemming the allergic response. By binding to both receptors simultaneously, GE2 halts the allergic reaction altogether. But this compound is not likely to be tested in humans for some years.

Interleukin-4 and -5 inhibitors Interleukin-4 and -5 are cytokines that play a role in the inflammatory process. Drugs to prevent the production of interleukin-5 are under investigation as a long-term treatment for asthma.

R112 This experimental drug, the first in its class, is being tested for treating allergic rhinitis. Unlike current allergy drugs, such as antihistamines and antileukotrienes that target only a single chemical involved in activating mast cells, R112 is thought to work by blocking all major chemicals from the mast cell response that contribute to inflammation. If it proves effective for allergic rhinitis, it may also be tested for asthma.

Genetic treatments

So far, researchers have identified more than 291 genes associated with asthma, paving the way for numerous new targets for drugs. One that has researchers quite excited is the gene responsible for the enzyme arginase, previously thought to be involved only in the liver. Today, some researchers believe that arginase plays a major role in asthma, appearing to be the molecule that 'kicks off' the chain of actions that leads to asthma symptoms.

More individualized treatments

Researchers have begun considering individualized asthma treatments, depending on the form of asthma you have. For instance, some people have asthma attacks predominantly when mast cells infiltrate the smooth muscle of the airways, while others are more affected by the inflammatory effects of eosinophils. Each requires a different treatment approach. In the future, you can expect doctors to spend more time determining the specific cause of your asthma attacks and what exacerbates them before prescribing medications.

More combination drugs

Look out for more combination therapies, such as Seretide and Symbicort, that bring beta2-agonists and corticosteroids together. The fewer drugs people have to take, the more likely they are to take them, improving overall asthma control. Both Seretide and Symbicort are available in three different strengths, reflecting the dosage of inhaled steroid needed by different asthmatics.

Into the future: beyond drugs

Drugs are not the only area that researchers are investigating in their pursuit of effective allergy and asthma treatments. Other novel approaches, include:

Genetically modified forms of grass, peanuts and soya beans For instance, researchers at the Plant Biotechnology Centre, Melbourne, Australia, genetically modified ryegrasses, used in lawns all over the world and the main hay fever culprit in Europe and Australia, to eliminate two common hay fever allergens. Additionally, soya beans growing in Hawaii have been genetically modified to eliminate a gene thought to trigger most allergic reactions.

Can asthma drugs make my asthma worse?

While this may seem like a silly question, it's not. And the answer is that yes, in some instances, certain drugs, particularly when overused, can aggravate your condition. Several studies have found that people who use short-acting bronchodilating beta2-agonist medications, such as salbutamol, several times daily can eventually develop increased symptoms of airway constriction, which worsens asthma. If you are using a short-acting beta2-agonist medication this frequently, your disease is not well controlled and you should make an appointment to see your doctor.

● **Nasal plugs for allergic rhinitis**

These plugs, developed by Australian researchers, come with sticky filters to catch pollen grains before they enter the nasal cavity and trigger an allergic reaction. The idea is that you would use them when you go outside on days with high pollen counts.

● **Preventing allergy sensitization**

In preliminary studies in Finland, pregnant women, breastfeeding mothers and newborns are given probiotics – a type of bacteria usually found in the gut that affects the immune system – to try to prevent allergy development in at-risk infants.

There is some research to support this approach. In a study published in the British medical journal *Lancet* in May 2003, researchers gave a group of pregnant women either probiotic capsules or placebos every day starting a few weeks before their due dates. Those who breastfed continued to receive either placebos or probiotics for six months, while bottle-fed babies received placebos or bacteria in their formula. By the age of four, those in the probiotic group were signi-ficantly less likely to have developed the allergic skin condition known as atopic dermatitis, often a precursor of allergic rhinitis and/or asthma.

Future preventive efforts may be more bold, says Dr Harold S. Nelson, professor of medicine at the National Jewish Medical and Research Center in Denver. For instance, some day doctors may give infants endotoxin or killed bacterial DNA to counteract the cleanliness believed to be related to the increasing incidence of allergies (the so-called hygiene hypothesis).

Beyond medications

The investments in finding new ways to treat and prevent allergies and asthma are huge; the stakes are high; and the number of doctors, researchers and laboratories working worldwide is probably in the thousands.

For the moment, however, the best thing you can do for yourself is to not need any medicine at all, and the best way to do that is to keep allergens at bay. So leaving the laboratories behind, the next chapter will enter a more toxic place: your home. Chapter 8 shows you how you can improve your personal environment to reduce your chances of allergies and asthma.

Chapter **eight**

The right
environment

Back in the 16th century, the Archbishop of St Andrews in Scotland invited the acclaimed Italian physician Gerolamo Cardano to his country for advice on treating his asthma. Cardano's diagnosis was simple and astute. The problem was the bed, and he recommended that the Archbishop get rid of his feather bedding. The result? A 'miraculous' recovery.

Some 400 years later, in 1927, Storm van Leeuwen created a 'climate chamber' in the Netherlands to make a similar point. He successfully showed that asthmatic patients improved when moved from their homes into the chamber. Van Leeuwen wrote: 'In our endeavours to find the cause of the attack...we utilized the known fact that the environment of the asthmatic patient is, as a rule, of primary importance in determining the intensity and frequency of his attacks.'

Cardano and van Leeuwen came upon truths that even the greatest medical advances of recent years haven't changed; if you want relief from allergies or asthma, you need to get rid of the triggers in your home.

It may not seem logical, but indoor environments are often worse for your allergies and asthma than the great outdoors. Your home, with its fabric-covered furniture and cushions, its carpeting, tightly sealed windows and warm, damp spaces – is like a field strewn with allergy land mines. Research shows that indoor air pollution can be up to 10 times greater than outdoor pollution and its effects much more intense, since we generally spend more than 80 per cent of our time indoors, at home or at work. And since we breathe about 22,000 times a day, just imagine what we take into our airways.

To be clear, people are rarely sensitive to the materials that make up the house itself – the bricks, concrete, steel, wood, and so on. It is the furnishings, such as carpets, MDF furniture, paints and wood treatment that can cause chemical sensitivity. And above all, it is the microscopic things that grow and accumulate inside the house that cause allergies and asthma attacks.

These unwanted occupants come in several forms. The most prevalent in-home allergens are dust and its components (primarily dust mite droppings), pet hair and dander, and moulds, although there is increasing evidence of the role of airborne chemical allergens. All of these are discussed in this chapter, as well as the places where they accumulate most: bedding, carpets and damp areas. Most importantly, you will discover how to make your home as all ergen-free and fresh as possible.

One caveat. Although diligent cleaning and removal of allergy triggers can still make a big difference even if there is smoke in the atmosphere, if someone in your home smokes it is best if they do it outside. Not only does smoking seriously damage the lungs of anyone who has allergies or asthma, but secondhand smoke is equally detrimental for a child or spouse who is an allergy or asthma sufferer.

Dust: the dirty truth

One of the biggest culprits in your home is often invisible. Dust. Studies have found that the average six-room home in the UK collects about 18kg (40lb) of dust each year. You think: 'I dust every few days, wash the floors, scrub the bath-rooms and change the linens weekly. How could I have that much dust?'

Some dust in your home is inevitable and would be there even if you scrubbed daily. It is composed of flakes of dead skin, pet hair and dander (even if you don't have pets, your shoes may bring hair and dander into the house), breakdown of fabrics, debris blown in from outside and so on. As if that were not bad enough, that layer of dust coating your coffee table or television screen or lying behind the sofa may also contain cockroach droppings, another potent allergy trigger found increasingly in our inner cities. Obviously, there *is* a correlation between cleaning and dust levels – the more you clean, the less dust you will have.

The problem with dust isn't only aesthetic – it provides a regular supply of food for dust mites. As we said in chapter 3, these microscopic bugs are literally everywhere in your home, munching away on teeny flakes of your skin that have sloughed off in the course of normal living. What is more, the UK is particularly badly affected. According to a 2004 report from the European Federation of Allergy and Airways Diseases 'The United Kingdom and Ireland appear to be the worst countries for house-dust mite asthma in Europe.'

Dust mites are a major source of allergies, with about 10 per cent of the population and 90 per cent of people with allergic asthma having positive skin tests to dust mites. Those figures are even higher in children, with recent studies suggesting that at least 80 per cent of children are allergic to dust mites.

Plenty of research has shown that if you remove patients with allergies from an environment with a high count of mites, their symptoms improve and, in the case of asthma, their breathing tubes are less 'reactive' or sensitive. So a radical reduction in mites will help some asthmatics at least.

However, in a normal, humid, household environment it is extremely difficult to achieve a significant and lasting reduction in mite levels, however hard you try. Killing live mites doesn't deal with the dead bodies or faecal pellets, which may persist for months or even years in hidden corners of house dust. And the mites quickly re-establish themselves unless pesticides are applied regularly or the humidity of the home is kept low all year round. That said, it's worth doing everything possible to reduce exposure to dust mites in your home.

Dust mites

There may be as many as 19,000 dust mites in a single gram of dust (about the weight of a paper clip). And each female can add another 25 to 30 mites to the population during her lifetime.

These tiny creatures thrive in normal household environments, when the relative humidity is 75 to 80 per cent and the temperature at least 21°C (70°F). Reduce the humidity and you reduce the numbers of mites, since they cannot survive in humidity of less than 40 to 50 per cent.

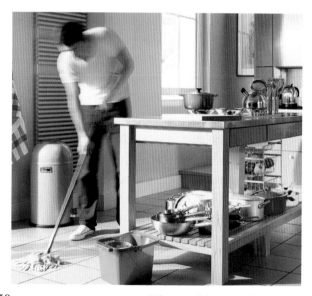

If you have mites, they are most prevalent in the room where you spend the most time – the bedroom, where we inhabit the bed for about one-third of our lives. They thrive in our beds: the 1g of skin cells shed daily and 300ml of water we sweat and breathe out provides all they need for their

The problem with dust isn't only aesthetic – it provides a regular supply of food for dust mites, and they are a major source of allergies.

What does hypo-allergenic mean?

It simply means that something is *unlikely* to trigger an allergic reaction. What it doesn't mean, however, is that the item *will not* cause an allergic reaction. Check the ingredients before using any hypo-allergenic products, particularly if you are highly allergic.

welfare and reproduction. And it is not worth trying to combat them with insecticides. They won't solve the problem, and those sold for mites, called acaricides, can cause skin or lung irritation. Instead, it is better to concentrate on other ways to reduce your exposure to mites in your home. It's a worthwhile goal.

One study found that reducing levels of dust mites in children's beds by one-third cut the number of days they wheezed and missed school by nearly a quarter (22 per cent).

As part of the Breathe Easy Plan, this book provides a step-by-step, room-by-room guide for making your home as allergy-free as possible. In the meantime, however, here are some ways to reduce the levels of dust mites (and dust) throughout your house.

■ **Cover your mattress and pillows** In past years, your only option for mattress and pillow covers was slippery, hot vinyl. Today, however, you can buy covers made of tightly woven fabric or semi-permeable polyurethane, both of which are as comfortable as regular covers. But forget so-called hypoallergenic covers and pillows; they still attract dust mites. Also, your problem is not solved once your bedding is safely covered. You still need to vacuum the mattress cover or wipe it with a damp cloth every month. Otherwise mites will simply begin multiplying on top of the cover as you shed skin flakes. You can also now buy waterproof mattress and pillow protectors with an upper surface of soft, absorbent cotton towelling and a light, breathable polyurethane waterproof membrane that, unlike that on a standard waterproof mattress, is a proven dust mite barrier. They are available, along with quilt and pillow covers, from **www.snugnights.co.uk**

Unfortunately, only one-third of people with allergies use these covers, although numerous studies find that they help to reduce medication use and asthma attacks in adults and children.

■ **Wash with hot water** Forget washing your sheets and covers with cool or warm water. The best way to kill those mites is washing in very hot water (60°C/140°F) at least once a week. Alternatively, an hour in a hot dryer will also kill most mites, or you can wrap items in a plastic bag and put it in the freezer overnight (but neither will get rid of mite by-products, namely eggs and faeces).

■ **Dry out the air** This is not much of a problem in the winter, when central heating tends to dry the air and reduce humidity. In the summer, though, it can be difficult to keep humidity levels, and thus dust mite levels, lower. If you are lucky enough to have air-conditioning at home, keep the fan running at all times so air constantly goes through the filter. If the humidity is still high despite air conditioning, or if you don't have air conditioning, try using a dehumidifier in any rooms that retain dampness, such as the bathroom and basement, or put one in your bedroom to ensure extra-dry air. You can buy an inexpensive instrument called a hygrometer to measure the level of indoor humidity, which should remain below 50 per cent but above 30 per cent, particularly in your bedroom.

Dust with electrostatic disposable cloths Available from supermarkets, these are far more effective than dusting with a dry cloth, which simply stirs up mite allergens. Be sure to dust *everything*. If you are particularly sensitive to dust, ask a non-allergic friend or family member to do the job. Each month, put your houseplants in the bath and shower off the dust; that's good for the plants as well as for your health.

Bag it right Use a vacuum cleaner with a double or triple-layered micro-filtration bag or a HEPA (high-efficiency particulate air) filter (see box, page 133) to trap any allergens that pass through the vacuum's exhaust. If you have your home professionally cleaned, make sure that the cleaners use your vacuum; otherwise they could unwittingly release allergens from other people's homes.

Go unnatural Replace wool or feather-stuffed cushions with synthetic materials that can be washed. Choose stuffed animals and other children's soft toys that are washable.

Clean your carpets If possible, remove all carpeting in the bedroom. Otherwise treat carpets every four to six months with a product to kill dust mites. Then vacuum carpets thoroughly to remove the dead mites, which can still cause allergic symptoms. Do not use chemical mite killers for surfaces or fabrics with which children have close or regular contact, such as soft toys or pillows.

Remove all carpeting from concrete floors. Such floors trap moisture allowing dust mites and mould spores to thrive. Seal the floor with a vapour barrier, and then cover it with a washable surface such as vinyl or linoleum.

Use steam Dry steam, available now in home carpet and floor cleaners, is most effective at removing dust mites and other

Breathe Easy tip: eucalyptus oil kills mites

A study published in the *Journal of Allergy and Clinical Immunology* found that when eucalyptus oil was used to pre-soak loads of bedclothes, it killed 95 per cent of mites that survived high-temperature water. The researchers mixed 1 part liquid detergent and 4 parts eucalyptus oil in a small container, then added 1 teaspoon of the mixture to a tumbler of water. They filled the washer with water, added the diluted detergent and eucalyptus mixture, and let the bedding soak for an hour before washing. You can buy eucalyptus oil at health-food stores and some chemist shops or wherever healing oils are sold.

allergens from carpets and upholstery. Use it on mattresses and pillows, too. And if you have your carpets professionally cleaned, make sure that the cleaner uses dry steam, not a wet shampoo method. The shampoo simply provides a more tasty meal for mites, and the dampness can bring on moulds

Carpet: put your foot down on allergens

People with allergies are in luck these days; after decades of wall-to-wall, thick pile carpeting representing the ultimate in home flooring, today's homes are more likely than ever to have flooring made of hardwood, laminate, tiles or vinyl.

Yet many people still prefer carpeting, at least in some of their rooms. The trouble is, carpet has fibres that easily trap indoor air pollutants, such as dust mites, moulds, fungi, pet hair and dander and other irritants. In fact, one study found that carpeting collects allergens at 100 times the rate of bare floors.

If you insist on having a fitted carpet, select a type that has a short pile; shag or deep-pile carpeting is the worst for anyone with allergies. And always use a vacuum with a HEPA filter (see box on page 133); or you will simply scatter the dust mites around the room.

Never lay your carpeting directly over concrete; this simply encourages dust mite growth. Instead, make sure you lay carpet and padding over a subfloor, usually made of plywood. It is also important to steam clean carpets every three to six months. Several studies in which carpeting and furniture were steam cleaned found significant improvements in levels of allergens and allergy symptoms. In one study, people with asthma whose homes were steam cleaned had a fourfold reduction in bronchial hyper-reactivity nine months after the cleaning, compared with no change in a group whose homes received 'fake' treatment. Another approach might be to treat carpets with tannic acid, which kills dust mites but has some toxic side effects. If you have basement accommodation, try using some type of laminated flooring instead of carpet. With just a little dampness, that carpet could become a breeding ground for moulds and fungi.

Pets: the most loving allergen source

As discussed in chapter 3, if you are allergic to your pet, don't blame the animal's hair or fur. What you're really allergic to are the proteins secreted by oil glands in the animal's skin, as well as proteins in saliva, which sticks to the fur when the animal licks itself. Another source of allergy-causing proteins is animal urine. When the substance carrying the proteins dries, they are free to float into the air. Obviously, if you are allergic to animal dander, the most effective solution is to find a new home for the pet, be it a gerbil or a German shepherd. But that may be easier said than done. The UK heads the European league when it comes to pets, with more than 14 million cats and dogs plus some 37 million small animals. Around 15 per cent of adults and more than 50 per cent of children are allergic to pets, yet many still have them in their homes. In such situations, you may want to consider allergy injections (a doctor would prefer you to avoid the pet), but there are also steps you can take to minimize the dander.

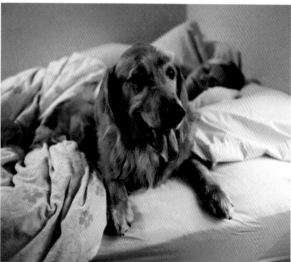

Keep pets out of your bedroom Keep them out at night and close your bedroom door during the day to stop them coming in. If possible, keep them out of the house altogether, in a warm bed in an outside shed or kennel.

Let someone else do the grooming Pets should be brushed regularly, but not in the house and not by you. Even cleaning a litter box is a chore best left to your non-allergic spouse, partner or child.

Treat dander like dust Many of the recommendations for managing dust mites and such hold true for pet-generated allergens. Use HEPA filters in your vacuum. Dust regularly with an electrostatic cloth. Whenever possible, choose smoother, harder surfaces for your floors and furniture: they are much less likely to harbour animal hair or pet dander.

Keep your pets out of your bedroom, not only at night time, but every minute of every day.

Wash your hands every time you touch your pet And invest in a non-perfumed moisturizing lotion to replenish your skin.

Bath your pet regularly Some studies find a significant reduction in the amount of pet allergens when dogs are bathed weekly. There is less evidence that bathing works for cats, however.

Change your pet's diet The right diet can minimize your pet's hair loss, reducing dander indoors. Talk to your vet about what kind of food will be most appropriate for your pet.

Consider using a product such as PetalCleanse Made from natural products including mild detergents, this Allergy UK award-winning solution removes allergens and dander from dogs, cats and small animals. You simply wipe it on your pet with a cloth. Studies show that after 2 to 3 weeks it reduces symptoms in more than 90 per cent of pet allergic people.

Sneezing? Blame the fish

Quite often, the only pets children and adults with asthma or allergies have are fish. Believe it or not, though, your fish tank could be contributing to your allergies, since the fish-food residue that accumulates on the inside of the tank above the water line is a magnet for dust mites.

Make sure that you wipe the inside of the tank once a week and check for leaking filters, a potential source of mould. Another hazard is dry fish food, which contains potent proteins that can adversely affect some people with asthma.

■ **Make extra-sure your pets are housetrained** If the cat is peeing in the corner of the living room or your dog has accidents when you're out at work, you probably have mould and fungus growing on your carpet, not to mention the allergens in the urine.

Indoor chemicals

With the ever-increasing amount of chemicals that are used in our environment, more and more people are developing a sensitivity to chemicals, even at very low concentrations. Although not yet fully understood, chemical sensitivity tends to occur in those with allergies or asthma, or with a family history of allergy, often aggravating symptoms. While exposure to outdoor chemical pollutants – exhaust fumes, industrial emissions, crop spraying, pesticides – is often beyond our control, we can at least limit the potential culprits we allow into our homes. And it's astonishing how many there are. In most modern homes air pollution is worse indoors than outside, largely because of chemicals known as volatile organic compounds (VOCs) given off by modern building and furnishing materials, synthetic fabrics, toileteries, cleaning materials, gas cookers and, of course, people who smoke.

Common VOCs and their sources include: formaldehyde (in chipboard, foam insulation, particle board and household cleaners); styrene (in disinfectants, plastics, paints); terpenes (scented deodorizers, polishes, fabric softeners); benzyl chloride (vinyl tiles); trichloroethane (aerosol sprays, fabric protectors, dry-cleaned clothes). Aerosols, window cleaners, paints, paint thinners, varnishes, lacquers, adhesives, soaps, cosmetics and perfumes are potential sources of acrylic acid esters, ketones and ethers. And, lighting a kerosene heater or a wood fire at home generates polycyclic aromatic hydrocarbons – as does smoking cigarettes.

Banning smoking at home is an obvious first step to take. In addition, the following measures will help to keep the number of potential chemical allergens in your home to a minimum.

■ **Keep your home well ventilated** to allow any pollutants to escape. If you have a gas-fired boiler or gas fire, make sure they are installed correctly and regularly serviced by a CORGI registered engineer: even a slight carbon

What is the best vacuum cleaner for allergies?

Well, that depends. The basic fact is that vacuuming often releases as much dust *into* the air as it picks up out of the carpeting.

For instance, one 2003 study compared five brand-new HEPA (high-efficiency particulate air) filter vacuum cleaners with an old, non-HEPA filter vacuum. Researchers tested the machines in five homes that had cats and then in an experimental (dust-free) chamber. Then they measured the amount of cat allergens in the home's air.

Rather than clearing the air, both types of vacuums significantly *increased* the amount of airborne cat allergens when used in the home. The HEPA vacuums worked better, however, in the experimental chamber. It seems that the force of vacuuming in the home increases levels of airborne cat hair by pulling it from clothes, skin and other surfaces.

The good news is that vacuums are improving all the time. A study found that 1999 models released far fewer allergens into the air than models from 1993, the previous time the researchers conducted the study. So if you have been using a vacuum that is more than three years old, consider replacing it with a new one.

You should look for a vacuum with a HEPA filter. This type comprises a core filter folded back and forth over corrugated separators, thus adding strength to the core and forming air passages between the pleats. The filter itself is composed of very fine submicron fibres in a matrix of larger fibres. It helps to prevent leaking, thus allowing fewer allergens to escape from the vacuum.

If you choose a vacuum that uses bags, buy high-quality, triple-thick types called microfiltration bags, which studies find are best at keeping dust where it belongs. And choose an upright vacuum in preference to a canister, since a 1999 study found that upright models leaked fewer particles into the air.

When it comes to brands, it is virtually impossible to tell you which work best in terms of ability to suck up (and keep down) allergens. Some brands carry the Allergy UK seal of approval – although the review protocol itself came in for criticism in a May 2005 Consumer Report article, and the seal of endorsement does not necessarily mean that a product will reduce an allergy sufferer's symptoms.

There is no impartial evidence to suggest that high-end, high-priced vacuums do a better job of corralling allergy-causing dust. So if you find yourself a good upright vacuum cleaner with a HEPA filter and triple-filtration bags, it is probable that you'll have the best that the limited research reveals.

monoxide escape can provoke chemical sensitivity. Ensure that your cooker has an appropriate, properly installed extractor and change the filter regularly. Be sure to use any extractors installed in interior rooms.

Check your household cleaning products Consider substituting natural products; see those listed in the box on page 134. A 2004 study at Bristol University, published in the journal *Thorax*, suggested that even prenatal exposure to cleaning products could be potentially harmful. Researchers discovered that children born to families who regularly used bleach, carpet cleaners and paint strippers were twice as likely to suffer wheezing, which can lead to asthma.

Natural cleaning products

Irritants such as the chemicals found in the majority of household cleaners can aggravate airborne allergy symptoms, so you should avoid them as much as possible. That is easier to do these days, given the recent trend towards more natural cleaning products. Yet for just a few pennies you can make your own natural cleaning products, thereby ensuring that you are protecting your own health and the long-term health of the environment.

Grease cutter Mix 1 cup lemon juice and 1 cup water.
Scouring powder Mix 1 cup bicarbonate of soda with enough water to form a paste.
Laundry stain remover Use 1 teaspoon white vinegar or bicarbonate of soda per machine load.
Toilet bowl cleaner Pour 1 cup vinegar into the toilet, leave overnight, and scrub with a toilet brush the following day.
Floor and furniture polish Mix 2 parts vegetable oil and 1 part lemon juice.
Metal cleaners (brass and copper) Mix lemon juice and salt until it forms a paste, use a lemon wedge dipped in bicarbonate of soda, or mix hot white vinegar with salt to make a paste. Believe it or not, hot ketchup applied with a rag also cleans these metals.
Glass cleaner Add 2 tablespoons vinegar to a small bucket of warm water. Dry with a clean cloth.
Carpet cleaner Rub a little baking soda on wet stains or baking soda dissolved in water on dry stains.
To remove and discourage mould When cleaning bathroom tiles or shower screens and the refrigerator or freezer, add 1 tablespoon of bicarbonate of soda to the final rinsing water. To remove mould on window frames or sills, use a bicarbonate of soda and water paste. Scrub with a stiff brush (an old toothbrush will do), then wipe clean.

Allergy UK's five-page fact sheet, 'Handy Hints for Chemically Sensitive People', has more information on a range of natural household cleaning products. Reusable, long-lasting E-Cloth Cleaning System cloths, which you simply dampen with water to use, have received the Allergy UK consumer award.

Choose environmentally friendly furnishings Fumes from plastics and vinyl can trigger allergic reactions, as can chemicals given off from MDF, a widely used component of furniture and flooring. Some carpets and underlays are now pre-treated against mould and dust mites with sprays containing potential chemical allergens.

Consider giving up perfumed soaps, powders and toiletries Instead, opt for unscented toiletries and soaps, and clean your teeth with herbal toothpaste; you can even use sodium bicarbonate alone or mixed with sea salt (2 parts to 1 water). You might also benefit from avoiding perfumed air fresheners.

When decorating Check paints for VOC content and when possible choose one of the growing number of water-based paints. Try to avoid vinyl wallpapers and wood varnishes.

Air quality

Double glazing, central heating and wall-to-wall carpeting all help to make our homes cosier. But modern, energy-efficient homes have reduced the intake of fresh air and air changes needed to remove airborne pollutants and allergens and to prevent condensation problems.

Good ventilation is crucial to a healthy indoor environment. Research suggests that the rate at which indoor air exchanged for fresh air is now 10 times lower than it was

30 years ago. So remember to open windows regularly – as little as 10 minutes a day will help – and to open your bedroom window at night. Most new windows have trickle vents, which allow air in and protect the building fabric from damp.

If you are an allergy or asthma sufferer and want to keep out pollens and outside pollutants, you might consider having a house ventilation system to bring in clean or filtered air and flush out used air. This is a major investment and will also need to be maintained and regularly serviced to stop dust, dirt or microbes accumulating in the system.

One problem that is strongly associated with poor ventilation is condensation, caused when water vapour produced by cooking or bathing hits cold surfaces such as windows and walls behind wardrobes. Traditionally associated with damp, poorly insulated, unheated environments, condensation facilitates the growth of mould spores and, over time can lead to wet or dry rot in floor-boards and joists. Yet it also commonly occurs in damp environments within well-insulated modern homes.

Several different types of air purifiers are also available, at prices from £30 to £600, which may help to reduce your risk of airborne allergens at home. But don't imagine that you can simply buy one for every room and say goodbye to your allergies.

First of all, whatever the advertisements say (and some claims have been shown to be exaggerated) air purifiers do little to curtail that greatest of all indoor allergens, dust mites. This is because, of course, living dust mites are not air-borne. They are present in furniture, curtains, carpets and mattresses (the average bed could be home to 1.5 million of them).

Secondly, the machines don't help much with either asthma or allergies. A January 2000 study of asthma and indoor air exposure by the US Institute of Medicine found that air cleaning 'is not consistently and highly effective in reducing [asthma and allergy] symptoms'. Other scientific studies have found

How to check products for allergen safety

Are you wondering whether that new laundry detergent could be making your allergies worse? Or if the wax you used to polish your car might be the reason for that asthma attack you had soon after you finished the job? The US Specialized Information Services of the National Library of Medicine have developed a vast database of common household products that includes the potential health effects and other safety and handling information for each. Simply go to http://hpd.nlm.nih.gov/ and click on the category of product you are interested in. For instance, you may find that your toilet bowl cleaner could be irritating your upper respiratory tract.

It is also a good idea for allergy sufferers to resist trying brand-new products that promise relief. For instance, S.C. Johnson AllerCare Dust Mite Carpet Powder and Dust Mite Allergen Spray, which claimed to rid homes of dust mites, were recalled in the USA when it turned out that their strong fragrance could cause – what else? – asthma attacks.

similar results. When researchers evaluated 10 studies on air-filtration devices and people with asthma, they found that the systems had no effect on medication use or morning PEFR values, although they were associated with fewer asthma symptoms. And the systems aren't much better for allergies. While some studies do find they are effective at removing animal hair and dander, they show minimal, if any, effectiveness in relieving allergic respiratory diseases.

Air ionizers, which remove pollutants by generating negative ions, are widely advertised and marketed as being of benefit to asthma sufferers, yet a 2004 Cochrane review also found insufficient evidence that they help to ease asthma symptoms or to improve lung function – and some studies even suggest that they can have an adverse effect.

Some types emit ozone, which is known to exacerbate asthma, and others (called ozone generators) even use an electrical charge to generate ozone, which may be called trivalent oxygen or saturated oxygen. The US Environmental Protection Agency advises that such devices should only be used in unoccupied spaces as ozone can damage the lungs and relatively low amounts can cause chest pain, coughing, shortness of breath and throat irritation.

Certain indoor plants, such as spider plants, act as natural air filters, especially against formaldehyde (found in insulation, paper products and cleaning agents) and benzene (in environmental tobacco smoke). Among the most effective are gerbera, English ivy, lady palm and bamboo palm. But avoid cultivating pollen-producing plants that might exacerbate allergies or asthma

How healthy is your local pool?

Going to the leisure centre or local swimming pool should be one of the healthiest things you can do. But there is mounting evidence that repeated exposure to the chemicals necessary for hygiene could actually harm your health. Some believe they could be triggering asthma in thousands of children every year.

The chlorine in our swimming pools is essential to kill disease-spreading bacteria but the engineering and the levels need to be constantly checked to make sure it is present in the right form and concentrations. The chlorine also deals with the nitrogen in people's skin, sweat and urine; the more it uses up in this way, the more has to be added. But when chlorine and

sweat or urine react, chloramines (and the characteristic swimming pool smell) are produced. It is these fumes which may damage children's lungs and leave them susceptible to allergens which can then trigger asthma, according to research in 2003 in Belgium and in 2002 at Birmingham's Heartlands Hospital.

Careful controls, changing the water frequently and more stringent requirements for bathers to shower before swimming can all reduce the risks and the general consensus is that the benefits of exercise outweigh the effects of chlorinated water. And while it is thought that chloramines may trigger asthma, they are not currently considered to be a direct cause.

and plants such as *Ficus benjamina*, which has been linked to skin allergies, allergic rhinitis and asthma. Change plant soil regularly to reduce the chances of mould spores.

Mould: minimizing the growth

Have you checked your shower curtain lately? Unless you take it down and clean it thoroughly every couple of weeks, it is likely to be incubating mould spores. At least 60 species of mould have spores thought to be allergenic, and 30 per cent of people with respiratory allergies seem to be particularly sensitive to moulds, with children appearing to be the most sensitive. There is also a strong link between moulds and asthma.

Moulds are present indoors almost all year round. They thrive in damp environments such as bathrooms and showers, and on window frames when there is condensation. Dehumidifier water reservoirs are a favoured breeding ground, as are the seals on refrigerator doors. And mould spores can hide under wallpapers and in the soil of houseplants. As you'll see when you work through the Breathe Easy Plan, nearly every room in your house can contain mould. But doing battle against it is not that difficult. An effective mould remover is 1 part bleach and 10 parts water, or about 1½ cups of bleach to 5 litres (1 gallon) of water. (Also see the box on page 134.)

What about the mould on those leftovers at the back of the refrigerator? Try to check the fridge regularly and be ruthless about discarding food that is past its best. If you're allergic to moulds, even cheese can be a trigger, because cheese is essentially mouldy milk. In particular, you should avoid fermented cheeses such as blue cheese, Brie and Camembert. The following simple measures will help to minimize indoor moulds.

Increase ventilation Open windows and close internal kitchen and bathroom doors when cooking, bathing or showering to prevent steam from entering other rooms. Always ventilate the kitchen, bathroom and utility room after thorough cleaning. From time to time, leave wardrobe doors ajar to ventilate the clothes, which should not be too tightly packed together.

Food management Do not allow food to decay (bread, fruit and vegetables are especially vulnerable to mould), and regularly clean and thoroughly dry the refrigerator, particularly around the seals.

Remove breeding grounds Throw out old foam mattresses and pillows and take any piles of old newspapers to be recycled. Keep houseplants to a minimum; remove any dead, dying or diseased leaves; change the soil or compost regularly, and keep the soil surface covered with gravel. Strip the wallpaper from any damp walls. If using a dehumidifier, empty the water reservoir every day and stop mould growth by rinsing with bleach at least every month. Do not use humidifiers. Don't bring in damp wood for the fire, or wood that has been kept in a damp shed.

Condensation Dry any condensation that occurs on windows, and clean any visible mould from window frames or sills.

Preparing for the Breathe Easy Plan

This chapter has offered plenty of advice on reducing allergens in your home. In Step 3 of the Breathe Easy Plan, beginning on page 197, you'll discover how to translate this into a simple, room-by-room personal programmme, complete with a checklist.

Chapter **nine**

The right
foods

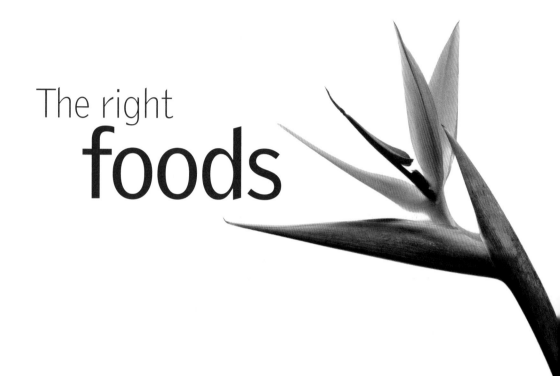

Millions of us in the UK, it seems, ignore official guidelines on how to follow a healthy, balanced diet based on a variety of foods. We tend to eat too little fruit, vegetables, complex carboyhydrates (such as rice, bread or pasta) and also fish. And most people consume too much fat, salt and sugar – partly as a result of our passion for prepared and processed foods.

We consumed two billion fast food meals in 2001; the sales of snacks and confectionery continue to rise, outstripping those in all other European countries; children eat on average only two portions of fruit and vegetable a day (instead of the recommended five); and young adults drink an average of six cans of fizzy drink a week. It's hardly surprising that two out of three people in the UK are overweight or obese.

Interestingly, the decline in the quality and nutritional health of our eating patterns closely parallels the rise in allergies and asthma in this country. Is this coincidence? An increasing body of evidence suggests not.

It has only been within the past decade or so, with the increase in allergy and asthma rates, that researchers have begun to examine a possible connection with diet. What they are finding is intriguing. For instance, who knew that whole milk could even protect some people against asthma? Or that eating margarine could increase your risk of developing asthma? Apples, it seems, can protect against asthma in some people – although there is also a high incidence of sensitivity to apples among patients with asthma and hay fever.

This chapter explores possible nutritional contributors to asthma and allergies and tells you about dietary changes that may help with your condition. Then, Step 4 of the Breathe Easy Plan puts it all together in an easy-to-follow 'Eat to Beat Allergies and Asthma' nutritional programme.

Watch your weight

Obesity and overweight have been linked with everything from heart disease to increased rates of cancer. Now you can add asthma to the list. Not only can being overweight (defined as having a body mass index, or BMI, of 25 or higher) increase your risk of developing asthma in the first place, it can also make existing asthma much, much worse.

First, the asthma development connection. When scientists from King's College, London, studied 15,000 children aged between 4 and 11 and found that 17 per cent were suffering from asthma, they also found that the heaviest children were the most likely to be at risk. Similar studies have found that the risk of developing adult-onset asthma also increases with obesity.

Although researchers do not fully understand the reasons for this, they do have various theories. When it comes to children, they suspect that it may have something to do with the fact that overweight children are less likely to be out-doors on the soccer field and more likely to be inside playing video games and watching television. All that indoor time may lead to a greater propensity for allergies because indoor air is significantly more polluted than outdoor air. And allergies, of course, are a strong trigger for asthma.

There are also physiological changes that occur when you are overweight. For instance, the more fat cells you have, the more inflammation you have, because fat cells are important sources of the chemicals that encourage inflammation. There is also some evidence that increased weight contributes to bronchial hypersensitivity, a hallmark of asthma in which the bronchial openings go into spasm with little provocation.

BMI defined

Body mass index, or BMI, is a well-established tool for indicating weight status in adults. It measures weight in relation to height. BMI is described in Step 4 of the Breathe Easy Plan (the chart is on page 209). If you are an adult over 20 years old, you can see from the chart how healthy your weight is with reference to the categories below:

BMI	Weight status
Below 18.5	Underweight
18.5–24.9	Normal
25.0–29.9	Overweight
30.0 and above	Obese

Milk: the pros and cons

The common myth that drinking milk produces mucus in the airways has prompted many people with asthma or allergies to cut down on dairy foods. Yet the worst milk does is to thicken your saliva temporarily – unless you happen to be lactose intolerant (see page 72).

In fact, some recent studies have suggested that consuming milk and butter *reduces* asthma risk. One Dutch study of 3,000 young children found that those who consumed full-fat milk and butter daily had far lower rates of asthma and wheezing than those who had them less often. The reason is not clear. It could be linked with other factors, such as a healthier diet – brown bread was also found to be protective – or avoiding more hazardous products: children who eat butter probably eat less margarine and omega-6 polyunsaturates (which contribute to inflammation). Further research is required.

Research into early nutritional influences suggests that breastfeeding protects against asthma whereas early introduction of cow's milk increases the risk, and Asthma UK recommends breastfeeding for up to a year if there is a family history of allergy and not introducing cow's milk into the baby's diet in the first year.

A recent Cochrane review confirms that cow's milk is best avoided in the first 12 months: it found that infants fed hydrolyzed rather than cow's milk protein formula have less asthma and wheeze in their first year. In addition, there is no doubt that many children (1-3 per cent) have early cow's milk intolerance, and that these children are more likely to go on to develop asthma or hay fever.

Dairy products contain selenium, thought to protect against asthma development, but there are richer sources (Brazil nuts, fish and meat).

Then, there are the effects of excess weight on existing asthma sufferers. When researchers in Australia compared medical data on 1,971 adults with asthma, they found that those who were severely obese (with BMIs above 40, about 45kg/7 stone overweight for men and 35kg/5½ stone for women) were significantly more likely to wheeze, have shortness of breath when they exerted themselves, and use much more medication to treat their asthma than those with lower BMIs.

The reasons are numerous. More fat around your abdomen prevents your lungs from fully expanding and your diaphragm from moving downwards because they have to fight all that fat. In other words, you simply can't get a good, deep breath. Furthermore, if you weigh more than you should for your body frame and height, you require more oxygen simply for everyday living. Getting enough oxygen is difficult enough when you have asthma and are not overweight; adding the extra pounds makes it much worse.

The good news? While being overweight may increase your risk of asthma or make your asthma worse, there is compelling evidence that losing weight can improve the situation. Researchers in Finland had 38 overweight or obese adults with asthma either enter a 14-week weight-loss programme or do nothing. Those in the weight-loss group slimmed down an average of 14.5kg/2¼ stone; the other half, predictably, remained the same or even gained a couple of pounds. Those who lost weight found that their lung function tests significantly improved compared with those of the control group. Better still, the changes held for an entire year, during which the thinner participants radically reduced their use of steroid medications and experienced far fewer asthma flare-ups.

What is the connection? Well, researchers speculate that losing weight reduces the incidence of early airway closing, especially while lying down. It also improves the ability to exercise, lowering the likelihood of asthma symptoms during exertion. And it's likely that reducing the amount of fat around the abdomen reduces symptoms of gastroesophageal reflux disease (GORD), which, as discussed in chapter 4, may make asthma much worse.

As part of the Breathe Easy Plan, we'll give you some easy-to-follow tips to lose some weight, thus relieving some of the worst aspects of your asthma.

The heartburn-asthma connection

So you went out for a big meal at the local Chinese restaurant, and later that evening, you had a pretty severe asthma attack. You probably blamed it on your sensitivity to MSG (monosodium glutamate), a common flavouring ingredient in Chinese dishes. But you may have simply overeaten, exacerbating your heartburn, or gastro-oesophegeal reflux, which in turn made your asthma worse.

The link between the two conditions – GORD and asthma – is still controversial but as many as 60 per cent of people with asthma may also suffer from GORD. If you do happen to be one of them, it is certainly worth treating as some studies have found that treating GORD symptoms in asthma sufferers also alleviates asthma symptoms.

While your doctor can prescribe antacids and proton pump inhibitors, such as omeprazole (Losec) and pantoprazole (Protium), that may help the symptoms, it is worth trying a dietary approach first.

Essentially, small meals that are rich in vegetables and include modest servings of complex carbohydrates and lean protein are – predictably perhaps – the order of the day. Meals like this are not only healthy for your heart and body but also the easiest on your digestive system.

When it comes to specifics, it's easiest to list the foods you should avoid. The following foods aggravate the acid reflux effect, in which stomach acid spurts up into your lower oesophagus. Some are otherwise healthy – particularly tea, onions and garlic – so avoid them only if they irritate your stomach.

■ **Fatty or fried foods** Instead of a high-fat hamburger, for instance, opt for low-fat chicken, fish or turkey. Bake chicken instead of frying it, and eat potatoes boiled or mashed, not fried.

Peppermint or spearmint You should stay away from peppermint herbal remedies for asthma, if you have GORD.

Whole milk Substitute low-fat or fat-free milk and opt for low-fat when you buy other dairy products.

Oils Foods cooked in oil or butter tend to linger in the stomach and can cause digestive problems.

Chocolate It interferes with the ability of the lower oesophageal sphincter to prevent stomach acids creeping back up the oesophagus.

Tomatoes The acid in tomatoes can aggravate heartburn.

Creamed foods or soups Too rich and fatty.

Most fast foods Ditto.

It is advisable to try to limit your intake of the following foods – or even consider cutting them out of your diet altogether – as they can irritate an already inflamed lower oesophagus. (Smoking has a similar effect, so you should give that up, too.)

Citrus fruits and juices (choose and apple or banana instead)

Coffee, decaffeinated and regular

Soft drinks, caffeinated and non-caffeinated (think how much you burp after downing a fizzy drink)

Tea

Alcoholic beverages

Garlic and onions

Vinegar

Spicy foods, especially curries

Junk food, particularly oily snacks such as potato crisps

Foods to focus on

Several studies show links between individual foods, such as salt and sugar, and asthma or allergies. Based on the research, here are some suggestions.

Stick to brown bread A large study evaluating 3,000 children in the Netherlands found a significantly reduced risk of asthma in those who ate brown (whole grain) bread instead of white bread. Whole grain bread is a good source of valuable antioxidants.

Limit salt Most of us eat far too much salt (sodium), partly because of all the processed foods we eat. Now, several studies point to an association between asthma symptoms and salt intake. For instance, in one study, 37 people with mild to moderate asthma stayed on either a low-sodium diet (1.92g a day) for five weeks or a high-sodium diet (4.8g a day) for one week. While on the high-sodium diet, their asthma symptoms and use of medications increased, while their lung function test results dropped. More research is needed to establish a strong association between high salt intake and asthma.

Eat plenty of fruit Apples, pears and citrus fruits significantly reduce the risk of asthma, as well as wheezing, in children.

Limit sugar and fat An Australian study found that children who showed signs of airway hyper-responsiveness (an early sign of asthma) ate 23 per cent more refined sugar and 25 per cent more high-fat foods than children who did not have such symptoms.

Drink coffee or tea It seems these beverages contain substances called methylxanthines, which act as natural bronchodilators. Several studies have found a reduction in asthma incidence and symptoms with consumption of black or green tea or of coffee. For instance, in one study, subjects who regularly drank coffee were nearly a third less likely to have asthma than non-coffee drinkers. However, if you have GORD and asthma, you should avoid coffee and tea because they may aggravate your symptoms.

Honey There is reasonable evidence that eating natural, unprocessed local honey (it must come from near where you live to have the right pollen mix) early in the season helps to reduce both the frequency and severity of subsequent hay fever.

GORD is a product not only of what you eat but also of how you eat it. Here are some recommendations that will help you to avoid heartburn and, possibly, associated asthma attacks.

▪ Eat several small meals throughout the day rather than just a few big meals. This alone can make a huge difference by keeping your digestive system from being overloaded at any one time.

▪ Start every meal with a glass of water or a bowl of healthy soup. The liquid not only dilutes stomach acid, it also helps fill you up so you eat less.

▪ Eat slowly and calmly. Put down your knife and fork after each mouthful. Sip water between mouthfuls. Intersperse eating with telling your dining partner about the amusing things that happened during your day. Heartburn can be

What to choose when eating out

It's worth following these guidelines from the National Heartburn Alliance at www.heartburnalliance.org to avoid an after-dinner bout of heartburn and asthma. If you are not sure how a dish is prepared, ask.

Italian restaurants

Avoid	Go for
Heavy tomato or cream sauces	Dishes with little or no cheese
Pizza toppings such as double cheese, sausage and pepperoni	Pasta 'en brodo' – a light, broth-type sauce
Lots of garlic (macaroni and bean) soup	Minestrone (vegetable) or pasta fagioli
Oil-based salad dressings	Veal or chicken in a light mushroom sauce
Rich, heavy desserts such as cheesecake or tiramisu	Biscotti and a fresh orange salad – for dessert

Mexican restaurants

Avoid	Go for
Hot salsa	Guacamole on a flour tortilla
Fried tortilla chips	Fajitas or other grilled items
Condiments such as jalapeño peppers, onions and hot sauces	Dishes flavoured with herbs such as cumin and coriander, which tend to be heartburn-friendly
Mole (chocolate) sauce	Low-fat refried beans and rice
Flan or other rich desserts	
Sangría and margaritas	

Chinese restaurants

Avoid	Go for
Egg rolls, spare ribs, and other high-fat dishes	Dishes made with vegetables in a light sauce
Breaded and fried entrées	Brown rice
Sauces thickened with eggs and butter	Sauces thickened with broth and cornflour
Overly spicy dishes	Dishes such as beef with broccoli, or prawn with mushrooms and bamboo shoots

caused by overloading your system with food faster than it can handle it. Plus, your brain follows your stomach by about 20 minutes when it comes to hunger signals. So if you eat slowly enough, your brain can catch up to tell you that you are no longer in need of food.

Choose the right fats

Understanding that high fat is bad and low fat is good is not all there is to know about dietary fats. People who have asthma and allergies also need to pay attention to the *kind* of fat they eat. A growing body of research suggests that the type of fat you eat, not the amount, may play a role in the rise and severity of asthma and allergies.

The culprit appears to be the large amount of polyunsaturated fats in Western diets. It's not that these fats are bad for you: for years, nutritionists have been telling us that these fats, found in vegetable oils and some nuts and grains, are good for us – or at least much better than the heart disease-promoting saturated fats found in animal protein and dairy products, or the industrially hardened trans fatty acids (so-called 'hidden fats') found in processed foods such as cakes, biscuits, pies and crisps.

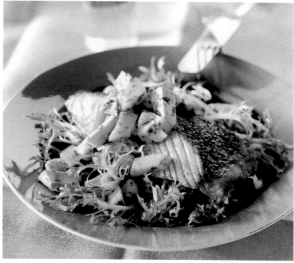

Salmon and other oily fish are rich in omega-3 fatty acids, which may reduce inflammation and lower the risk of developing asthma.

The problem is balancing the types of polyunsaturated fats we eat. There are two main types of polyunsaturated fatty acids: omega-6 fatty acids, which are abundant in most vegetable oils, and omega-3 fatty acids, found in high amounts in so-called 'oily' fish such as mackerel, salmon, sardines and swordfish, as well as in soya beans, walnuts and some dark green vegetables.

If we consumed equal amounts of omega-3s and omega-6s, all might be well. But the average UK diet with its emphasis on processed foods and vegetable oils, includes more omega-6 fatty acids. These fats, it turns out, may increase inflammatory reactions that lead to asthma and allergies. Omega-3 fatty acids, on the other hand, may reduce inflammation, which is why a 1:1 ratio, instead of the 6:1 ratio in the typical UK diet, would probably be beneficial. In fact, researchers attribute the lower rates of cancer, heart disease, asthma and autoimmune diseases in parts of the world where people eat far more omega-3s, such as Greece and Greenland, to the consumption of these beneficial fats.

In studies, researchers have found that children who eat oily fish rich in omega-3s more than once a week have only a third the risk of developing asthma than children who eat no fish. Other studies find that adults with asthma who regularly eat oily fish have better lung function, less wheezing and breathlessness and fewer episodes of waking up with chest tightness.

Additionally, when 29 children with bronchial asthma received either fish-oil capsules containing 84mg of EPA and 36mg of DHA (both forms of omega-3 fatty acids) or placebos (dummy pills), those receiving the fish oil had fewer asthma symptoms and responded better to beta2-agonist medications such as salbutamol (Ventolin) than those who were given the placebos. Similar results have been found in adults, where a study of people with allergic asthma who took daily fish-oil supplements for a month found that participants had reduced levels of leukotrienes. Those are the molecules, remember, that are released by mast cells and are to blame, in part, for the increased mucus production, airway constriction and inflammation of asthma and the runny, stuffy nose of allergies.

Olive oil and rapeseed oil (canola oil), although good sources of omega-6s, are composed mainly of omega-9, or monounsaturated, fatty acids, making them an ideal choice for cooking. But it is best to avoid cooking with rapeseed oil: research suggests that at high temperatures it turns into the most unhealthy of all fats, trans fatty acids, which are linked to heart disease and other ailments.

Another polyunsaturated fat to watch out for is arachidonic acid, found in relatively high amounts in beef, pork, lamb, dairy products and shellfish. It also contributes to inflammation, suggesting a further reason for getting plenty of omega-3s, which counteract its action. This could be why one long-term trial of a vegan diet, in which all animal products were eliminated, found that 92 per cent of the 25 asthma patients who completed the study significantly improved. The response didn't happen overnight, however; participants had to stay on the diet for a year before the 92 per cent success rate was achieved.

You don't have to go that far. Instead, as we'll show you in the Breathe Easy Plan, reducing your intake of red meat and sources of omega-6 fatty acids while boosting your omega-3 fatty acid intake should give you the relief you crave.

Probiotics: powerful anti-asthma nutrients

If you have ever eaten live-culture yoghurt, you have eaten probiotics. These are 'friendly' bacteria, similar to those that are naturally present in the gut, which protect against harmful bacteria. They stimulate your body to produce certain white blood cells and antibodies, as well as various growth factors that

The elements of an anti-asthma diet

When researchers in the UK evaluated the diets of 1,471 asthma sufferers aged between 15 and 50 and 864 people who didn't have asthma, they found some interesting correlations.

- The more fruit and vegetables participants ate, the less likely they were to have asthma.
- People who ate apples (a rich source of phytochemicals called flavonoids) two or more times a week were 32 per cent less likely to have asthma.
- People who ate onions (rich in the anti-oxidant quercetin) two or more times a week were 18 per cent less likely to have asthma.
- People who drank tea (another excellent source of flavonoids) two or three times a day were 17 per cent less likely to have asthma than those who didn't drink tea.
- People who drank one to two glasses a day of red wine (also rich in flavonoids) were 18 per cent less likely to have asthma; in those who had asthma, symptoms were likely to be less severe.

The study is a good example of why food works better than dietary supplements. As the researchers note, there are numerous phyto-chemicals in foods that could be responsible for their beneficial effects. The most likely ones are flavonoids. These chemicals have antioxidant, anti-allergenic and anti-inflammatory properties; prevent the release of nitric oxide (implicated in asthma) and histamine; and interfere with arachi-donic acid metabolism and cytokine production. So it's all the more important to ensure you have your five portions a day of fruit and vegetables.

A word of caution Eating more apples and having a glass of wine with your meal may not suit everyone. Along with their protective nutrients, apples also contain salicylates (used in aspirin, and also occurring naturally in berries, oranges, paprika, tea and almonds), which may trigger asthma attacks in susceptible people – as may certain elements in red wine. Sulphur dioxide is released when a bottle of red wine is uncorked, and the wine itself contains histamine.

are important for preventing allergies and asthma and keeping your body from over-reacting to allergens. But numerous things, ranging from stress and antibiotics to fluoridated water and chlorine, can kill off these helpful organisms, contributing, it is now thought, to allergies and asthma. For instance, studies suggest that lactobacilli (a form of probiotic) are less common in the intestines of Westerners than in those of people from the Third World and are also less prevalent in children who suffer from allergies than in those who are not allergic.

It turns out that probiotics are critical in helping to stem inflammation and control your immune response to stimulants such as allergens, particularly when it comes to food allergies. In fact, probiotics have been found to be beneficial in controlling and preventing food allergies, as well as atopic dermatitis (eczema), an allergy-related skin condition.

And, in the most exciting study to date on the role of probiotics in allergies and asthma, a group of Finnish researchers is following 132 children at high risk of developing allergies or asthma. Their mothers took probiotics during pregnancy and, if they breastfed, for the first six months of breastfeeding. The infants who were bottle-fed received their probiotics in their formula. Four years later, the researchers found that children in the probiotic group had half the rate of atopic eczema, often a first sign of asthma or allergies, when compared with the placebo group.

You can obtain probiotics (another form is bifidobacteria) from live yoghurt (look for 'bio' or 'acidophilus' on the label), or from supplements.

Fruit and vegetables: always healthy

Every time you breathe, eat or run (or walk, watch TV, make love or sleep), your body's cells are affected. Through a process called oxidation, many of the activities of daily living actually have the power to harm cells, leading to disease (including asthma) and ageing. It happens when rogue molecules called free radicals roam around your body trying to snatch electrons from healthy molecules, thus harming cells.

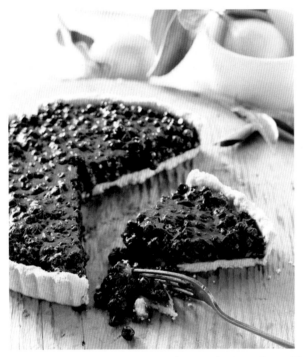

Antioxidants, found in fruit and vegetables, help to prevent free radical damage, a suspect in exercise-induced asthma.

But oxidation is not all bad news. Powerful antioxidants, chemicals found in certain foods that also occur naturally in your body, act as scavengers, passing on one of their electrons to free radicals and thereby disarming them. This process helps to prevent cell and tissue damage that could lead to disease.

Both oxidation and free radicals play a role in asthma. For instance, some researchers think that exercise-induced asthma attacks may be partly due to the free radical damage that occurs during exertion. To test their theory, Israeli researchers gave 38 people with exercise-induced asthma 64mg a day of natural beta-carotene (a powerful antioxidant supplement) for one week. Fifty-two per cent had no exercise-induced asthma.

A Norwegian study found that young adults with asthma who smoked (a major contributor to free radical development) but who also consumed large amounts (at least 395mg) of the antioxidant vitamin C from food had much less wheezing and coughing than smokers who didn't get as much vitamin C. (Their symptoms would, of course, probably improve even more if they gave up smoking.) Other studies have found lower levels of vitamin C in the blood and sputum of people with asthma. In fact, studies show that vitamin C is effective in treating asthma and in reducing the severity of asthma symptoms.

The antioxidants coenzyme Q_{10} (CoQ_{10}) and vitamin E may also be important when it comes to asthma. One study of 77,866 women found that those with the highest vitamin E intake from food (whole grains, sunflower seeds, wheat germ and spinach) had half the risk of asthma compared with those who had the lowest intake. But a recent Asthma UK-funded study at Nottingham University found no benefits for people with asthma in taking a daily 500g vitamin E supplement. The researchers suggest that possible reasons for the apparent conflict between these results and earlier studies could be linked to other dietary and lifestyle factors, and also that vitamin E may need to be taken with vitamin C for it to be most effective.

Then there is the antioxidant quercetin. Found in many vegetables and fruits, it controls inflammation by reducing the release of histamine and other chemicals involved in allergic reactions and stabilizing cell membranes so they are less reactive to allergens. Although there have been few clinical trials with humans, a Japanese study in which mast cells from the nasal mucus of people with perennial allergic rhinitis were treated with quercetin found that the supplement significantly inhibited the release of histamine, with an effect twice that of sodium cromoglicate at the same concentration. Dietary sources of quercetin include apples, onions, and green and black tea.

Vitamins and minerals

A healthy diet is critical. For those with limited diets and certain types of bowel disease, taking a good-quality multivitamin/mineral supplement may also be a good idea, and one that is part of the Breathe Easy Plan. That's because, in addition to the benefits of the antioxidants mentioned above, numerous other links between vitamins and minerals and asthma have been found. Specifically:

Magnesium This mineral, which is plentiful in seafood, pulses (especially soya beans), nuts, whole grains and dark green, leafy vegetables, is often given intravenously in the hospital during an asthma attack. It relaxes the smooth muscles that line your airways, minimizing the spasms characteristic of an attack. Magnesium levels are frequently low in people with asthma, which has given rise to the as yet unproven suggestion that such patients should take a

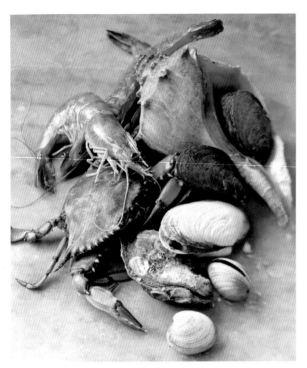

Shellfish are rich in asthma-fighting nutrients such as magnesium and selenium, as well as iron, zinc and omega-3 fatty acids.

daily magnesium supplement of 200mg to 400mg.

Selenium A trace mineral found in the soil, selenium is absorbed by plants as they grow. But because levels of selenium differ dramatically depending on where plants are grown, it is difficult to estimate the amount of selenium in fruits and vegetables. What *is* known is that selenium is a valuable antioxidant, that people with low levels of this vital mineral have an increased risk of asthma, and that people with existing asthma have very low selenium levels.

So what happens when you take a selenium supplement (and this is one nutrient that is best obtained via a single supplement or a daily multivitamin/mineral)? Well, when researchers in Sweden gave 24 adult asthma patients either a placebo or a supplement of 100mcg of selenium daily for 14 weeks, the selenium group had significant improvement in their asthma symptoms.

Vitamin B$_6$ This vitamin is often called the 'energy' vitamin, and it's often low in people with asthma. Plus, the asthma drugs theophylline (Nuelin SA, Slo-Phyllin, Uniphyllin) and aminophylline (Phyllocontin) can depress B$_6$ levels. Adding B$_6$-rich foods (bananas, avocados, chicken, beef, fish, brown rice) to your diet or taking a supplement could improve your asthma. That was the finding of researchers in one study of 76 asthmatic children who received 200mg of B$_6$ daily for five months. Their symptoms improved and their use of bronchodilators and cortisone decreased. In another study in adults, taking 50mg of vitamin B$_6$ twice daily decreased the frequency and severity of asthma attacks.

Molybdenum You don't hear much about this trace mineral but, if you have asthma, it is one you should know about. Found primarily in pulses, leafy vegetables and cauliflower, this nutrient helps the body to detoxify sulphites, chemicals added to foods that often provoke asthma symptoms.

Although there have been few studies on its use in people with asthma, one anecdotal 1989 report in a medical journal described how three months of daily molybdenum injections reduced one woman's wheezing and allowed her to reduce her use of inhalers from four times daily to twice daily. In an Australian study of 1,750 asthma patients, 41.5 per cent were deficient in molybdenum. When molybdenum was added to their diet, their symptoms improved.

There is an evident need for more solid research into the possible effect of diet, vitamins and minerals on allergic diseases such as asthma. For the moment it is probably more advisable to concentrate on eating a balanced diet and maintaining a healthy weight.

Elimination diets

Many people with allergies and asthma, and particularly parents of asthmatic or allergic children, swear by elimination diets, in which they cut out certain foods they think make their conditions worse, such as dairy products, meat, wheat and sugar. It's not that they are allergic to these foods but rather that they think they have food sensitivities that trigger asthma or allergy attacks.

It is true that food allergies can trigger or exacerbate bronchial constriction in asthma and that food allergies are often underdiagnosed in children with asthma. But it's also true that food alone will *not* trigger an asthma or allergy attack unless you have a bona fide food allergy, as described in chapter 5.

Nevertheless, people have very strong emotional feelings about foods, and if someone truly believes that a food is problematic, it is very hard to convince them otherwise. For instance, if you eat a piece of chocolate, and an hour later you have an asthma attack, the two become forever linked in your mind.

If you do try an elimination diet, you should eliminate one food at a time, then wait at least two weeks before either putting it back into your diet or eliminating another food. Track your asthma and allergy symptoms before and after the food is eliminated, using the chart in Step 4 of the Breathe Easy Plan. If you don't notice any consistent, long-lasting improvement, there is no sense in depriving yourself of that food.

Also, never put a child on an elimination diet. Severely restrictive diets are especially dangerous for children, who need a careful balance of vitamins, minerals and other nutrients to ensure healthy growth and development.

No way around it

There's simply no way around it: you *are* what you eat. Following a healthy diet can help to protect you and your children from developing asthma in the first place as well as help to keep symptoms of existing asthma under control.

In the next chapter, we'll look at some alternative therapies designed to help you both relax and de-stress and target your asthma/allergy symptoms.

Chapter ten

The right
alternative
choices

Looking for something new to treat your asthma? How about tiny live sardines swallowed whole with secret herbs – a 'miracle' asthma cure supplied free of charge by an Indian family to thousands of asthma sufferers who flock to their house in Hyderabad every year on an astrologically significant day.

While this may sound ludicrous (the fish convey aromatic herbs into the stomach, which allegedly clear phlegm from the system) it's just one in a long list of alternative remedies that people use to treat allergies and asthma.

One in 10 people in the UK use some form of alternative medicine each year and half of us use it at some point during our lifetime. Open-minded people with asthma and allergies are trying everything from herbal remedies such as ephedra and grapeseed extract to yoga, acupuncture, breathing exercises and homeopathy. Some asthmatics even spend hours a day in subterranean caves or salt mines in the course of a treatment called speleotherapy.

Some of these efforts work, some don't, and some should be avoided because they may even be dangerous. In fact, one study found that people with asthma who had self-treated with herbs, coffee and black tea had higher rates of hospitalization than those who followed more standard medical advice.

The reality is that there is little scientific evidence to either support or disprove many of these alternative therapies. It is hard to find funding for even well-designed research on alternative remedies, and often difficult to design such studies. And the studies that have been conducted often appear to have methodological flaws that limit their interpretation and application to contemporary medical practice.

Yet increasingly people with allergies and asthma are trying so-called CAM (complementary and alternative medicine) therapies. However, because something is natural doesn't necessarily mean it is safe. Some herbal remedies can have dangerous interactions with prescription or over-the-counter medications. Others can seriously exacerbate allergies or asthma.

You should never *substitute* alternative remedies for conventional medicine. If you stop taking your asthma drugs, for instance, you could end up very ill in hospital, regardless of any alternative therapy you are trying. Instead, talk to your GP about integrating such therapies into your medical treatment: the GP's practice may even employ alternative practitioners to offer a service to patients.

The goal of this chapter is to set the record straight, presenting what is known (and what isn't) about the available alternative therapies and their efficacy for asthma and allergies, as well as any special cautions.

Clinical trials defined

Throughout this chapter, you will see references to clinical trials performed to determine the effectiveness and safety of alternative treatments. Here is a glossary of clinical trial terms.

Blind A randomized trial is blind if the participants don't know whether they are being given the treatment being tested, a placebo or standard therapy; also called masked.

Single-blind study A study in which one party, either the investigator or the participant, is unaware of what medication the participant is taking; also called single-masked.

Double-blind study A clinical trial in which neither those taking part nor the study staff know who is getting the experimental drug and who receives a placebo (or another therapy). Double-blind (also called double-masked) trials are considered objective, as the expectations of the researchers and the participants about the experimental drug do not affect the outcome.

Controlled trials Control is a standard against which experimental observations may be evaluated. In clinical trials, one group of participants is given an experimental drug, while another group (the control group) is given either a standard treatment for the disease or a placebo.

Placebo A placebo is an inactive pill, liquid, powder or procedure that has no treatment value but is used as a control. In clinical trials, experimental treatments are often compared with placebos to assess the effectiveness of the treatment. In some studies, the control group participants receive a placebo instead of an active drug or treatment.

Placebo effect A physical or emotional change occurring after a substance is taken or administered that is not the result of any special property of the substance. The change may be beneficial, reflecting the participant's expectations and those of the person giving the substance.

Deciding on a complementary health care provider

In the UK, much of complementary medicine is still largely unregulated and practised without recognizable training, qualifications, professional standards or insurance. Practitioners can set themselves up in a wide variety of healthcare professions, provided they do not claim to be registered medical practitioners and do not practise protected disciplines such as supplying medicines limited to prescription, dentistry, veterinary medicine, midwifery or physiotherapy.

However, recent Acts of Parliament have established the General Chiropractic Council (GCC) and the General Osteopathic Council (GOsC) for the statutory self-regulation of these professions. Now, only practitioners registered with these bodies may use the titles chiropractor and osteopath, respectively. Acupuncture, herbal medicine and homeopathy are likely to follow suit soon. In March 2004, the Department of Health published a consultation paper setting out its proposals for the regulation of acupuncture and herbal medicine. The report on the consultation paper is at **www.dh.gov.uk** The Council of Organizations Registering Homeopaths (CORH) has also begun a consultation process around regulation. For details see **www.corh.org.uk**

How to find a qualified CAM practitioner

- *Complementary healthcare: a guide for patients*, published by the Foundation for Integrated Health, is designed to help people choose a suitable therapy and find a properly trained, qualified and registered practitioner. Go to **www.fihealth.org** (downloadable free).
- The Institute for Complementary Medicine, **www.i-c-m.org.uk** The ICM administers the British Register of Complementary Practitioners, a database of practitioners who have achieved a high level of competence in their discipline that can be searched according to geographical area.
- NHS Directory of Complementary and Alternative Medicine lists all practitioners who

have elected to work either in NHS practice or from their own practice on a referral basis but their details are only available to NHS staff, who need to register (free). The directory can be found at: **www.nhsdirectory.org** which also has general notes for patients about accessing complementary healthcare through the NHS.

On-line resources on CAM

- CAM on PubMed (Medline): www.nlm.nih.gov/medlineplus/alternativemedicine.html is a US site with access to 270,000 references. Best used for specific questions or specific health conditions.
- Herbal safety news (MHRA): www.mca.gov.uk/ourwork/licensingmeds/herbalmeds/herbal-safety.htm Provides safety information on herbal medicines. The MHRA is also setting up a Herbal Medicines Advisory Committee to provide expert advice to the MHRA on the safety and quality of herbal medicines. The Committee will look at both unlicensed medicines and those registered from 2005 onwards under the new EU Directive on Traditional Herbal Medicines.
- Quackwatch, www.quackwatch.org. A guide to quackery and health frauds, including questionable products and services.
- Research Council for Complementary Medicine (RCCM), www.rccm.org Aims to develop the evidence base for CAM; has general information on CAM, including reports and newsletters.
- University of Maryland Medical Center (complementary medicine): www.umm.edu/altmed/ Has a database on ingredients, therapies and interactions. The section on asthma is at: www.umm.edu/altmed/ConsConditions/Asthmacc.html#Herbs

Other websites • www.acupuncture.org.uk
- www.medical-acupuncture.co.uk
- www.chiropractic-uk.co.uk • www.gcc-uk.org
- www.trusthomeopathy.org • www.nimh.org.uk
- www.hypnotherapists.org.uk

Acupuncture

If there's any CAM therapy that has gained credibility in the past decade, it's acupuncture, which has traditionally been used for asthma treatment in China. In the UK, a survey found that 7 per cent of 3,837 people with asthma had tried acupuncture, with most of those (71 per cent) saying they thought it was helpful. But long-term benefits to people with asthma have yet to be shown. And although there is some evidence that acupuncture may be of help in asthma and rhinitis, there is still very little research into how it may affect allergic disease.

You may think of acupuncture as needle therapy, but that's just one very small part of it. The underlying principle of acupuncture is that vital energy, or Qi (pronounced *chee*) flows along invisible pathways in your body called meridians. When Qi is blocked, pain and illness result. Acupuncturists unblock Qi by inserting hair-thin needles at specific points in the body. Sometimes, they use a laser beam that doesn't break the skin or apply strong pressure with their hands.

Each illness relates to certain specific acupuncture points that tend to be areas of decreased electrical resistance, which may be part of the scientific basis for acupuncture's effects. In addition, acupuncture is believed to release certain brain chemicals such as endogenous endorphins (think runner's high) that reduce pain and discomfort.

What the studies show One study found that acupuncture during an acute asthma attack increased lung function by 58 per cent in one test and 29 per cent in a different form of test, both significant improvements. Overall, studies of acupuncture during asthma attacks have found that it improves airflow about half as much as an inhaled beta2-agonist, such as the prescription inhaler salbutamol (Ventolin).

Several small, controlled trials found that a short-term programme of acupuncture (one to twelve weeks) positively affected lung function, enabling patients to reduce their use of medication. But one well-designed study, in which adults and children with moderate to severe asthma received four weeks of biweekly acupuncture or sham acupuncture (the placebo), found no significant effect on symptoms, medication use, or pulmonary function during the treatment period or for several weeks afterwards. Yet another study comparing the effect of five weeks of biweekly electro-acupuncture therapy in adults with moderate to severe asthma, found a significant improvement in lung function and a significant decrease in beta2-agonist use compared with the control group. So the results are mixed. One review of seven well-designed studies stated that 'no recommendation can be made one way or the other to patients, their physicians, or acupuncturists on the basis of available data.' In other words, it's up to you.

Precautions Although complications from acupuncture are rare, make sure your acupuncturist follows strict sterilization procedures and inform the practitioner of any medications you are taking or medical problems you have. Also, go to only well-trained, certified acupuncturists.

Cost This varies depending on the practitioner, where you live and length of session: £25 to £100.

Bottom line Acupuncture is safe and will not interact with medications or make your asthma or allergies worse. But there is no clear evidence that it makes a significant difference in asthma.

Chiropractic

You probably think about chiropractic for back pain or other muscle or joint aches but people are increasingly turning to it for asthma and allergies. Typically, chiropractic includes joint manipulation, use of physical therapy tools such as ultrasound to strengthen muscles and reduce inflammation, and rehabilitative exercises.

What the studies show As with many alternative therapies, the studies are few and their findings are mixed. One study, published in the *New England Journal of Medicine*, compared chiropractic spinal manipulation for children with mild or moderate asthma with simulated chiropractic (the placebo). Although symptoms of asthma decreased, use of short-acting beta2-agonists was reduced, and quality of life increased in both groups, there was no significant difference between the two. Another study, on 36 children aged 6 to 17, found that after three months of combining chiropractic therapy with optimal medical treatment, the children rated their quality of life substantially higher and their asthma severity substantially lower – and the bene-fits were maintained at a one-year follow-up. But, objective lung tests showed little or no change.

Precautions Serious complications are rare, with some short-term discomfort being the most common side effect. Beware, however, of chiropractors who immediately recommend several visits a week for several weeks or months.

Cost Most private health insurance plans cover chiropractic, and sometimes the NHS pays for it, although it is not widely available on the NHS. Cost varies, from £20 to £50.

Bottom line Again, there is no clear answer. There is very little evidence showing any objective physiological improvement in asthma as a result of chiropractic. Most of the improvement was subjective.

Homeopathy

Homeopathy works on the principle that 'like cures like'. Thus homeopathic remedies contain a minute amount of the substance that, in much higher doses, would be expected to cause symptoms similar to those being treated. Within limits, the more dilute the medicine is, the more therapeutically active it is considered to be. Sometimes a dilution is so high that few molecules of active material remain, yet it is believed the body's own natural healing powers can still be stimulated and promote recovery.

Most of the thousands of remedies are available without prescription in various solid and liquid forms. They are produced according to methods set out in homeopathic pharma-copoeias by licensed manufacturers and pharmacies that are subject to regular inspection by the MHRA. Some practitioners dispense their own remedies. Under a recent EU directive designed to create harmonization across the EU, pre-packaged homeopathic medicines will be allowed to include a list of authorized efficacy for minor self-limiting conditions.

In the UK, homeopathic hospitals have been part of the NHS since its inception in 1948. Although homeopathic therapy is generally only available privately, GPs may in certain cases be able to refer patients through the NHS. Consult your doctor if you are interested.

What the studies show A few studies have shown positive effects of homeopathic remedies on allergic rhinitis. In one randomized, double-blind, placebo-controlled study of 28 people with moderately severe allergic asthma, treatment with a homeopathic preparation of the diluted allergen for four weeks significantly reduced the severity of symptoms compared with a placebo. But a large double-blind, controlled trial examining homeopathic immunotherapy in 242 asthmatic adults allergic to house dust mites found no significant differences between those given the remedy and those given a placebo.

Precautions Homeopathy is considered to be safe, although in the short term it may aggravate your existing allergic condition. It should not be confused with herbalism, where larger dosages are used and there is the potential for dangerous interactions between different herbs and between herbs and orthodox medicine.

Cost Homeopathy is available on the NHS, but most people have private treatment. Ask about the cost of a consultation before making an appointment. Homeopathic preparations sold in pharmacies or health stores, of course, tend to be much cheaper than those mixed individually by a specialist.

Bottom line Although more robust evidence of its effectiveness is needed, there is preliminary evidence that homeopathy may help allergic rhinitis, but clear scientific evidence that it does *not* help asthma. Talk to your doctor about using homeopathy along with your regular treatment.

Relaxation therapies

Hypnosis, yoga, meditation, visualization, controlled breathing. They all fall under the rubric of relaxation therapies – and relaxation is critical when it comes to asthma. While we no longer think asthma is 'all in your mind', there is evidence that your levels of stress and anxiety can trigger attacks or make existing symptoms worse. That is why it is worth exploring the remedies described below. When used in conjunction with your medical treatment, they may result in your using less medicine and having fewer symptoms overall than if you only took your medicine.

Jacobson's progressive relaxation

This exercise teaches you to discriminate between states of tension and relaxation by tensing and relaxing each of the 15 muscle groups, paying close attention to the sensation. Also referred to as progressive relaxation, it is often used to help people with insomnia to fall asleep by helping them become especially aware of the parts of their bodies that are particularly tense. Eventually, they learn to become more sensitive to rising tension levels before the tension becomes so great that it causes distress. The technique is named after Dr Edmund Jacobson, who pioneered it in the 1920s.

What the studies show Studies are fairly positive, with one study of 44 children with moderate to severe asthma finding that lung function significantly increased in a group of children who learned progressive relaxation as compared with others who just sat quietly. Another study of 20 asthmatic boys who received either Jacobson's relaxation training or assertiveness training found that by the end of the training, lung function measurements in the relaxation group improved by 17.7 per cent and remained far superior to those in the assertiveness training group even one month after treatment ended.

Precautions None; this is a great way to relax and is often used at cardiac rehabilitation centres. **Cost** Most cardiac rehabilitation centres offer training in this technique. Fees vary.

Once you receive the necessary training from a class or audio tape, you can practise the technique on your own wherever and whenever you like. **Bottom line** Who couldn't do with some help relaxing? Try out a tape or sign up for a class.

Biofeedback

Biofeedback is a therapeutic technique that claims to teach you how to control physical responses, such as breathing, hand temperature, muscle tension, heart rate and blood pressure, which are not normally controlled voluntarily. The way you achieve this control is by learning how to focus on and modify signals from your body. For instance, in the case of asthma, biofeedback could help you to learn to control your breathing and bring down your anxiety level when your symptoms start to flare up. **What the studies show** One study of 20 children with non-steroid-dependent asthma who received either biofeedback for facial tension or were in a control group found that the perception of asthma severity decreased significantly in the biofeedback group as compared with the control group, although there was no effect on lung function. **Precautions** None; biofeedback is safe when performed properly.

Cost Biofeedback can be expensive, and you may require 20 or more sessions. Be sure to check the cost before you start the therapy.

Bottom line Biofeedback may help you to control stress, which tends to make people more aware of any chronic illness. There is little good evidence that it improves asthma or reduces the need for medications.

Strengthen your breathing muscles

Take a deep breath in. Now take another. See how your chest rises and falls? Well, it isn't doing it on its own. There are muscles in there called inspiratory muscles (or intercostal or subcostal muscles). They lie between and under your ribs and work by reflex, expanding as you breathe in and contracting as you breathe out. You are probably quite unaware of them until you have trouble breathing.

If you have problems inhaling or can never completely fill your lungs with air, those unused-muscles grow weak. Taking corticosteroids for asthma can weaken them further. The idea behind a technique called inspiratory muscle training is that by strengthening those muscles, you can enhance your ability to breathe.

Inspiratory muscle training occurs in two ways, either by taking a deep breath and holding it for as long as you possibly can, or by using an ingenious device called POWERbreathe. Invented at Birmingham Universiity by a team led by Dr Alison McConnell, a leading authority on breathing and exercise, the drug-free device looks like a large inhaler and contains a fan and a valve. As you breathe through the mouthpiece, your respiratory muscles are forced to work harder because air is released through the fan only when you build up enough pressure within the device to open the valve.

An Israeli study published in 2002 compared 15 patients who received inspiratory training with others given sham training, evaluating the perception that they were short of breath and their use of beta2-agonists. Researchers found that the stronger the patients' inspiratory muscles became, the less shortness of breath they reported and the less medicine they used.

POWERbreathe is available at all Lloyds pharmacies and branches of Boots and Argos, or via the internet at **www.powerbreathe.com**.

Everyone knows how to breathe. But the chances are that your breathing is too shallow and you do not take the deep breaths that your lungs really need. Breathing correctly can also help with asthma; anecdotal evidence suggests that asthma responds well when you control the associated hyperventilation (over-breathing) that causes you to lose too much carbon dioxide. Breathing retraining can help you to stop hyperventilating.

Breathing retraining takes several forms. One form is Buteyko breathing (named after the Russian physician Konstantin Buteyko), in which you learn exercises to reduce the frequency of your breaths. These include breath-holding exercises, yoga breathing and physical exercises, as well as deep diaphragmatic breathing designed to build up your diaphragm muscles. The stated aim is to increase the diameter of the thoracic cage – and thus chest capacity – for maximum lung efficiency. In fact, nothing increases chest capacity – not even running 20 miles a day – and any benefit is related to relief of anxiety. Step 7 of the Breathe Easy Plan shows you how to breathe properly to help reduce your asthma symptoms.

What the studies show In one study, 67 asthmatic adults participated in a 16-week programme in which they received diaphragmatic breathing training or physical exercise training or were put in a waiting-list control group. Those receiving deep diaphragmatic training significantly reduced their use of medication, experienced far less intense asthma symptoms and found they could spend nearly 300 per cent more time in physical activities than before they learned the breathing technique. In another study, 36 adults with asthma were either trained in the Buteyko breathing technique via a video or received a placebo video to watch at home twice a day for four weeks. Those in the Buteyko group significantly improved their quality of life (based on a scientifically designed survey) and significantly reduced the amount of inhaled bronchodilator medication they used. But more research is needed into the possible benefits.

allergy & asthma **sufferers ask**

Why do people turn to alternative therapies?

The reasons are numerous, according to Prof. Edzard Ernst, Director of Complementary Medicine at the Peninsula Medical School, Universities of Exeter and Plymouth.

1 Frustration with conventional medications. Face it, many medications for asthma and allergies have side effects and take a while to work. They can also be expensive, and natural remedies may provide a cheaper alternative.

2 They want something 'natural'. Some people are uncomfortable taking medicines that were conceived in laboratories and manufactured on assembly lines. Their mistake, however, is to conclude that 'natural' means safe or effective. That's not always the case.

3 They want a cure. Unfortunately, there is no cure for asthma or allergies, whether you try traditional medicine or alternative medicine.

4 They want to be in control. Because alternative remedies don't require prescriptions, patients can decide what to take.

5 They want to address what they perceive as the underlying cause of their illness. Many alternative therapies claim to reduce stress or 'bolster' a weak immune system.

6 They are following cultural beliefs. Many cultures have a long tradition of using natural remedies and other alternative therapies; to them, it's the modern world of pharmaceuticals and scientific research that is 'alternative'.

Precautions None; it is safe and painless.

Cost The cost of training varies depending on whether you receive it from a private practitioner or from a video or CD-ROM.

Bottom line It's as harmless as breathing. Some studies show improvement, so it may be worth a try.

Hypnosis

Widely regarded as a means of treating emotional problems (depression, anxiety) hypnotherapy is increasingly used in pain management, to help treat conditions ranging from irritable bowel syndrome, to allergies and asthma. It is even employed to improve wound healing in surgical patients.

This is not new. The use of hypnosis in medical healing dates back nearly 300 years, with published reports noting that patients who were hypnotized before surgery in the days before anaesthetics were not only more likely to survive the operation but also healed faster and with fewer complications. The core of hypnotherapy lies in the complex connection between the mind and the body. It is known that illness can affect your emotional state (consider the correlation between heart disease and depression), and that your emotional state can affect your physical state (think of the dozens of medical conditions caused or made worse by stress).

Hypnosis carries that connection to the next logical step: Deliberately harnessing the power of the mind to affect physiological systems in the body. Essex-based hypnotherapist, Richard Wells, had an 11-year-old patient who came to him with breathing difficulties and severe wheezing. The boy was on medications in the form of injections, daily pills and an inhaler, which seemed to help but did not cure his condition. The boy's GP had agreed to hypnosis. Wells formed the opinion that there was an emotional element in his condition, and used regression therapy to establish that his asthma came on after a fight with another boy at school. Over the next few weeks Wells used hypnosis to raise the

Not worth trying

Throughout this chapter, we've told you about remedies and therapies for which there is little concrete evidence of efficacy but which can't hurt to try. But the following *can* be harmful, either physically or to your pocketbook, and there is really no evidence of their efficacy. Skip them.

Ozone therapy This newest addition to alternative treatments for asthma involves either exposing a person's blood to ozone gas and then reinjecting it or directly introducing ozone either rectally or vaginally. It could have serious adverse effects, since ozone is a well-known trigger for asthma.

Enzyme-potentiated desensitization This treatment, popular in the UK, involves mixing an allergen with beta-glucuronidase, a common enzyme in the body, and applying it to the body in very low doses. Studies find no significant benefits to this treatment.

Urine autoinjection This treatment involves injecting freshly collected, sterilized urine back into the donor. There is no clinical evidence it works, and it may cause kidney problems.

boy's self-confidence and self-esteem, and also used suggestions of deep breathing and relaxation of the airways, associated with feelings of safety and security.

Two months later the boy's asthma had reduced to 10 per cent of previous levels, which the boy, his GP and his parents considered satisfactory.

What the studies show Results are mixed, with one study of 252 children finding that those who received hypnotherapy had a 4.3 per cent improvement in one measure of lung function, a small but significant increase. Another study, this one over a one-year period, found that those who received training in hypnosis and self-relaxation were able to reduce their use of beta2-agonists.

Precautions None, provided that you use an experienced hypnotherapist with good credentials.

Cost Varies widely, based on the practitioner, the type of hypnosis, and where you live.

Bottom line Hypnotherapy could be a good healing option provided that it is integrated into your orthodox medical treatment.

Yoga

These days, yoga classes are increasingly popular and the number of yoga studios is growing. The practice itself, which originated in India, is more than 5,000 years old. It involves a combination of physical and breathing exercises and meditation and is considered to be an excellent stress-reducing technique. There are indications it can improve asthma as well. Any yoga practice includes *pranayama,* or breath-slowing exercises, and meditation. Thus, yoga's benefits may be related to its relaxing effects on those who practise it, reducing stress hormones that can lead to inflammation, the bane of anyone with asthma.

What the studies show Numerous studies show beneficial effects from yoga, regardless of the type practised, on asthma symptoms. In one study, 53 people with asthma trained for two weeks in an integrated set of yoga exercises, including breathing exercises and meditation, and then were told to practise the exercises for 65 minutes daily. Compared with a control group that did no such exercises, the yoga group significantly improved in terms of fewer asthma attacks, scores for drug treatment, and peak flow rates.

In another study of 17 adults with asthma, nine were taught yoga and relaxation exercises, including breath-slowing exercises, physical postures and meditation, three times a week for 16 weeks; the rest received no training. The yoga group used fewer beta2-agonists even though pulmonary function in both groups did not differ significantly. But the yoga group had a greater level of relaxation,

a more positive attitude, and better yoga exercise tolerance than the control group, leading the authors to conclude that 'yoga techniques seem beneficial as an adjunct to the medical management of asthma'. A larger study of 287 subjects found that those who practised yoga had a statistically significant increase in vital lung capacity over time.

Precautions Be sure to tell your instructor about your asthma, allergies or any other medical conditions and about any medication you are taking.

Cost Varies depending on area, class size and length of session.

Bottom line Yoga seems to offer significant benefits – at least in terms of relaxing, breathing and exercise tolerance. It is safe, is an excellent relaxation therapy, and provides a good workout for flexibility and muscle strength. Try it – but do not give up your regular medical treatment.

Massage

Far from being simply a self-indulgent luxury reserved for special events and five-star resorts, massage is increasingly popular and available at alternative therapy centres. A centuries-old healing technique, its many medical benefits are now being shown for a variety of different conditions.

What the studies show In the only study that has been done to date on the effects of massage on asthma, 32 children aged 4 to 14 received either massage therapy or relaxation therapy from their parents 20 minutes before bedtime each night. The younger children who received massage showed an immediate decrease in behavioural anxiety and levels of cortisol (a stress hormone) afterwards. Also, their attitudes towards asthma and using their peak flow meters and other pulmonary function tests improved throughout the study. The older children also reported reduced anxiety levels after receiving massage as well as improved attitudes towards asthma, but only one measure of lung function (FEV1) showed improvement.

But can you prove it works?

Although many complementary therapies have been around for thousands of years, there are often few, if any, solid clinical studies proving they work. This is partly because it is quite difficult to get funding for such research and also because designing a traditional prospective, double-blind, placebo-based study with therapies such as massage or meditation is difficult at best.

But conventional, academic institutions are beginning to take more interest. In the UK, for instance, Professor Edzard Ernst is Director of Complementary Medicine at the Peninsula Medical School of Exeter University where his work involves evaluating clinical trials with an emphasis on efficacy and safety. In the States, the National Institutes of Health's Center for Complementary and Alternative Medicine is becoming increasingly prominent and attracting new funding for clinical trials.

Of course, it is also true that we don't always know exactly how conventional therapies and drugs work, either, although all medical drugs undergo stringent testing before they are licensed. That is likely to become increasingly true for herbal medicines and supplements in the future as new EU regulations come into force.

Meanwhile, in this chapter you'll find many techniques that can benefit anyone, whether or not they have asthma or allergies. We can all use ways to help us to cope better with the stress in our lives, and most of these relaxation strategies have been shown to lower levels of stress hormones such as cortisol.

Plus, don't discount the power of the mind. If you take a herb, smooth on an aromatic oil or have a massage and then find you are breathing more easily, so much the better. The bottom line is that *you feel better*. Never forget that the mind is one of the most powerful medicines.

Precautions You may feel sore the day after, but there is little risk of other adverse effects.

Cost Varies depending on area. Massages last from 30-90minutes and cost from £25-£60 an hour.

Bottom line Massage therapy may be viable to decrease anxiety and increase positive attitude but it's role in asthma treatment seems to be minor.

Meditation

Meditation is a mental discipline often described as deep thought or contemplation of a single thing (such as a symbol, sound or object). The practice aims to produce a state of inner calm, peace and heightened awareness, bringing physical, emotional and spiritual benefits.

For people with asthma, meditation can be a valuable adjunct to medication in terms of helping you to cope with stress in your life that could exacerbate your condition.

What the studies show Little research has been conducted on meditation and asthma (much more has been done on yoga postures and asthma), but one six-month study of 21 patients trained in transcendental meditation found that the practice was a 'useful adjunct' in treating asthma. Although not directly relevant, it is noteworthy that many major medical centres and cancer clinics have added meditation and yoga centres to their services in recent years, and urge patients with serious chronic disease to enrol.

Precautions None; mindful meditation is safe and non-invasive.

Cost Usually per course and very variable – from £10-£20 a session.

Bottom line As a relaxation therapy for asthma and other medical conditions you may be coping with, meditation is a beneficial adjunct to conventional medical therapy.

Herbs and supplements

There has been something of an explosion in the supply and availability of herbal remedies and other supplements in the UK in recent years. Almost every pharmacy and health food store now sells pills and powders that promise to improve everything from your memory to your sex life, so it's no surprise to find many claiming to improve your asthma and allergies, too.

But before you go on a spending spree, you need to find out a bit more about the world of herbs and supplements.

At present some over-the-counter herbal remedies are regulated as food supplements and are not permitted to list what conditions they might treat. Others, labelled with the letters PL (product licence) are regulated by the Medicines and Healthcare products Regulatory Agency (MHRA) and must meet criteria of quality, safety and efficacy.

In October 2005 the EU directive on traditional herbal medicines was implemented. Now, manufacturers who want their products registered must produce bibliographic or expert evidence of the product's medicinal use for at least 30 years prior to application. (But traditional herbal medicinal products already on the market when the directive came into force have a transitional period until 2011 to fulfil registration requirements.)

In the course of their practice, however, herbalists will still be allowed to sell relatively untreated herbs (dried, crushed) labelled with only the name of the plant. Herbal food supplements do not fall under medicines law and are therefore not covered by the directive.

Supplement warning

There are some supplements you should avoid taking at all if you have asthma, because they may exacerbate your condition.

Glucosamine-chondroitin People with arthritis or ageing joints often turn to this dietary supplement compound for pain relief and to strengthen joints and bones. Indeed, it is now often recommended by orthodox medical specialists. But a report published in late 2002 described the case of a woman whose well-controlled asthma suddenly became much worse when she began taking a glucosamine-chondroitin sulphate compound to treat her arthritis-related pain.

Once she stopped taking the supplement, her asthma improved within 24 hours. Doctors suspect that her reaction was related to an allergy or sensitivity to seafood, as chondroitin is made from shark cartilage. Anyone who has asthma and is allergic to shellfish should be especially cautious.

Melatonin A study in the September 2003 issue of the *Journal of Allergy and Clinical Immunology* found that people whose asthma becomes worse at night have higher levels of the sleep hormone melatonin, which may induce the release of inflammatory chemicals, and make asthma worse.

Melatonin supplements, though not readily available in the UK, are sometimes taken to aid sleep or offset jet lag, but should be avoided if you are asthmatic as they could exacerbate your condition.

Bee pollen (royal jelly) This can trigger a severe allergic reaction in people with allergies or asthma, who should avoid it – along with propolis, sometimes known as bee glue.

Lobelia Sometimes known as asthma weed, this herb, which is used in homeopathic asthma medicines, can be poisonous if it is not taken as prescribed by a professionally qualified herbal practitioner.

Speleotherapy

In Armenia in Eastern Europe, people with asthma descend nearly a fifth of a mile beneath the Earth's surface to a salt mine to reach Republican Speleotherapeutical Hospital, an underground medical clinic specifically designed for the treatment of asthma and other respiratory illnesses.

Practitioners of the treatment, called speleotherapy, believe that the salt environment, with its dry air and consistent temperature, has a healing effect on the respiratory system. They also believe that the low carbon dioxide/oxygen ratio in mines and caves leads to deeper, more intensive breathing. Similar clinics can be found in mines and caves throughout much of Eastern Europe, and there are internet guides to help you to locate speleotherapy caves.

There is even some slight evidence that it may have some benefit. Although available studies are few and far between, at least one scientifically designed study conducted in 1994 found a slight improvement in lung function after three weeks of speleotherapy.

With all that in mind, here are some practical steps you should follow when you are considering taking herbal remedies, medicines or supplements.

Talk to your doctor Be sure to tell your doctor about any supplement that you are considering taking – even if it's only a vitamin.

Talk to a pharmacist Registered pharmacists often have more information about and knowledge of potential drug interactions than doctors, and an increasing number of pharmacies today have access to databases that warn of potential interactions.

Find a qualified herbal practitioner Members of the National Institute of Medical Herbalists undergo a lengthy training before they can register as qualified medical herbalists. Practitioners train for at least three years and adhere to a strict code of conduct before they gain MNIMH or FNIMH after their name.

Know how to find out more There are thousands of supplements and hundreds of brands on the market. The MHRA, the government body overseeing both over-the-counter and professionally prescribed herbal medicines, has a useful website (see box, page 154) for more information on UK legislation.

Remember that supplements are still drugs Just because they have the word 'natural' on the label doesn't mean that they are any safer to use than pharmaceutical drugs. They are still chemicals that will have an effect in your body. You should never take higher-than-recommended doses, and don't take supplements for more than the recommended time period.

Be sceptical If you hear something about a supplement that sounds too good or too bad to be believed, it probably is. To separate the truth from the fiction, check out websites such as **www.quackwatch.org**

Do your homework If you take supplements, you should keep up with the growing body of scientific research about their effects. A good place to start is the US National Institutes of Health's National Center for Complementary and Alternative Medicine at **www.nccam.nih.gov**

Proceed with caution What works for your neighbour or friend may not work for you. Know what you're taking and why you're taking it; don't rely on a recommendation alone. If pregnant or breastfeeding, avoid herbal remedies unless your doctor recommends them.

The following list is not complete. There are numerous mixtures of herbs, particularly in Chinese, Korean, Japanese and Indian medicine, that purport to help with asthma and allergies. If herbal remedies interest you, consult a qualified medical herbalist from the National Institute of Medical Herbalists (NIMH) – see **www.nimh.org.uk** – who is trained in herbal therapies, particularly Chinese medicine, but inform your doctor first.

Bromelain

Bromelain is an enzyme derived from the stem of the pineapple plant. It works as a decongestant, drying up mucus and other secretions.

What the studies show Research shows that bromelain works by reducing swelling and mucus production, but no studies show its effectiveness in people with allergies. In fact, there are several reports of bromelain-related allergies.

Precautions Allergic reactions may occur if you are sensitive to pineapple.

Bottom line Don't bother with this one.

Butterbur

Extracts of this herbaceous plant have been used to treat asthma and allergic rhinitis.

What the studies show In one study of 125 people with seasonal allergic rhinitis that compared butterbur with cetirizine (Zirtek), both groups showed improvements in quality of life assessments. But 12 per cent of those receiving Zirtek reported sedative effects, compared with no such reports from those who received butterbur.

Precautions The plant's pyrrolizidine alkaloids are thought to cause liver damage and be carcinogenic in animals, so only buy extracts from which these substances have been removed.

Bottom line Consult your doctor before trying it.

Dried ivy extract

This is not a remedy you can prepare yourself from home-grown ivy; if you want to try it, buy the preparation from a health food store or seek treatment from a qualified medical herbalist.

What the studies show In a double-blind, randomized clinical trial, 24 children with asthma received about 35mg of dried ivy extract for three days. There was no significant improvement in lung function, but there was a significant decrease in airway resistance when compared with a placebo.

Precautions None.

Bottom line Present evidence of its efficacy is inconclusive; ask your doctor before trying it.

Chamomile

Chamomile tea has anti-inflammatory properties, and chamazulene, an active ingredient in chamomile, is a leukotriene inhibitor.

What the studies show German studies have found that chamomile reduces the release of histamine from mast cells (at least in rats) and may slow allergic reactions by increasing the adrenal glands' production of cortisone, which reduces lung inflammation and makes breathing easier.

Precautions None.

Bottom line There is no clinical evidence that it improves allergies or asthma but chamomile tea before bed can help promote relaxation and sleep.

Echinacea

This herbal remedy is often used to treat upper respiratory tract disorders.

What the studies show While at least one trial has shown a reduction in the number of upper respiratory infections, a known trigger for asthma exacerbation, other studies have not confirmed this.

Precautions Avoid echinacea/goldenseal combinations, since one of the active ingredients in goldenseal, hydrazine, causes constriction of blood vessels and high blood pressure. Do not take echinacea with other drugs nor if you have any form of autoimmune disease, such as rheumatoid arthritis, MS, lupus, as it can exacerbate symptoms.

Bottom line It may have some benefit but allergic reactions have been reported.

Ginkgo biloba

Ginkgo is a traditional Chinese herbal treatment. Its alkaloids have anti-inflammatory properties and are claimed to help relieve asthma by reducing airway hyper-responsiveness and bronchial spasms.

What the studies show In one study, those given 15g of concentrated ginkgo leaf liquor three times a day, had a significantly greater improvement in their lung function tests after eight weeks than a placebo group. But many other clinical studies have failed to confirm the herb's benefits.

Precautions If you are scheduled to undergo any type of surgery or dental work, you should stop using ginkgo for at least 14 days before the procedure. Ginkgo biloba may have anticoagulant (blood-thinning) effects.

Bottom line If your doctor agrees, ginkgo biloba is worth a try as part of a conventional medical treatment plan but has no proven benefit.

Grapeseed extract

Believed to work as a natural antihistamine, grapeseed extract is often touted as a natural remedy for allergies and asthma.

What the studies show A US study of 54 adults, aged 18 to 75, with diagnosed ragweed allergy recorded their symptoms while taking either 100mg of grapeseed extract or a placebo twice daily. After eight weeks, there was no difference in the reported symptoms or use of medications.

Herbal blends: are they safe?

Few people are well versed in healing herbs, a fact not lost on the supplements industry. Many entrepreneurial companies have created complex blends of herbs with name such as Sinus Clear and Breathe Easy that promise a natural solution to your allergy or asthma woes. Now under review by the Medicines and Health products Regulatory Agency (MHRA), some herbal blends have licences and from 2005 the EU Traditional Herbal Medicines directive has set minimum standards for quality and product claims. But this does not cover internet purchases. So the National Institute of Medical Herbalists (NIMH) warns:

• Each blend may have a different underlying approach. One product we looked at was a blend of mostly homeopathic medicines. Another was mostly Chinese herbs. One was all Western herbs. Others bring together all of these. Don't even consider a blended supplement if you don't understand and agree with its approach.

• Some include herbs like ephedra (under investigation by the MHRA), which should only be prescribed by medical herbalists, or obscure herbs, barely known by natural healing experts.

• Is it worth paying to test an unproven herbal blend from a little-known company?

• If you're prone to allergies, you may react to the herbs and other product ingredients as they do have side effects for some people, or could interact with your more standard medicines.

Consult your doctor if a supplement interests you. It's advisable to see a qualified herbal practitioner if you are on medication and want to try herbal blends. Do not self-prescribe.

Precautions Grapeseed may enhance the effect of drugs affecting coagulation or platelet aggregation, such as aspirin, warfarin and clopidogrel (Plavix).

Bottom line There is little evidence as to its efficacy, but it is relatively safe. It has some antioxidant and anti-inflammatory effects, so you could try it with your doctor's knowledge.

Datura

The datura family includes devil's weed and jimsonweed, commonly found along roadsides and in cornfields and pastures. When smoked, datura has mildly hallucinogenic properties, which, in 1968, prompted the USA to ban over-the-counter preparations containing it. Still, it has a long history as a herbal medicine for asthma. In fact, people with asthma smoked cigarettes made from this herb throughout much of the 20th century, and it is still a common ingredient in many over-the-counter 'natural' asthma preparations available from other countries, such as Asthmador, Barter's Powder, Kinsman's Asthmatic Powder, Green Mountain Asthmatic Compound and Haywood's Powder.

What the studies show One small study of 12 patients with asthma found that inhaling the smoke of one jimsonweed cigarette substantially decreased airway restriction in 11 patients to the point that even inhaling albuterol afterwards caused no further improvement for most of them.

Precautions This herb is known to cause hallucinations, and an overdose can be fatal. Don't take it if you have glaucoma, a blockage in your gastrointestinal tract or myasthenia gravis. Also avoid it if you are using anticoagulant (blood-thinning), diabetes or anti-anxiety medication.

Bottom line Skip this one. It's too risky.

Ma huang (Ephedra)

This Chinese herb has been used for thousands of years to treat asthma and other respiratory conditions, including allergic rhinitis. It contains various forms of ephedrine, used in over-the-counter and prescription decongestants, which is why it's so good at drying up a runny nose and leaky eyes. It is often the primary ingredient in Chinese herbal mixtures for asthma, including Minor Blue Dragon (xiao-qing-long-tang, or XQLT). In 2004, ephedra was banned for over-the-counter sale in the USA by the FDA. It is currently being assessed in the UK by the Medicines and Healthcare products Regulatory Agency (MHRA).

What the studies show Of all the herbal remedies used for allergies and asthma, ma huang has the strongest basis of scientific support, which is not surprising when you consider that its active ingredient – ephedrine – is the one used in most decongestants.

Precautions Ma huang should never be self-prescribed. Taken in large doses or by people with high blood pressure or certain heart conditions, ephedra can cause strokes or heart attacks and even be fatal. There is also evidence that it interacts with certain prescription asthma drugs.

Bottom line It is not advisable to experiment with the Chinese herb. You derive the same benefits from prescription and over-the-counter preparations, without the worries.

Peppermint

Peppermint has a long history of use in healing and to treat the common cold. Peppermint oil contains menthol, a powerful therapeutic agent used in numerous over-the-counter and prescription drugs. It acts as a muscle relaxant, particularly in the digestive tract (hence the custom of sucking a peppermint after a big dinner), and it can reduce inflammation of the nasal passages, thus making it a common antidote for nasal congestion. It has also been found to prevent the release of histamine from mast cells in allergic rats, decreasing their sneezing and nose rubbing.

Flush away your allergies

What if you could simply rinse away those allergens? Well, with a small gadget called a Neti Pot, you can. Resembling a palm-size Aladdin's lamp and available over the internet, it is designed to flush water from one side of your nose to the other. Here's how it works.

- Fill the pot with warm saltwater (about 1 teaspoon of salt per cup of water).
- Lean over a sink, tilt your head to the left and tip the spout into your right nostril. The liquid should trickle out the opposite nostril, 'power washing' your nasal passages.

- Continue until the pot is empty, then blow your nose and repeat on the opposite side.

Sterimar, a seawater nasal spray, works in a similar way. Alternatively, make your own nasal rinse with 1 teaspoon each of salt and bicarbonate of soda dissolved in a pint of water: close one nostril, sniff up the solution from the palm of your hand; repeat on the other side. It's simple, and it works. Studies on children and adults who used nasal irrigation found that their symptoms significantly improved, and they used fewer antihistamines than those who did not irrigate.

What the studies show No studies have been published on the effect of peppermint on allergies or asthma.

Precautions People with chronic heartburn problems should avoid peppermint.

Bottom line A soothing cup of peppermint tea may help to relieve congestion although there are no human studies to confirm its efficacy for allergies or asthma. But it certainly can't hurt.

Pycnogenol

Pycnogenol is an extract of the bark of pine trees that grow near the sea in France. Studies find that it appears to inhibit the release of histamine. Pycnogenol has some anti-inflammatory effects, inhibiting production of pro-inflammatory chemicals such as leukotrienes, cytokines and adhesion molecules. It also relieves swelling, supporting easier breathing and reducing hives.

What the studies show In one study, 22 adults with asthma received either 1mg of Pycnogenol per pound of body weight each day (up to 200g per day) or a placebo for four weeks. Lung function values in the Pycnogenol group rose significantly, from an average of 60 per cent to 71 per cent. At

the same time, the number of leukotrienes in the participants' blood dropped, as did the severity of their asthma.

Precautions None.

Bottom line Try it but ask your doctor first.

Saiboku-to (TJ-96)

This herbal preparation, approved by the Japanese government for the treatment of asthma, contains 10 herbs, including ginger, Korean ginseng, magnolia, Baikal skullcap and liquorice. It is, in fact, quite effective, primarily because it appears to reduce eosinophilic inflammation, a hallmark of asthma, by interfering with the production of leukotrienes.

What the studies show In a double-blind, placebo-controlled study conducted in Tokyo, researchers gave subjects either 2.5g of TJ-96 or a placebo three times a day for four weeks. While on the herbal preparation, the participants' symptoms and levels of eosinophils in their blood and sputum significantly decreased. In another study, 40 asthma patients were treated with Saiboku-to for 6 to 24 months, and all were able to greatly reduce their use of steroidal asthma medications.

Precautions TJ-96 may interact with allergy and asthma medications. It may also increase and prolong effects of steroids when taken with them.

Bottom line May be worth trying; inform your doctor as your medication may need adjusting.

Stinging nettle

A common weed found throughout the world, stinging nettle can leave you with a nasty stinging sensation if you brush up against its prickly leaves. But those leaves contain a plethora of chemicals and vitamins that give the plant its anti-allergy and anti-asthma properties. For one, they are high in quercetin, the flavonoid we discussed in chapter 9 that helps to reduce the release of histamine and blocks inflammation. The leaves are also high in the antioxidant vitamins A and C, and vitamin C acts as a natural antihistamine. The plant's history as an asthma remedy dates back to the 1st century AD when Greek physicians used it to treat the disease.

What the studies show In one randomized, double-blind study, 98 participants with allergies were given either 1,300mg of nettle leaf or a placebo. Overall, 58 per cent rated nettle leaf higher than the placebo, reporting a slight reduction in hay fever symptoms, including sneezing and itchy eyes.

Precautions None, but don't take it if you are allergic to it.

Bottom line It doesn't hurt.

Tylophora

This plant is indigenous to India and is reputed to provide relief for people with bronchial asthma.

What the studies show In five double-blind trials on the herb, results were mixed. Three studies showed improvement; two showed no differences between the herbal group and the placebo group.

Precautions None.

Bottom line If tylophora interests you and you want to give it a try, talk to your doctor first.

Buyer beware

As you can see, when it comes to alternative therapies, it really is a 'buyer beware' world. Unlike pharmaceutical drugs, for which we know we have government oversight as a protection, there is little or no oversight when it comes to these remedies. Be sure to follow these four main rules when using alternative therapies.

1 **Discuss your interests** and plans with your doctor.
2 **Integrate them** into your conventional medical treatment. You should never stop taking prescribed medication or seeing a doctor simply because you are using alternative therapies.
3 **Avoid remedies** that have been proved useless or dangerous.
4 **Follow directions** carefully.

Up to now, we have talked mostly about remedies and therapies that require clear thought, expert advice and good planning and judgment. In the next chapter, we offer advice for those moments – and we hope they are rare – in which you need to make an immediate decision about your asthma or allergies.

Chapter eleven

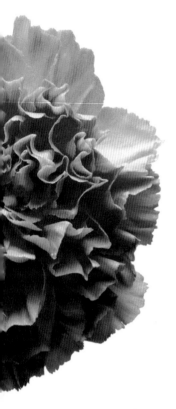

The right
responses

Choose the right doctor. Use the right medications. Purge your home of allergens. Improve your diet. Choose appropriate dietary supplements. Learn to relax. These are all part of sound, intelligent management of an ongoing fight against allergies and asthma; they are also crucial steps in the Breathe Easy Plan.

But there is also another side to these diseases: dealing with an attack. At that moment, all the long-term solutions fade away and the only thing on your mind is, 'What do I do *now* to cope with this?'

The following pages provide guidelines and all sorts of practical advice for that most unwelcome event – a strong allergy or asthma attack. A sequence of differents kinds of scenarios are described because, as all sufferers know, such reactions take on many forms and intensity levels and can occur at the most inconvenient of times and places.

One key and very basic aspect of your coping mechanism is to ensure that you always take your medications. The best thing you can do is to keep the right rescue medicines with you at all times so that when an attack occurs, you have the appropriate weapon to halt it. That applies regardless of the form and cause of your allergies or asthma.

In many of the scenarios presented here, something to the effect of 'and by accident, your medicine was left at home' has been included. It's in such circumstances that knowing what to do is of crucial importance. As these examples were put together, certain themes quickly emerged.

1 **If the reaction is strong** and you lack the correct rescue medicine, get to a doctor straight away. Don't feel guilty, don't feel ashamed, and don't feel that you are being overly cautious. A strong asthma attack is serious.
2 **Staying calm always helps** It not only keeps those around you sane, it also helps to mitigate the effect of the attack. Most important of all, it helps you to focus on the right things to do rather than panicking.
3 **If possible, immediately move** far away from the allergen or asthma trigger. Continued exposure will only make the attack worse.

All of the following 10 scenarios are based on real-life cases.
If you recognize yourself in any of them, you should pay close attention to the proper response. If you're lucky, you will never need to use this wisdom but, if you are less fortunate, you will be glad you had it.

Keep your doctor informed of what medications you are taking, regardless of whether it's a prescription or non-prescription preparation.

1 You wake up in the morning with your head stuffed, your nose running and your eyes streaming and red from allergies. You feel dreadful, but you have an important meeting at work in two hours' time at which you have to give a critical presentation.

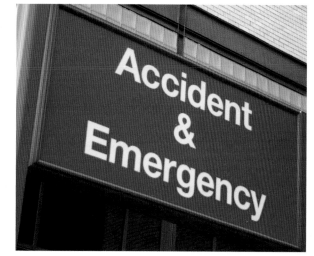

You don't want to turn up half asleep and groggy for an important presentation, so here's what to do.

▨ **Take a non-sedating antihistamine** If you have a prescription medicine, take it; if not, buy a non-sedating over-the-counter antihistamine such as Boots Hayfever and Allergy Relief All Day, Benadryl Allergy Relief, Aller Tek, Piriteze Allergy, Zirtek Allergy or Clarityn Allergy.
▨ **Try a decongestant spray,** such as oxymetazoline (Otrivine) for nasal relief.

A strong asthma attack is a serious matter. If you lack the correct rescue medicine, don't worry about being overly cautious – get to a doctor straight away.

Use a nasal steroid but take it regularly to clear congestion effectively. Using the decongestant first will help the steroid to get into the nose.

Take some paracetamol (regular or brands such as Panadol) to ease the death-warmed-up feeling. *Don't* take aspirin or other non-steroidal anti-inflammatory drugs such as ibuprofen (Nurofen); they may exacerbate your symptoms if you are allergic to them.

Eat the right breakfast to give you an antioxidant boost for the day. Start with some cut-up fruit or a glass of orange juice to provide vitamin C. Then choose some wholemeal toast or a bowl of high-fibre, fortified cereal for a vitamin E boost.

Use eyedrops to reduce the swelling and redness. Another option is to sit with a cold compress on your eyes for a few minutes to relieve the itching and swelling.

2 You have no known food allergies, and you have even had skin tests in an allergy clinic that showed no reaction. At a restaurant, you order a prawn cocktail, which you have eaten dozens of times. Thirty minutes after eating it, just after finishing your main course, you develop hives on your abdomen that quickly spread all over your body. At the same time, your face begins to swell and you have difficulty swallowing and severe nausea. What should you do?

We know that certain foods – particularly prawns – can cause your body to release inflammatory chemicals such as histamine even without an IgE reaction. Thus, an allergy skin test may not indicate an allergy because those tests show only the presence of IgE antibodies.

If your reaction is as severe as described above, you are in a life-threatening situation, particularly if you're having trouble swallowing. Ask someone to take you straight to casualty or dial 999 for an ambulance immediately.

Even if you're experiencing only hives, it's possible that they are only the first part of the reaction. It could get much worse very quickly. Be particularly watchful for difficulty with swallowing. Also, be aware of any tingling in your lips or eyelids. Because the skin is thinnest and has lots of blood vessels in these two areas, they are likely to swell the most.

If it is clear that your reaction is not progressing beyond a few hives or itching – and that's the typical case – you should still excuse yourself from the table and quickly find the nearest chemist or supermarket to buy one of the many over-the-counter antihistamines. Take it as directed.

No matter how severe the reaction is, *do not try to vomit.* You will have already absorbed part of the culprit food into your bloodstream, and vomiting simply increases the risk that you could inhale, or aspirate, particles of vomited food, which would make a bad situation much, much worse.

3 Your four-year-old son has severe atopic dermatitis (eczema), and in the past couple of days, has had a cold and a slight cough. He wakes up wheezing in the night. What should you do?

Atopic dermatitis, an allergic skin rash, is very often the first sign of other allergic diseases, such as asthma and allergic rhinitis. Your child may have infection-induced asthma. Viral infections are the number one triggers of asthma in young children. Consult your GP as soon as possible. Meanwhile:

▥ **Keep him hydrated** The rapid breathing that comes with an asthma attack can be very dehydrating, so try to push liquids, preferably warm ones. Warm tea, which contains caffeine (a bronchodilator), may help. Also, if you happen to have some, you could try chicken broth. The rich soup contains homocysteine, a chemical that helps to break up and thin mucus. If neither of these is available, warm water will do – it mustn't be cold.

▥ **Give paracetamol for fever** A high fever can also cause dehydration. Do *not* use aspirin. Not only can it stimulate an allergic reaction in some people, but aspirin given for fever in children can lead to a dangerous condition called Reyes' syndrome.

▥ **Keep your child sitting quietly** Read a book together, have him sit in your lap while you rock him, or play a favourite video or DVD or get him to listen to a story tape. Activity can increase bronchial spasms, making the asthma worse.

▥ **Do *not* give him a cough suppressant** It will simply make him retain mucus, and you want him to cough. It's a normal physiologic mechanism to get the mucus out of his lungs.

▥ ***Never* give your child medicine containing codeine** (which many cough syrups contain) if he is breathing rapidly, which is a necessary defence. Codeine will slow his breathing, which will result in retention of more carbon dioxide.

If the attack gets worse and the child suddenly begins breathing very rapidly, is distressed and having difficulty getting enough breath in, you must get him to the emergency room IMMEDIATELY. Just go straight to the hospital or dial 999 to call an ambulance.

▥ **Don't give your child any food** While he is breathing so rapidly, he could easily aspirate food into his lungs, leading to serious pneumonia or other lung problems.

▥ **Be a source of calm** Your child will be quick to sense and mirror your emotions, particularly if you show anxiety, fear or lack of control. You should be reassuring and loving and make it seem to him that you know exactly what you are doing, no matter what is going on inside you.

4 You are scuba diving on holiday when you suddenly become short of breath. You didn't bring your asthma medication with you because you haven't had any problems for four years. Now you are underwater and having problems breathing. What should you do?

▮ **Signal to your diving partner and get to the surface,** but don't go any faster than you are trained to go. You don't want to initiate a bad case of the bends on top of the asthma attack.

▮ **Get out of the water as quickly as possible,** because the cold water may be making your breathing worse. Wrap yourself in a warm blanket. If there is hot coffee or tea on board , try sipping that; the caffeine has a bronchodilating effect, and the warmth will relax constricted airways. Ask the captain if, by chance, anyone on board has a short-acting brochodilator or even if there is any adrenaline (epinephrine); on some boats, it is included in emergency medical kits and, though not a recognized asthma treatment, it may help in an emergency. Try to stay calm. It's at times like these that knowing a formal relaxation method, such as those discussed in chapter 10, is most useful.

▮ **Cut the trip short** if the warming and calming don't curtail the attack within a few minutes. Even if you recover, get to a doctor as soon as you reach shore. Gasp out your apologies to your diving companions as best you can and, if you are out in a boat, get them to turn back. And next time, take your inhaler. Asthma is as unpredictable as the weather.

5 You have been diagnosed with allergies and asthma and are on a treatment regimen to control both. You're on a plane home from a wonderful holiday when, all of a sudden, you develop chest tightness and shortness of breath. You mistakenly packed your medications in your luggage, which you checked in so they are now out of reach. What should you do?

The bottom line is that you should never, ever check in your medication with your luggage, no matter what kind of medication it is or what disease it is for. Having said that, there are a few things you can do if you don't have your medicines with you.

▮ **Let the flight attendant know** what is going on. Some airlines carry medical kits that include adrenaline, which may help in an emergency.

▮ **Ask the flight attendant** if the pilot could make an announcement to ask if there is a doctor on the plane. The doctor may be able to assess the seriousness of the situation better than you can and make an objective determination about whether it is serious enough to call for an emergency landing. The doctor may also have a medical kit on board.

■ **Ask the pilot to make an announcement** to find out if anyone has a short-acting bronchodilator medication available. Given that more than 8 per cent of the population has asthma, it is fairly likely that someone is sitting on the plane with their own rescue medication close at hand.

■ **Try sipping hot coffee or tea** Caffeine acts as a mild bronchodilator, and the warmth itself can often help relax airway spasms. Avoid iced drinks; they will only make the spasms worse.

■ **Practise a relaxation exercise** Close your eyes, visualize yourself in a safe, quiet place, and focus on your breathing, visualizing it gradually becoming slower and deeper.

6 Your asthma has been fairly well controlled for several months, but lately, you have been under a lot of stress at work and at home. Suddenly, you wake up in the middle of the night fighting to breathe. You're having an asthma attack but you haven't renewed your prescription and there is no medication in the house. What should you do?

■ **Make yourself a pot of coffee or a cup of hot tea** The caffeine and warmth will help to open constricted bronchial passages.

■ **Don't eat** Forget that leftover doughnut. Eating when you are in the midst of an asthma attack could result in you inhaling particles of food into your lungs, which would make things worse.

■ **Practise some of the relaxation techniques** that you learned about in chapter 10.

■ **Don't take a cough suppressant** That will only keep the mucus down in your chest and you *want* to cough it up, no matter how horrible it sounds or feels.

■ **If you're still struggling to breathe after 5 minutes, you need medical help** But don't be tempted to drive. Ask someone to drive you to the hospital casualty department or doctor's surgery or dial 999. Carbon dioxide builds up in your lungs and bloodstream during an asthma attack; if the levels become too high, there is a risk that you might pass out at the wheel.

In this case, the stress you are under has exacerbated your underlying condition and suddenly there you are in the midst of an attack. But it shows that you can't stop taking your medicine just because your asthma is well controlled. Too many people tend to do this when they feel better but the reality is that the medicine is *why* they're feeling better.

Asthma is a chronic condition, as are high blood pressure or diabetes, and you wouldn't stop taking insulin just because your diabetes was well controlled. Yet some of the worst cases seen in casualty are people who stopped taking their asthma medication.

7 You've just moved from London to Oban, on the west coast of Scotland, where you thought the air would be beneficial for your allergies and asthma. Yet it's only your first week there, the packing cases are virtually untouched, and you've developed some terrible wheezing. You don't want to move again. What should you do?

This is advice that far too many people with asthma and allergies receive. Move to a low-pollen area, and your condition will improve. But it's not true. If you have allergies in London, the chances are you will have allergies in Oban: you may simply be responding to different allergens.

So, once you've unpacked, make some local enquiries and then:

▒ **Sign on with a new GP** and ask for a referral to a new allergy or asthma specialist in Oban.

▒ **Make an appointment** with the new doctor as soon as possible for a complete evaluation and medication check.

▒ **Consider having your new home professionally cleaned** As we have discussed in earlier chapters, cat hair is ubiquitous and almost impossible to get rid of even with regular vacuuming and cleaning. In addition, all the commotion of moving may be stirring up massive amounts of dust and allergens, be it those left behind in your former home or those that you imported in the possessions you are unpacking. A professional cleaning may be what is needed to make your new home ready for you to live in.

▒ **Begin making environmental changes** to your surroundings, such as those described in Step 3 of the Breathe Easy Plan, in the meantime – before the doctor's appointment and before the cleaners turn up.

8 You are visiting your sister in Hayward's Heath. She has a cat but has given it to a neighbour during your visit because she knows that you are severely allergic. Within 10 minutes of sitting down on her sofa, you begin sneezing, coughing and dripping. What should you do?

The cat may be elsewhere but remnants of its presence are everywhere. The antigen causing your reaction comes from the cat's saliva, urine and dander. Because cats lick themselves so much, their hair is very sticky, so no amount of vacuuming will remove it from carpet and upholstery. Here's what to do.

▒ **Tell your sister how much you appreciate her** trying to make your visit more comfortable for you. Explain exactly what we just told you about cat allergens and how difficult it is to get rid of them.

▒ **Ask her to recommend** a nearby hotel.

- Check in at the hotel.
- **Buy your sister a really nice dinner** to soothe any remaining hurt feelings.

9 You are doing your Christmas shopping, and the shops are crowded and overheated. As you walk into a department store, the strong scent of perfumes from the cosmetics counter hits you like a brick wall. You begin to wheeze and feel your chest tightening. What should you do?

- **Get far away from any asthma trigger** Either leave that part of the store or go to another store. If it's cold outside, don't go out; the cold air will simply make your asthma worse.
- **Take your rescue medications or try to enjoy a hot cup of coffee or tea** Relax with the soothing warmth of the liquid as you begin to feel the bronchodilating effects of the caffeine.
- **Take the afternoon off if possible** Go home and change into your most comfortable clothes, pop in a DVD or video and remember what the season is *really* about while you sip hot chocolate. You were probably also stressed by the pre-holiday commotion and pressure. A crowded, overheated shopping environment can do that. Later that evening, when you're calm and your asthma has subsided, go online and finish your Christmas shopping the dot.com way.

10 It's a November weekend, and you're having a football game with some friends when you suddenly feel as if you can't breathe. You have never been diagnosed with asthma. What should you do?

Exercise is a trigger for a majority of people with asthma. That's why you should use your bronchodilator 15 to 30 minutes *before* you exercise, especially if you are exercising in cold outdoor air.

- **If you have never been diagnosed** with asthma, though, you probably don't have an inhaler. In that case, you should try to get inside into warm air as quickly as possible, as the cold air is probably making the exercise-induced asthma worse. At the very least, sit in someone's car with the heater running. Also, ask if anyone in the game has an inhaler you can borrow.
- **If your condition doesn't improve** after you warm up and your body relaxes from the exertion of the game (this should take 5 to 10 minutes), ask someone to drive you to the nearest hospital. And first thing Monday morning, make an appointment with your GP for a complete evaluation. Even if exercise turns out to be the only trigger for your asthma, you still may need to be on inhaled steroids.

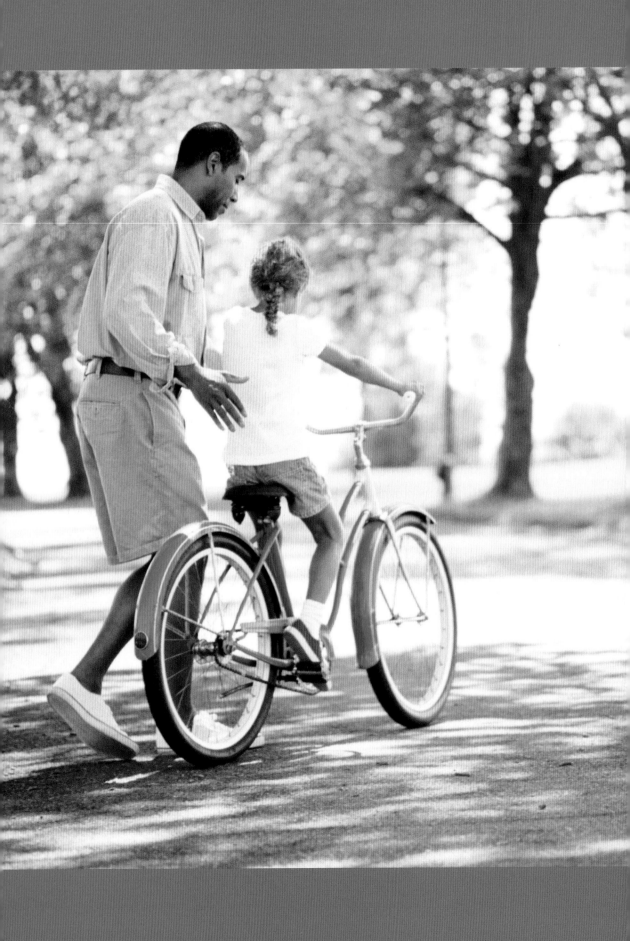

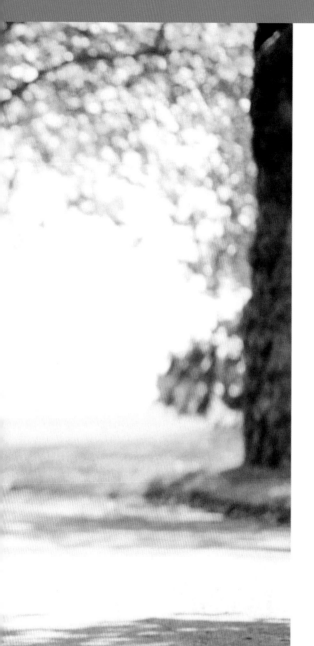

PART THREE

The **Breathe Easy** Plan

By reading this far, you have gained the knowledge you need to control allergies and asthma. Now, with the seven-step Breathe Easy Plan, you will also have all the specific steps, advice and wisdom required to use that knowledge in order to end the attacks and fully control your condition.

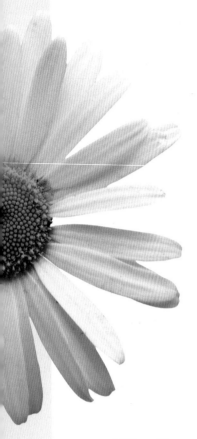

Welcome
to the plan

The Breathe Easy Plan to beat allergies and asthma is spelt out in detail in this section. It has been created by medical experts with the goal of offering you the most thorough and effective action plan available for taking control of the allergies or asthma that have been troubling you or your family.

It is evidently true that there is no such thing as a one-size-fits-all plan. Not only do the nature and intensity of allergies and asthma vary from one individual to the next, so do schedules, family commitments, financial resources and levels of motivation. But these issues need not deter you. This plan has been intentionally devised to be easily adaptable to almost any scenario. In essence, it takes the seven most important components of allergy and asthma control and gives you the tools, tips and directions to master each, based on your own needs and resources.

How we recommend that you do the plan

- **Quickly review all seven steps** so that you understand what you will be doing.
- **While we would prefer that you follow the steps in order**, it is not essential, with the exception of step 1. It is best to complete that step first, regardless of where you turn next. It provides a road map to help you to understand where your priorities should lie and which steps you should focus on.
- **Think through what is involved and plan for it** Step 2, for example, requires a visit to your doctor. So you will obviously need to make an appointment in advance. Likewise, step 3 involves some intense housecleaning, reorganization and a potential financial investment. It may make sense to keep a few days clear in your diary to do the work.
- **Understand that there are no time limits for each step** This is not one of those weight-loss programmes designed to help you lose a target number of pounds a week over a 12-week period. Rather, the Breathe Easy Plan is intended for a lifetime of allergy and asthma control. Complete each step fully, and you will have taken control of your condition.
- **In many cases, we give you a menu of tips to consider** Read them all, then select those that make the most sense for your situation and condition. The trick is to *always do something*. Reading sensible advice is one thing, but the Breathe Easy Plan won't deliver on its promise of better health unless you act on that advice.
- **Enlist your family and your doctor** Don't hide the fact that you are reading this book and following the plan. You have decided that you have had enough of your allergies and asthma and are taking action. Ask for their help. Let your family know that the benefits stretch far beyond allergies and asthma; everyone in the household will be much healthier as a result of these steps.
- **If you wish to follow the plan for a spouse or child, that's fine** However, the chances of success are far greater if the other person is actively involved in the process. Their motivation and participation not only makes it much easier to follow the plan but also gives them the incentive to make it succeed. Plus, there is only so much you can do for someone else, as some of the steps require skills and strategies (such as new breathing techniques) that are entirely personal.
- **Finally, this is not a do-it-once-and-be-done programme** You should return to this section of the book every six months or so in order to fine-tune, implementing suggestions that may not have worked for you earlier but may fit better with your life now. Make copies of the charts and questions included throughout the section and keep them after you fill them out so you can see your progress.

Determine your situation

If you have read this far, your suspicions about allergies and asthma have probably been confirmed. Both come in many forms, for many reasons, which makes them particularly difficult to diagnose.

Our goal in step 1 of the Breathe Easy Plan is to help you to come to a clear and correct assessment of your situation. What is the most likely trigger for your allergy? How serious is your asthma? When do symptoms tend to flare up?

This book is not advocating self-diagnosis. As said repeatedly, it takes a trained, experienced doctor to make the official diagnosis of a medical condition. But armed with evidence that you will glean from this part of the plan, you will be able to explain your condition and help your doctor to make an accurate diagnosis.

What you will be doing

Filling out five forms to reveal all aspects of your allergies and/or asthma. This provides useful information for you to keep and summarize for your doctor.

How you should prepare

Before starting the forms, talk to people who know you well about their perceptions of your allergies and/or asthma. Good candidates are your work colleagues, your partner, your children and good friends (particularly those with whom you spend time outdoors). They may have noticed certain things of which you are not aware. For instance, maybe your eyes always water when you visit Aunt Mary and her cat. Or perhaps your asthma seems much worse in the spring (a clue that you may have allergic asthma).

What to have on hand

Copies of the forms. (You could write in the book, but then the forms can only be used once and you might want to pass the book on to other sufferers.) A folder to keep them together.

Could it be allergies?

Answer these 10 questions to help ascertain whether you do indeed have allergies.

1 My nose often runs with a thin, clear discharge.   YES ☐   NO ☐

2 I regularly have itchy, watery eyes, often with uncontrollable sneezing fits.   YES ☐   NO ☐

3 I am frequently kept awake at night by nasal congestion or an unproductive, hacking cough.   YES ☐   NO ☐

4 I breathe through my mouth because my nose is too blocked up.   YES ☐   NO ☐

5 I often have a tickling or itching feelingin my nose, leading me to rub the bottom of my nose for relief (the so-called allergic salute).   YES ☐   NO ☐

6 My symptoms occur only in certain places, such as the office   YES ☐   NO ☐

7 I develop symptoms after dining out at a restaurant.   YES ☐   NO ☐

8 Windy days, especially in spring and autumn, cause coldlike symptoms.   YES ☐   NO ☐

9 After touching certain things like cats, grass or various foods, I sometimes develop unexplained, itchy skin rashes.   YES ☐   NO ☐

10 Cold-like symptoms appear or worsen when I vaccuum, garden or clean the cat litter box.   YES ☐   NO ☐

THE RESULTS A positive answer to questions 2, 8, 9 or 10 would make you seem a likely candidate for allergies. The more *yes* answers, the more likely that you have the problem. The next form will help to determine the nature of your allergies.

Seasonal or perennial?

The frequency of your allergic reactions can help to determine both the cause and the treatment. If you have symptoms for only a week or two out of the year due to a specific pollen, you may be able to get by with over-the-counter antihistamines and decongestants. However, if you are like the majority of patients with allergies who have ongoing symptoms that worsen during certain times of the year, you might be a good candidate for a fuller regimen of medicine and preventive care.

Complete the tracking log on the following page in order to determine the timing of your allergies. For each month, tick off the symptoms you experience and the time of day when they are most prevalent. If they seem to last all day and night, you should tick in each box accordingly.

continued

Task 2 (continued)

Month (time of day)	Runny nose	Stuffy nose	Hives or rashes	Red, itchy eyes	Teary eyes	Sneezing fits	Difficulty breathing	Itching	Scratchy throat	Chronic cough	Wheezing
January											
Day (6am to 6pm)											
Night (6pm to 6am)											
February											
Day											
Night											
March											
Day											
Night											
April											
Day											
Night											
May											
Day											
Night											
June											
Day											
Night											
July											
Day											
Night											
August											
Day											
Night											
September											
Day											
Night											
October											
Day											
Night											
November											
Day											
Night											
December											
Day											
Night											

THE RESULTS With this log, which you may want to summarize for your GP, your doctor should be able to make some good guesses as to what types of allergens are causing you the most trouble. But what can you learn from it? First, if you have five or more boxes marked, or if there is a clear pattern to your ticks, you probably do have an allergy that requires medical treatment. If most of the ticks are in the 'night' boxes, it is likely that allergens in your house are causing the problem. Daytime symptoms suggest that work, leisure or outdoor allergens are responsible.

Allergy responses and triggers

Think about where you were, what you ate, and what you were doing when your attacks occurred.

Tick each box that applies and list specific items where applicable.

Allergy trigger	Runny nose	Stuffy nose	Hives or rashes	Red, itchy eyes	Teary eyes	Sneezing fits	Difficulty breathing	Swelling of face and throat	Facial flushing	Abdominal pain or cramping	Diarrhoea
Foods											
Shellfish (list)											
Peanuts											
Eggs											
Wheat											
Soy											
Nuts											
Dairy products (list)											
Other (list)											
Beverages											
Alcoholic beverages (list)											
Fruit juices with dyes (list)											
Other (list)											
Medications (list specific drugs or types)											
Antibiotics											
Pain medications											
Anaesthetics											
Other (list)											
Indoor environment											
Dust											
Mould											
Cleaning products (list)											
Other (list)											
Outdoor environment											
Weeds, trees or grasses											
Windy days											
Other (list)											
Animals											
Dogs											
Cats											
Insect stings (list)											
Other (list)											

THE RESULTS This form should also help to provide a clearer picture of the irritants that trigger your allergies. Explain what they are to your doctor who can then decide which allergens to test for.

Could it be asthma?

Now it is time to determine whether your symptoms are related to asthma. Your answers to the following questions will provide a good indication.

1 When I walk or do simple chores, I often have trouble breathing, or I cough.
YES ☐ NO ☐

2 Whenever I do something a little more strenuous, such as walking up hills and stairs or doing chores that involve lifting, I find that I have trouble breathing, or I cough.
YES ☐ NO ☐

3 Sometimes I avoid exercising or participating in sports such as jogging, swimming, tennis or aerobics because I have trouble breathing.
YES ☐ NO ☐

4 I am sometimes unable to sleep right through the night because I am woken up with either coughing attacks or shortness of breath.
YES ☐ NO ☐

5 Sometimes I find that I can't take a good, deep breath.
YES ☐ NO ☐

6 Sometimes I have wheezing sounds in my chest for no obvious reason.
YES ☐ NO ☐

7 Sometimes my chest feels very tight for no obvious reason.
YES ☐ NO ☐

8 Sometimes I find that I cough a lot for no obvious reason.
YES ☐ NO ☐

9 Dust, pollen and any contact I have with pets seem to make my coughing or breathing problems worse.
YES ☐ NO ☐

10 My coughing or breathing problems tend to become worse during cold weather.
YES ☐ NO ☐

11 My coughing or breathing problems become worse when I breathe tobacco smoke, or if there are any fumes or strong odours.
YES ☐ NO ☐

12 I find that whenever I catch a cold, more often than not it goes to my chest.
YES ☐ NO ☐

THE RESULTS Each *yes* answer is consistent with symptoms of asthma. The more *yes* answers you have, the greater the need to seek a professional evaluation.

How well controlled is my asthma?

Effective control of your asthma should be your key target. With today's medications most people should aim to manage their condition so that it has a minimal impact on their daily lives. Your answers to the following questions will indicate how well you are doing.

Do you never …

1 Have symptoms (cough, wheeze, shortness of breath) during the day or at night?   YES ☐   NO ☐

2 Have to limit your daily activities in any way
or take time off from school or work?   YES ☐   NO ☐

3 Have to resort to quick relief medications?   YES ☐   NO ☐

If you answered *yes* to most of these questions, you probably have **good control** of your asthma.

Do you …

1 Have symptoms more than twice a week but less than
once a day, and night-time symptoms no more than twice a month?   YES ☐   NO ☐

2 Experience excessive breathlessness when you exert yourself
(running, playing sport, carrying shopping up the stairs)?   YES ☐   NO ☐

3 Need quick-relief medication as often as once a day?   YES ☐   NO ☐

If you answered *yes* to some of these questions, you have **moderate control** of your asthma.

Do you …

1 Have daily symptoms and symptoms at night more than once a week?   YES ☐   NO ☐

2 Have to avoid certain daily activities because of symptoms?   YES ☐   NO ☐

3 Need quick relief medication once a day or more frequently?   YES ☐   NO ☐

If you answered *yes* to any of these questions, you probably have **poor control** of your asthma.

Do you …

1 Experience continuous day-time symptoms and frequent night
and early morning symptoms?   YES ☐   NO ☐

2 Have to constantly limit your activities and take time off school or work
as a result of your symptoms?   YES ☐   NO ☐

3 Need to use quick-relief medications more than once a day despite intermittent
increased doses of preventer medication and steroid tablets?   YES ☐   NO ☐

4 Have to consult your GP or attend A & E because of
unexpected severe attacks?   YES ☐   NO ☐

If you answered *yes* to these questions, you probably have **very poor control** of your asthma.

Concluding step 1

It is sometimes said that you can't find the right solution if you don't know what the problem is. Armed with all the information that you have acquired by filling out the forms, you should have a much better understanding of the scope and nature of your allergies and/or asthma.

That will be useful in many ways. First, you have a wealth of data that will help your GP to carry out the right tests, prescribe the best medicines for your situation, and direct you to appropriate lifestyle changes. Secondly, you now know enough to target your own efforts against allergies or asthma. After all, it's up to you to wash your sheets, monitor your food choices and vacuum your carpets – although a letter from your doctor could strengthen your case if you have poor ventilation at work.

If you have never consulted a doctor about your allergies or asthma, now is the time (see step 2). If you have already visited a GP about your condition and are taking prescription medications, your findings here may surprise you or shed new light on your condition.

In that case you may decide to make a new appointment and tell your doctor that after doing a thorough review of your symptoms and attacks, you realize that you have not provided the full picture.

Explain that you have been learning about allergy and asthma medicines and would like a fuller discussion about what medication you are taking and whether it should change. Once you do this, you have probably taken the biggest step of all towards breathing more easily.

STEP TWO

Create your arsenal for relief

Without question, there are many important and effective ways to manage allergies and asthma that don't involve medicine. In fact, the next five steps of the Breathe Easy Plan will detail them clearly. But not even the most extreme alternative healers would deny that modern medicine should play a significant part in your battle against allergies and asthma.

In this step of the Breathe Easy Plan, you will achieve three crucial things:
- Find a doctor to treat your particular condition
- Learn to understand the best medications for your condition
- Make sure that you are managing your medicines effectively

This step is especially useful if you have not yet seen a doctor about your condition, but even if you have, you should go through the entire process. With your new knowledge of your condition and how the medicines for it work, along with a renewed commitment to improve your situation, a review of your medicinal arsenal – as well as your effectiveness in deploying it – is extremely valuable.

What you will be doing

First, you will set up a doctor's appointment. Then you and your doctor will determine the best medicine for your particular needs. (Do you need preventive medication? Should your prescriptions be changed?) Next, you will work out a plan to help guarantee that you take your medicine optimally. Finally, you will consider the possibility of any other approaches.

How you should prepare

Re-read chapters 7 and 10. Be ready for your visit to the doctor's surgery and then a visit to the pharmacy.

What to have on hand

All the forms that you filled out in step 1 (or summarized versions). A list of all the medicines and supplements you are taking, not only for allergies or asthma but for any other conditions as well (fill in the form on page 191).

Finding a doctor

If you have recently moved house and have not yet registered with a new GP, you should do so without delay. Your GP is the first person to consult about your allergies or asthma. If you are already registered, but it is a while since you saw your GP, make an appointment to review your condition. Regular monitoring is important. Your medication may need to be adjusted. Or it may be appropriate for your GP to refer you to a specialist. Answer these questions to find out.

1 I have had a life-threatening asthma attack at some time in my life. YES ☐ NO ☐

2 I am not meeting the goals of my asthma therapy after three to six months of treatment, or my doctor believes I am not responding to current therapy. YES ☐ NO ☐

3 My symptoms are unusual or difficult to diagnose. YES ☐ NO ☐

4 I have other conditions such as severe hay fever or sinusitis that complicate my diagnosis. YES ☐ NO ☐

5 I have never had any diagnostic tests done to determine the severity of my asthma and what causes my symptoms. YES ☐ NO ☐

6 I would like to consider immunotherapy. YES ☐ NO ☐

7 I have severe persistent asthma. YES ☐ NO ☐

8 I use continuous oral corticosteroid therapy or high-dose inhaled corticosteroids and/or have taken more than two bursts of oral corticosteroids in one year. YES ☐ NO ☐

9 I have made one or more emergency visits to a doctor or casualty ward due to asthma or breathing problems during the past year. YES ☐ NO ☐

10 I have had one or more overnight hospitalizations due to asthma or breathing problems in the past year. YES ☐ NO ☐

11 I feel that I use my asthma inhaler too frequently. YES ☐ NO ☐

12 Sometimes I don't like the way that my asthma medicine(s) make me feel. YES ☐ NO ☐

13 My asthma medicines don't control my symptoms. YES ☐ NO ☐

THE RESULTS If you answered *yes* to one or more questions, your GP may want to carry out diagnostic tests and/or review your medication(s). If you answered *yes* to any of the following questions – 3, 4, 5, 6, 7, 8, 9 or 10 – he or she may consider referral to a specialist. Show your doctor your answers to these questions and discuss the options. If appropriate, you may be referred to a specialist allergy clinic for treatment.

Take the completed forms from step 1 along to your appointment, together with a copy of the completed medication log on the opposite page.

The Breathe Easy medication log

Use this log to list all medicines and supplements that you take regularly. It's a good idea to copy the list and post it on your refrigerator or somewhere where you will see it every day, so you can update it.

Medication	What is it for?	Date started	Dose	Times per day	Prescribing doctor	Side effects? (yes or no)

Daily vitamins/supplements

Frequently used over-the-counter (OTC) medicines

Asthma/allergy medicines

Other prescription medicines

Allergy medicines

Although only your doctor can prescribe the appropriate medication for allergic rhinitis, this chart explains which medications are best for which symptoms, providing you with the information you need to have a discussion about your treatment. Take the chart with you to your doctor's surgery so that you can refer to it during your discussion.

Medication class	Brand name (prescription)
Sneezing	
Topical corticosteroid nasal sprays	Beconase, Betnesol, Vista-Methasone, Rhinocort Aqua, Dexa-Rhinospray Duo, Syntaris, Flixonase, Nasonex, Nasacort
Antihistamines	Rhinolast, Livostin (nasal sprays), Neoclarityn, Telfast, Xyzal, Loratadine, Mizollen
Mast cell stabilizer	Rynacrom, Vividrin
Leukotriene modifier	Singulair
Itchy nose and throat	
Topical corticosteroid nasal sprays	Beconase, Betnesol, Vista-Methasone, Rhinocort Aqua, Dexa-Rhinospray Duo, Syntaris, Flixonase, Nasonex, Nasacort
Antihistamines	Rhinolast, Livostin (nasal sprays), Neoclarityn, Telfast, Xyzal, Loratadine, Mizollen
Mast cell stabilizer	Rynacrom, Vividrin
Leukotriene modifier	Singulair
Runny nose	
Topical corticosteroid nasal sprays	Beconase, Betnesol, Vista-Methasone, Rhinocort Aqua, Dexa-Rhinospray Duo, Syntaris, Flixonase, Nasonex, Nasacort
Antihistamines	Rhinolast, Livostin (nasal sprays), Neoclarityn, Telfast, Xyzal, Loratadine, Mizollen
Mast cell stabilizer	Rynacrom, Vividrin
Anticholinergic spray	Rinatec
Leukotriene modifier	Singulair
Nasal congestion	
Topical corticosteroid nasal sprays	Beconase, Betnesol, Vista-Methasone, Rhinocort Aqua, Dexa-Rhinospray Duo, Syntaris, Flixonase, Nasonex, Nasacort
Decongestants	Ephedrine (nasal drops)
	Sudafed Decongestant, Otraspray, Otrivine,
Mast cell stabilizer	Rynacrom, Vividrin
Antihistamine nasal spray	Rhinolast, Livostin
Allergic conjunctivitis	
Antihistamine eye drops	Optilast, Emadine, Relestat, Zaditen, Livostin Direct, Alomide, Opatanol
Combination antihistamine/decongestant eye drops	Otrivine-Antistin
Mast cell stabilizer eye drops	Hay-Crom Aqueous, Opticrom Aqueous, Vividrin, Rapitil
Nonsteroidal anti-inflammatory eye drops	Voltarol Ophtha

Brand name (OTC) products include	Best way to use
Beconase Allergy, Beconase Hay Fever, Nasobec Hayfever, Boots Hayfever Relief, Flixonase Benadryl Allergy Relief, AllerTek, Piriteze Allergy, Zirtek Allergy, Clarityn Allergy	Daily as a preventative. Ensure nose is clear enough for spray to penetrate. Start 2 weeks in advance of pollen season. Take 2 to 5 hours before exposure to allergens. If you are constantly exposed, take daily. Start 2-4 weeks before exposure to allergens. Frequent use essential. Less effective than corticosteroid nasal spray. Daily preventatively. Not as effective as corticosteroid nasal spray.
Beconase Allergy, Beconase Hay Fever, Nasobec Hayfever, Boots Hayfever Relief, Flixonase Benadryl Allergy Relief, AllerTek, Piriteze Allergy, Zirtek Allergy, Clarityn Allergy	Daily as a preventative. Ensure nose is clear enough for spray to penetrate. Start 2 weeks in advance of pollen season. Take 2 to 5 hours before exposure to allergens. If you're constantly exposed, take daily. Start using 2 to 4 weeks before exposure to allergens. Use often. Daily as a preventative. Less effective than corticosteroid spray.
Beconase Allergy, Beconase Hay Fever, Nasobec Hayfever, Boots Hayfever Relief, Flixonase, Benadryl Allergy Relief, AllerTek, Piriteze Allergy, Zirtek Allergy, Clarityn Allergy	Daily as a preventative. Ensure your nose is clear enough for the spray to penetrate; you may need to use a decongestant first. Take 2 to 5 hours before exposure to allergens. If you are constantly exposed, take daily. Start using 2 to 4 weeks before exposure to allergens. Useful adjunct to corticosteroid nasal spray and antihistamine when runny nose is a major problem.
In most of these sprays the active ingredient is beclometasone; in Flixonase it is fluticasone. *Oral forms:* Phenylephrine (found in numerous OTC products), pseudoephedrine (Sudafed) *Nasal sprays:* Afrazine, Dristan, Non-Drowsy Sudafed, Tixycolds Nasal Spray , Vicks Sinex	Daily; best treatment to prevent nasal congestion. Make sure your nose is clear enough for the spray to penetrate. Be especially careful with nasal decongestants; don't take them for longer or more often than the recommended dosage schedule or you may end up with rebound congestion provoked by overuse of the decongestant. Start 2 to 4 weeks before exposure to allergens. Use frequently. Less effective than corticosteroid nasal spray. Can be used regularly; antihistamine tablets often better.
None	Use regularly in peak pollen season in addition to other medicines.
None Clariteyes, Opticrom Allergy, Optrex Allergy None	Short-acting relief of symptoms Start 2 to 4 weeks before exposure to allergens. Use regularly. Not recommended for hay fever symptoms.

Asthma medicines

Here are the therapies used for different levels of asthma severity (you determined yours in step 1).
Your doctor will aim to treat you with the minimum medication required to control your symptoms.

Recommended Medications							
Daily medication needed?	Daily inhaled cortico-steroid	Leukotriene modifier	Inhaled cromolyn	Theo-phylline	Daily long-lasting beta2-agonist	Oral steroids	Short-acting beta2-agonist
Mild intermittent							
No	Possibly*	No	No	No	No	No	As needed
Mild persistent							
Yes	Low or medium dose	Possibly	Possibly**	Possibly	No	No	As needed
Moderate							
Yes	Medium dose	Possibly	No	Possibly	Yes	No	As needed
Severe							
Yes	High dose	Possibly	No	Possibly	Yes	Possibly	As needed

* low dose and only if symptoms occur more than twice a week
** very rarely in lieu of inhaled corticosteroid

Managing your rescue medications

Your 'rescue medications' are the inhalers, pills or liquids that you use when an asthma or allergy
attack occurs. Having them immediately available is essential for controlling the attack. Yet, as we
are all aware, you never be sure when or where the next allergen will set off an attack and leave you
gasping for breath. So where should you keep your rescue medications? Follow the advice below to
ensure that you always have them at hand.

Keep them everywhere If you can afford extra supplies of rescue medicines, in particular inhalers, store one of each wherever you spend significant amounts of time. In addition, place one of each in your most frequently used purse, briefcase, computer case or gym bag.

Let's say, for example, that you are a businessperson who regularly works out at a gym and occasionally goes on business trips. You may wish to keep five sets (or partial sets) of rescue medications in the following places:

- At home
- At work
- In your car
- In your gym locker
- In your travel toiletry case

Other places that you should consider include:

- With your gardening supplies
- In your home workshop
- In a bag or belt used during walks or exercise
- In a drawer in your bedside table

The alternative remedies programme

In chapter 10, we provided a thorough review of the many vitamins, minerals and herbs purported to help manage allergies and asthma. Where no harmful effects are indicated and there is some evidence to suggest possible benefits, you could try them and see if they help. But only ever use them to complement (not replace) your medicinal remedies.

- **A daily multivitamin/mineral supplement** Be sure that it includes magnesium, selenium, vitamin C, vitamin E, beta-carotene and all the B vitamins (thiamin, riboflavin, niacin, B_6, B_{12}, folic acid, biotin and pantothenic acid).
- A cup of **peppermint or chamomile tea** each night before bed.
- Your choice of one of the following herbal supplements: **butterbur or Pycnogenol**.
- A daily dose of **echinacea** (follow the directions on the package) taken two weeks on, two weeks off. However, if you have any form of autoimmune disease, you should avoid echinacea.

Always be sure to check with your doctor before taking these or any other supplements, no matter how innocent they appear, because they may interact adversely with prescription or over-the-counter medications that you are taking.

Stock other supplies, too Often during attacks, you need tissues, water or other personal items. So it's worth keeping tissues wherever you spend a fair amount of time, be it the car, the office or the living room. You should also make sure that you keep bottled water with you in the car, at work and in the workshop.

Create a kit If it's not feasible to have more than one set of medicine, create a single but truly effective kit that fits into a small carrying case. Make it small enough not to be burdensome but large enough not to be easily lost or forgotten. Think of the kit as you do a mobile phone – something you need to keep near you as you go through your day. Probably, it will fit into a handbag or briefcase. Be sure to include your name and phone number in case you inadvertently leave it somewhere.

Also include a set of instructions for exactly what to do when you have an attack: the order in which to use the medicines, the dosages, how quickly you should get relief, and any other things to do or watch for.

Track its use Each time you get a new inhaler, stick on a piece of masking tape. Mark the tape whenever you use the inhaler so you have a sense of when it is time to replace it.

Remember wintertime When the cold air arrives, keep an inhaler or other rescue medicine in the pocket of your coat or jacket.

A medication strategy

Of course, no amount of medicine will help you if you forget to take it or if you take it at the wrong time. There is no single foolproof system for managing your medications, so instead, read the following advice and from it create a personal plan that you feel confident will work for you.

Update the medication log on page 191 to include your new medicines and supplements. Place a copy where you will see it every day.

Associate taking a medication with an activity. For instance, when you brush your teeth in the morning, use your nasal corticosteroid. When you eat dinner, take your antihistamine.

Use alarms on clocks, watches, mobile phones and computers to remind you when to take your medications. You can even buy electronic medicine organizers that beep at pre-programmed times. Check at pharmacies or visit **www.medicalarm.co.uk**

Use pill boxes or special holders to organize your medicines by hour, day and week. Then you can easily see if you have missed a dose.

Keep your medications in obvious places, such as the bathroom counter (out of reach of any children), so you see them first thing each morning. If you need to take them with meals, keep them on a shelf in the kitchen.

Use a medication diary, available from chemists or online at numerous websites.

Take your medications together, if possible. For example, if you are taking some in the morning and some at night, ask your doctor if you can take them all at one time.

With your medication log in hand and the preceding tips fresh in your mind, answer the following questions, then give yourself 48 hours to put your system in place.

1 Times I need to take my medicines

2 Routines I would like to establish for taking my medicines

3 Reminders I will use to take my medicines

4 Places I will keep my medicines

5 Tools I will use to help manage my medicines

6 A reward I will give myself for doing a good job

Adapt your home

Now that you have completed the first two steps of the Breathe Easy Plan you know that you have achieved the right diagnosis of your condition and are taking the most appropriate medicines to treat it. It is time to address the lifestyle and nutrition aspects of the plan. Starting with this step and continuing throughout the rest of the plan, it is largely up to you to take responsibility for the decisions and actions, although your doctor will, of course, monitor your condition and treatment.

Arguably the greatest challenge to your condition is your home. In this step, you will systematically examine your home for allergy 'hot spots' and do everything in your power to eliminate them. Be prepared, though: there is a great deal of cleaning involved, and you may wish to set aside a reasonable amount of money for a new vacuum cleaner, some better bedding and other allergen-fighting aids. For those with serious allergy or asthma problems, it may be time to tackle more radical projects as well, such as getting rid of carpet and replacing it with hard flooring. All of this will take time, effort and money but the reward may be considerable.

What you will be doing

First, you will carry out a top-to-bottom inventory of your house to determine where allergens may be congregating. Then, room by room, you will do a thorough clean-up to get rid of existing allergens and make the rooms less hospitable to allergens in the future.

How you should prepare

Schedule at least one full day to do nothing but a major house inspection and cleaning. Wear comfortable clothes that you won't mind getting dirty. Be prepared to commit to follow-up projects over the next few weekends as well.

What to have on hand

Copies of the logs, questions and charts in this step of the programme. A pen or pencil. Cleaning supplies. A torch.

Home inventory

Go into each room and use this inventory to mark off which allergen-harbouring items and conditions you find there, then use it to determine which rooms to concentrate on and which to tackle first.

Room	Carpet	Wallpaper	Clutter	Mould	Fabric furniture	Odour
Bedroom 1						
Bedroom 2						
Bedroom 3						
Bedroom 4						
Bathroom 1						
Bathroom 2						
Bathroom 3						
Living room						
Family room						
Kitchen						
Dining room						
Home office						
Laundry room						
Attic						
Basement						
Other						

The big clean-up: our best advice

Your task over the next few days or weeks is to clean out allergens in your home, attacking one room at a time. In general, your tasks include:

- Doing a thorough clean to get the room as close as possible to being allergen free.
- Assessing which items in the room are most likely to harbour allergens (use the inventory that you have just filled out) and taking preventative action to keep the allergens at bay. This could be as simple as changing your sheets more frequently or as radical as replacing carpet with tiled, wood, laminate or linoleum flooring.
- Adding accessories, rearranging furniture, and doing other tasks that can greatly aid you in your fight against allergens.

Each house, flat and maisonette is different, and since we can't honestly say whether this project will take two days or two months, we recommend the following. Read all the advice on cleaning your rooms, then go back to your inventory and think through what needs to be done in each room.

Air vents   **Light fittings**   **Dust**   **Dampness**   **Insects**   **Wall hanging(s)**   **Window coverings**

Entrance

You probably don't think much about the entrance to your house in relation to allergies, but it is the gateway to your home and whatever is outside is dragged inside. Here are some suggestions.

- Use a **doormat** made of synthetic material. A mat made out of natural material (such as rope or other fibre) can break down and become a home for mites, mould and fungus, which then become tracked into the house. You should wash all mats weekly.
- Clean out any **dead insects** from your porch lights. As the bodies decompose, they can easily become a source of allergens.
- Put a **shelf or rack** by the front door for footwear and encourage your family and guests to remove their shoes when entering.

This will reduce the amount of dust, mould and other allergens that are brought in on the soles of shoes.
- Keep some **soft slippers** in a basket by the front door for people who don't relish going shoeless, whether it's because they have holes in their socks, they are self-conscious about their feet or the floors are cold.
- If you have **carpeting** in your entrance hall, consider removing it or lay a disposable mat over it and replace it frequently. Ideally you should have a hard floor for easy cleaning.

continued

Bedrooms

First, make sure that your bedroom is in the right place. If your bedroom is in a basement, even one that is properly converted and well insulated, it may be too damp for the amount of time you spend there.

Next, take a look at all the items listed below. They are the worst things to have in your bedroom if you have allergies or asthma.

- **Wall-to-wall carpeting** Wherever possible, replace it with hard flooring and 100 per cent wool rugs that can be washed or dry-cleaned. If you must have fitted carpet, be sure to have it cleaned once a year.
- **Curtains** are dust magnets. Consider replacing them with wipe-clean blinds.
- **Down-filled duvets**
- **Feather anything** (dust mites love feathers).
- **Stuffed animals**
- **Pets** Don't allow dogs or cats into the bedroom at any time, and remember to keep your bedroom door shut so they can't inadvertently get in when you're not around.
- **Overstuffed cupboards** It's time to stop hoarding and have a thorough clear-out (see below for tips).
- **Plants** Ficus (fig) trees in particular may cause allergies in previously nonallergic people.
- **Upholstered headboard** Switch to a metal or wooden bedstead.
- **Piles of pillows and cushions** They look pretty but they are dust-mite magnets. If you keep a few, make sure the filling is synthetic.

Now, start cleaning

- **Tackle the dust** behind the bed and dressers, under the bed, and on top of the ceiling light. Always use a damp cloth; dry cloths simply spread the dust around.
- **Wipe every item** in your room, including books, ornaments, perfume bottles and jewellery boxes, with a damp cloth.
- **Wipe down the walls** and woodwork.
- If you are keeping the **curtains**, wash them in 54°C (130°F) water.
- **Strip the bed** and wash everything, including the duvet or blankets, in 54°C (130°F) water.
- **Vacuum the bed** with a vacuum equipped with a HEPA filter and wipe down the mattress with a damp rag.

And don't forget to...

- **Ventilate** your bedroom on a regular basis to minimize mould growth.
- Use **dust mite barrier** covers on mattresses and pillows in *all* bedrooms, even those whose occupants are not allergic, to keep down the dust mite population in your home.

Wardrobes and cupboards

If you are embarrassed to open your cupboard doors in front of guests, you are likely to be harbouring not only a lot of unnecessary clutter but also a host of allergens.

- Store all your clean clothing in **zippered plastic bags**.
- **Declutter** Give away coats and other clothing that you have not worn in the past year. Put sports equipment where it belongs. Slip shoes into hanging shoe bags, shoeboxes or a shoe rack. When you finish, you should be able to see the cupboard's floor and back wall.
- **Give up mothballs** in favour of cedar chips, or store clean woollens in sealed plastic bags

or airtight containers. You can also place garments in the freezer for several days to kill adult moths and larvae.

- Check **corners and walls** for mould; you may have a leak you have never noticed because it is at the back of a cupboard.
- Check for mould on any **boxes** and other containers stored in the cupboard.

Before switching your clothes each season, **wash or dry-clean** the new season's clothing to get rid of any dust mites that have taken up residence.

If dampness is a problem, and your cupboard has an internal light, put **a 75-watt bulb** in the light fixture and leave it on for long stretches to fight off mould and mildew.

Bathrooms

Hot steam, flushing toilets, soggy toothbrushes – bathrooms are persistently warm and wet, making them the perfect home to mould and mildew.

- Check under and **behind toilets** to make sure there is no mould growing as a result of condensation. Make sure that toilets are installed properly so water doesn't leak into the walls or floors, encouraging mould.
- Check **under the basin** for any leaks and mould. Throw out any damp items.
- Wash the **shower curtain** in hot water once a month or use an inexpensive shower curtain liner that you can replace every couple of months.
- Watch out for the slime that can accumulate in **shower door tracks**; make sure the tracks are cleaned at least every week.
- Check **window sashes** for any mould.

Wash the **bath mat** every week in hot water. The dampness from stepping onto it wet from a shower can attract dust mites and cause mould growth.

Always run the **extractor fan** and/or leave the window and door open when you are having a shower or a bath. You should also check regularly to see whether the duct from the extractor fan is clear.

Check the ceiling If you see any mould appearing, you may not have enough ceiling insulation.

Check your bathroom tiles regularly and regrout as necessary to **prevent leaks** that could lead to mould growth.

Living room and family room

Your everyday living spaces are often filled with fabrics, rugs, curtains and pillows, all of which attract dust. Piles of newspapers, magazines, catalogues, books and toys are also dust and dirt magnets.

- If you have a **wood-burning fireplace** and have asthma, you are better off converting it to electric or using it for decoration only. However well the chimney works, some smoke enters the house, irritating your lungs. Plus, the wood could have mould on it. When it is burned, millions of spores are free to enter the house. Ensure that any gas fireplaces are vented and burning properly to avoid a build-up of soot.

Watch out for candles Although they are romantic and lovely, they can also irritate supersensitive airways (this is especially true of scented types). If you must have candlelight, try electric window candles that use low-wattage bulbs instead of wax and wicks. Or stick with natural, unscented beeswax candles, and be sure they have lead-free wicks. Also,

continued

Task 2 (continued)

avoid candles in jars, which tend to burn unevenly, leaving more soot deposits on walls and floors and thus more potential allergens in the air.

Get rid of your **overstuffed, comfy sofa** and replace it with leather or vinyl. Otherwise, all those hours spent lying on the sofa playing video games, watching TV, reading or dozing will be like pouring petrol on the fire of your allergies.

Follow the advice for cleaning the bedroom, including cleaning under the furniture, dusting all ornaments, wiping down the walls and cleaning the curtains or blinds.

Kitchen and dining room

The problem with these rooms is that there are so many places for allergens to make themselves a home: underneath appliances, inside cabinets and drawers, in nooks and crannies of the floor, around the sink and in the waste bin. It is worth doing all you can to keep your kitchen clean and dry.

Put the contents of all **open boxes of food** in your larder into airtight containers to discourage insects.

Clean out **the refrigerator** regularly using a dilute bleach solution; a refrigerator is a potential mould magnet. You should also try to clean under and behind the refrigerator; any food trapped there can quickly become mouldy. Each time the refrigerator's compressor goes on, the mould spores are blown into the kitchen.

Check **under the sink** as water can leak through fittings and drip under the sink, soaking everything down there and creating a perfect environment for mould.

If you have any **evidence of cockroaches**, contact your local environmental health department who should be able to direct you to a domestic pest control service.

Clean the sides of the **doors of your oven, dishwasher and refrigerator** with a bleach solution. It's surprising how quickly mould

In every room...

- Use a **bright torch and a mirror** to check under furniture and in the corners of cupboards.
- Wipe around any **air-conditioning and heating vents** with a damp cloth.
- Do away with **air fresheners and other fragrances**, which can exacerbate asthma symptoms. If you have unwanted odours in your home, try placing bowls of vinegar in out-of-the-way spots; opening the windows on cool, wind-free days; or leaving a cottonwool ball soaked in vanilla extract in a saucer to absorb odours.
- **Check your houseplants** If you are overwatering them, you may be contributing to mould growth. Often, water leaks through a pot onto the carpet, creating a perfect environment for mould. Also, put pebbles or gravel on top of the soil to prevent mold spores from becoming airborne too easily.
- **Consider replacing any carpet** with solid-surface flooring such as laminate, vinyl or wood.
- Seriously **consider replacing curtains** with blinds that you can wipe clean with a damp cloth.

and grime can accumulate unseen around the edges of your kitchen appliances.

- If you leave a **tablecloth** on your dining room table, replace it weekly, even if you haven't used the table during that time. The cloth gathers dust even if you can't see it.
- Be particularly mindful of dust in the dining room, especially if it is not used very often.

Be sure to dust inside any **china cabinets** as well as outside and underneath.

- **Wash your sponge, kitchen towels and cloths** Their moistness makes them allergen magnets. Kitchen towels should be changed every two days and washed in hot water. Sponges should be bleached or put through the dishwasher every three or four days.

Laundry room

Washing machines generate moisture, and dryers generate steam, dust and heat. Together, they make laundry rooms dirty fast, even if you work hard at neatness.

- Always use **unscented laundry products.**
- Take out any carpet **under the washing machine.** Any leaking will encourage mould that can irritate allergies and asthma. Check and tighten plumbing fittings if necessary.

- Make sure that your **dryer is vented** to the outside. For every load of laundry you dry, 9kg (20lb) of moisture has to go somewhere. If your dryer is vented to the garage or basement you are simply encouraging mould.

Basement or cellar

Each time you enter your basement or cellar, air from it enters your house, particularly warm air, which rises. If they contain mould, those spores can get into the rest of the house. (This is also true if you have an adjoining garage.) The goal is to get rid of any dampness that could lead to mould and mildew growth.

- **Carefully inspect** every part of your basement or cellar for signs of dampness or mould. If you find any, clean the area with a bleach solution. Also try to track down the source of the water.
- Consider **better drainage** for your house if it is located so that rainwater flows down towards it. Creating a gully to drain away the water may be all that is required.
- Check all **fittings around pipes** to make sure that none of them leak, and insulate any that show any condensation.
- Check any **visible insulation** Is it wet or damp? If so, tear it out, find the cause of the dampness, repair it and install replacement insulation. Exposed insulation is also a magnet for pet dander and dust mites. If possible,

cover with foil-covered sheet foam insulation, which absorbs less moisture.

- At least three times a year, **clean the walls** and flooring thoroughly with a brush or cloth. Dust can accumulate in the basement just as easily as in any other part of your house and may be brought, tramped or blown up into the rest of the house.
- Check all **belongings stored in the basement** every month or two. Anything that is placed directly on a concrete floor – such as boxes, newspapers or wood – is subject to mould and rot from condensation. Whenever possible, your should store belongings on shelves or in cupboards.

continued

Task 2 (continued)

Don't store any items of clothing in a bare cellar, even inside containers, if there are any signs of dampness.

If you have **dehumidifiers**, which are an effective way to remove mould-causing moisture from the air, make sure that you periodically vacuum and clean off the coils, which can become dust traps.

Measure the humidity with a hygrometer, available from most hardware stores. You want a reading below 50 per cent.

Make sure that underfloor voids are **well ventilated by air bricks** to prevent floor timbers from being affected by wet or dry rot. These fungal growths release spores, which may trigger an allergic reaction.

Attic/loft

Don't ignore the loft in your whole-house inspection.

Check for any possible **roof leaks** that could eventually soak the inside of interior walls, causing mould. The problem could be individual slates or tiles that have slipped out of position or flashing torn off or dislodged in high winds.

Make sure there is **adequate ventilation** to prevent the build-up of condensation. Check that your insulation is not blocking the eaves.

Check for invaders such as squirrels, mice and their dirt, which could contribute to allergies.

Heating and air-conditioning units

You undoubtedly have a heating system. A few people may have central air conditioning and more of us are using portable units. Make sure that anything that affects the air in your home is clean and efficient.

Cobwebs behind all your radiators The area behind central heating radiators inevitably accumulates cobwebs, which trap dust, dead insects and fine debris that can easily give rise to mould spores and other allergens.

The 'fins' at the back of modern radiators are particularly tricky to clean and these are also areas where dust and dead insects can collect. You may be able to suck out some dust with one of the attachments on your vacuum cleaner or you could try fashioning your own spiral brush cleaner by twisting strips of cloth around a coat hanger.

Keep the thermostat at 18°C (65°F) or higher in winter as heat prevents mould. Turning off heating at night can encourage mould growth in the damper air and may also

prove a false economy in very cold weather as the system has to work harder to reheat the house when it has cooled right down.

If your house has a **central air-conditioning** unit, have it inspected and cleaned regularly. These units are perfect breeding grounds for mould and fungus.

If buying a portable air conditioner, **ensure you get the correct size** for the area you wish to cool. If it is too big, your home could feel damp and humid (which can encourage mould) instead of cool and refreshing. Take advice from the manufacturer about the cooling capacity of different models.

Check the instructions on your portable air-conditioner and ensure you maintain it properly and keep all the vents dust free.

Outside your home

Finally, make sure that the outside of your house is not contributing to allergies. Below are a few tips. Also check for mould, rotted wood, perpetually wet spots and holes or cracks in the foundations.

Keep **gutters clear** to stop water penetrating the walls which can encourage mould. Ensure they all have downpipes with the shoe pointing outwards so that water flows into the gully.

Check the gutters when it rains You shouldn't see water leaking out of the end caps, flowing on the outside, or dripping behind the gutters – all of which could indicate damage or blockages.

Minimizing allergens in your home: a planning guide

Use this log to help you to plan and organize your tasks. 'Projects' refers to major efforts such as removing carpet, reupholstering furniture or hiring an expert to leakproof your basement. 'Purchases' could range from new bedding or window blinds to a shoe rack by your front door. 'When?' is the column in which to target when you intend to start the work.

Room	Cleaning time needed	Project(s)	Purchases(s)	When?
Bedroom 1				
Bedroom 2				
Bedroom 3				
Bedroom 4				
Bathroom 1				
Bathroom 2				
Bathroom 3				
Living room				
Family room				
Kitchen				
Dining room				
Home office				
Laundry room				
Attic				
Basement				
Other				

Eat to beat allergies and asthma

Health and nutrition are inextricably linked, and the relationship is both negative and positive. Improper eating habits can cause health problems or make most health problems worse. Perhaps more important, eating the right foods can help to alleviate many health problems, including asthma and allergies.

This chapter explains how to change your diet to include more of the foods that can improve your condition, either directly or indirectly, and fewer foods that studies suggest may exacerbate allergies and asthma. However, this is not an eating plan for anyone with food allergies. If you have food allergies, or even sensitivities, as described in chapter 5, you need to eliminate the problem foods from your diet.

The general plan

First, you will assess whether your diet is helping or aggravating your condition. Next, you need to consider your weight. Do you need to lose a few pounds? If so, we explain how to do so. Then you will look at what's in your cupboards and refrigerator, and make sure you are stocking foods that can help your asthma and allergies. Finally, we explain the basic tenets of healthy eating and how to integrate them into your daily life.

How to prepare

Re-reading chapter 9 will certainly help. And since you will be cleaning out unhealthy foods from your kitchen and replacing them with healthier alternatives, you should set aside a day to clean out your larder and refrigerator. Most of all, you need an open mind and a positive attitude. Food habits are difficult to change, and the results are not always tangible or measurable. You need to be committed: the benefits are real.

What to have on hand

Copies of the questions and lists in this chapter. A pen or pencil. A dustbin for collecting any foods you no longer need. A budget for buying new, healthier food staples.

Assess your eating habits

In chapter 9, we discussed five primary ways that food and dietary habits can aggravate or improve allergies or asthma. They include:

1 **Weight** Studies have found that carrying extra pounds may trigger asthma symptoms and make asthma worse.

2 **Heartburn** Studies have also shown a clear link between asthma and heartburn, known as gastro-oesophageal reflux disease (GORD).

3 **The right fats** Certain polyunsaturated fats (omega-6s) promote inflammation; others (omega-3s) fight inflammation. Inflammation is a major problem in both allergies and asthma.

4 **Probiotics** Research suggests that having the proper level of digestive bacteria can help your body to create cells important in the battle against asthma.

5 **Antioxidants** Finally, studies show that antioxidants help to fight inflammation inside your body, an important factor in controlling allergies and asthma.

So how does your diet fare in these five categories? The answer, for most people, is hardly obvious. Not many of us can say which foods contain probiotics or which cooking oils have omega-3 fats rather than omega-6 fats. Answering the questions below will help you to sort it out.

Is my diet aggravating or helping my allergies or asthma?

Answer each of these true/false questions, then look at the end of the quiz for the healthier answers and the reasons why they are healthier.

1 You ate yoghurt at least three times last week.   TRUE ☐   FALSE ☐

2 You ate at least two servings of red or purple foods yesterday.   TRUE ☐   FALSE ☐

3 You have eaten salmon at least once in the past week.   TRUE ☐   FALSE ☐

4 The last three times you sautéed any food, you used olive oil   TRUE ☐   FALSE ☐

5 You can't remember the last time you bought a bottle of antacids.   TRUE ☐   FALSE ☐

6 You can no longer wear a favourite old belt because it has become too small.   TRUE ☐   FALSE ☐

7 Your idea of a balanced meal is a fried steak with chips followed by a couple of bought almond slices.   TRUE ☐   FALSE ☐

8 You count fried onions and chips as vegetables.   TRUE ☐   FALSE ☐

9 You drink more carbonated drinks than water each day.   TRUE ☐   FALSE ☐

10 You can count on one hand the number of green vegetables you enjoy eating.   TRUE ☐   FALSE ☐

continued

Task 1 (continued)

11 Part of your afternoon routine at work is a trip to the vending machine for a snack. TRUE ☐ FALSE ☐

12 Your breakfast is usually built around a Danish pastry, doughnut or croissant. TRUE ☐ FALSE ☐

THE RESULTS Hopefully, your answers match ours below. If not, you have some work to do, and you should read this chapter very carefully.

1 True Studies suggest that gut-friendly, live bacterial cultures contained in natural or bio yoghurt may have a beneficial effect on asthma.

2 True Red peppers, tomatoes, radishes, red onions and other colourful vegetables are particularly rich in the antioxidants you need to help fight the inflammation so common with asthma and allergies.

3 True Omega-3 fatty acids, which have strong anti-inflammatory properties, are particularly abundant in oily fish such as salmon, mackerel, swordfish and tuna.

4 True If you used other oils, such as sunflower and rapeseed oil, they are rich in omega-6 fats, which may spark inflammation.

5 True If you are taking antacids on a regular basis you may have gastro-oesophageal reflux disease (GORD), which is known to exacerbate asthma. Pay special attention to the section on heartburn-free eating.

6 False If you are replacing belts and other clothing because you have gained weight lately, pay special attention to the section on weight loss. Studies have found that being overweight can significantly exacerbate asthma.

7 False If you are really eating like this, you are consuming too much fat and omega-6 fatty acids, which are known to increase inflammation. A nutritionally balanced diet that includes plenty of fruits and vegetables has been shown to improve asthma symptoms.

8 True Of course both are vegetables but both are fried. For maximum nutritional benefit, the vegetables you eat, which should include green leafy vegetables as well, should be as close to their natural state as possible.

9 False Carbonated drinks are filled with sugar, making them very high in calories, and carbonation (even in diet sodas) can upset your stomach. They also cost a lot. Water is the perfect liquid for health – and from a tap, it's almost free.

10 False This is a difficult one. The average UK diet includes only a few green vegetables: peas, broccoli, green beans, lettuce, and perhaps some slices of green pepper. From artichokes to courgettes, from pak choi to chard, there are so many vegetables that most of us don't eat, and they're among the most healthy foods.

11 False As we will discuss later, too many of us eat out of habit or boredom, not hunger. Habitual eating is one of the big contributors to the UK's weight problems. There are better ways to take an afternoon break than eating a chocolate bar. Try taking a brief walk outside, for example.

12 False This is another difficult one. While a carbohydrate food should form part of a healthy breakfast, it should be wholegrain and high in fibre. Instead, the breakfast foods listed in this question are made with refined wheat, and many are filled with inflammatory omega-6 fatty acids, dangerous trans fatty acids and calorie-boosting sweeteners.

Address your weight

The next phase in this step of the Breathe Easy Plan is to determine whether you need to lose weight. One way to do this is to use the Body Mass Index (BMI), a method of classifying body fat content based on height and weight. Your BMI number, essentially indicates whether you are carrying a healthy or unhealthy level of body fat and is a more useful and accurate measure than weight alone.

To find your BMI number on the chart below locate your weight in the column on the left. Then scan the horizontal row of numbers to find your height (or the number closest to it). Then look at the shaded areas to discover within which range your number comes.

A BMI of 25 to 29 means that you could be up to 20 per cent overweight, and a BMI over 30 indicates medical obesity, which is considered a disease that should be treated by a doctor. Your goal should be to have a BMI below 25.

Although it provides a useful guide to levels of excess body weight, the BMI is not foolproof. It gives you a very wide target range for your weight, since it does not factor in different body types.

Body Mass Index (BMI) Chart

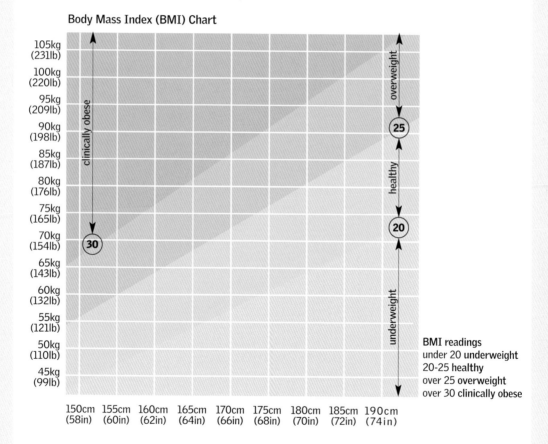

BMI readings
under 20 **underweight**
20-25 **healthy**
over 25 **overweight**
over 30 **clinically obese**

REMEMBER Losing even a few pounds when you are overweight will make you healthier. Not only can it alleviate your asthma or allergies, it can also reduce your risk of conditions such as heart disease and diabetes. If you have a long way to go to reach a BMI of 24, set some milestones for the road ahead. And don't forget to reward yourself along the way. Every lost pound is significant.

The golden rules of weight loss

Weight loss can be reduced to a simple formula: burn more calories in a day than you consume. One pound of fat equals about 3,500 calories (or, more strictly, 'kilocalories'). So for every 3,500 calories you eat above the amount you burn, you gain a pound. The reverse is also true: If you burn 3,500 more calories than you eat, you lose a pound.

Popular diet programmes such as the Atkins Diet tend to be based on the deeper science of how the body digests, burns and stores different nutrients. At the end of the day, however, they all come back to the fundamental truth: burn more calories than you consume. The main ways to do that are by increasing your activity levels and by taking in fewer calories. The best weight-loss efforts combine both..

Here are 10 rules to start you off on the path to permanent weight loss.

1 Increase physical activity

Most people find it easier to cut down on calorie intake than to burn calories. And in truth, it takes a lot of exercise to lose a pound. Rigorous exercise burns about 500 calories an hour. Cut out a few snacks, and you have achieved the same calorie deficit as you would if you spent an hour on a bicycle. But exercise is also well worth the effort as it brings huge benefits. It reduces appetite. It builds muscle that burns more calories around the clock. It strengthens your heart and lungs. It makes you look and feel better. It's fun. It makes you more energetic. It lifts your mood. And yes, it definitely helps you to lose weight. So if you put away the biscuits and go for a walk instead, you skip hundreds of calories of unneeded food and burn off a few hundred calories as well. That's a double win.

2 Halve all portions

Whether you eat at home or in a restaurant, immediately halve the amount on your plate, in the takeaway bag, and so on. Arguably, the worst food trend of recent decades has been the explosion in portion sizes on our dinner plates (and breakfast and lunch plates, too). We eat far, far more today than our bodies need. Indeed, studies have found that if you serve people more food, they will eat more food, regardless of their hunger levels. This is another reason to avoid self-serve buffets. Remember, too, that portion sizes on food labels are only a guide and are sometimes over-generous.

3 Stick to water

Soft drinks are a major source of extra calories. In 2004 UK soft drink consumption totalled 13.7 billion litres, a 10 per cent increase on the previous year. Fizzy drinks are a major hidden source of calories: a single can contains seven teaspoons of sugar, equivalent to 142 calories – although 'diet' or 'light' versions have significantly fewer. Given that it takes 3,500 calories to gain or lose a pound of fat, if you are a regular soft drink consumer you could probably lose several pounds a year simply by switching to calorie-free water instead of soft drinks.

4 Eat at home

You are more likely to eat more – and eat more high-fat, high-calorie foods – when you eat out than when you eat at home. Restaurants now tend to serve much larger portions than they did 20 or 30 years ago.

5 Feast on fibre

High-fibre foods – beans, vegetables, fruits and whole grains – fill you up faster and keep you full for longer than simple carbohydrates such as doughnuts, ice cream and potato chips. Make high-fibre foods the centrepiece of your meals and save the sugary snacks for infrequent special occasions.

6 Avoid white foods

There is some scientific legitimacy to today's lower-carbohydrate diets. Large amounts of simple carbohydrates in your diet can wreak havoc on your blood sugar levels and lead to weight gain. But don't go to the extremes that some protein-based weight-loss diets call for. Instead, follow a simple rule. Avoid the most popular 'white' starches – refined sugar, white rice, refined flour and pasta – and instead eat whole grain breads, brown rice and, in general, fewer sweet foods.

7 Plan, plan, plan

If you plan your meals, you are less likely to tear open a package of crisps an hour before dinner. This goes for when you are out and about as well. Stock your desk at work with healthy snacks and carry a small cool bag in your car with cut-up fruit and vegetables and low-fat cheese sticks so you won't be tempted by sweets at the petrol station when hunger pangs hit.

8 Eat when you are hungry

It's surprising how much we all eat out of boredom, nervousness, habit, frustration or even celebration. Likewise, we eat (and drink) as a social activity, as a way to show love, and as a social custom. What these situations too rarely involve, however, is hunger. Arguably, the best thing you can do to consume fewer calories is to eat for fuel and health and skip all those other eating opportunities. After all, you don't need food to calm yourself, enjoy a party, show your love or make a problem go away. You are strong enough to do all that on your own.

9 Track what you eat

Studies have found that people who keep food diaries of everything that they eat or drink are more likely to lose weight and keep it off than those who don't. Just remember, if you cheat and don't write down what you are eating, the only one who loses out is you.

10 Think life, not diet

The best weight-loss efforts are those that are sustainable for a lifetime. They include habits such as eating more vegetables, taking exercise and eliminating habitual snacking. The problem with 12-week crash diets is the 13th week. If you haven't learned sensible long-term habits, you are almost certain to regain your lost weight.

The Breathe Easy Eating Plan

By now, you have probably realized that eating well for allergies and asthma is similar to following a normal healthy balanced diet. The Breathe Easy eating plan is essentially about eating reasonable portions of whole grain foods, lean proteins, and fruits and vegetables. The primary addition to a standard healthy diet is an emphasis on probiotic foods, as well as foods containing omega-3 fatty acids.

The plan is divided into three parts: A cupboard and refrigerator clean-up, a restocking, and 12 guidelines for making food decisions. But there is one final matter that you may have to deal with before you can begin.

You are probably not the only person eating in your home. You and your family need to decide whether your change to a healthier diet is a solo effort or one that involves everyone. Don't make assumptions. This should be discussed with everyone who is affected. At the first opportunity when you're all eating together, try to explain how important this is to you. Tell them that your bid to change your eating pattern is part of your battle against your allergies and asthma and (if necessary) is also an attempt to lose some weight. Tell them all what this will mean – less junk food, more vegetables, and so on. And, most importantly, invite the rest of the family to join your personal crusade.

Once that issue has been decided, apply the following steps to either the whole household's food supply or just yours.

1 Clean out your kitchen

Plan to do this on the day before your rubbish is collected. Bring a dustbin lined with a strong bin bag into the kitchen for food you are going to throw out, along with a sturdy box or two in which to put unopened cans and packages that you can give away. Start with your larder, then move to the refrigerator and freezer. Throw out or give away:

High-salt processed foods, including canned soups and stews, prepackaged rice dishes, frozen vegetables in sauce, and so on. Check the labels for salt or sodium content.

Packaged snacks and sweets This includes biscuits, potato crisps, sweets, cheese crackers, and other such foods.

Any and all food that you have kept in your larder, refrigerator or freezer for more than six months. Make no exceptions.

White breads and any other baked goods made with bleached or refined flour.

Margarine It contains trans fatty acids.

Large containers of vegetable oil You will be using olive oil as your primary cooking oil, so keep only enough sunflower or other vegetable oil on hand for those few recipes in which it is really necessary.

Carbonated and other sweetened drinks, such as bottled juices and iced tea.

When you have finished your major clear-out, tie up the garbage bag and take it out to the dustbin. Load the box of food that you plan to give away into your car boot. Consider spending an hour or two thoroughly cleaning your larder and refrigerator now that they have been purged of unwanted food.

2 Go shopping

It's time to refill the space that you cleared out. This is an opportunity not only to stock up on healthier foods but also to begin a meal-planning effort. Before you go shopping, take a pencil and paper and answer the following questions, then add your own items to our recommendations.

- How many dinners do you need to buy supplies for on this shopping trip? Be sure to pick up a lean protein food and at least one vegetable for each dinner.
- What raw vegetables will your family eat? One of the best tricks for healthier meals is to put a plate of them on the table at every meal. Stock up on cucumbers, carrots, sweet peppers, celery and tomatoes. Add a bowl of low-fat dressing for dipping, and you will be astonished how quickly those carrot sticks and pepper strips disappear.

- If each person in your home eats three, four or five servings of fruit a day, how many apples, pears, bananas or other fruits do you need to buy? And don't forget citrus fruits, a good source of the antioxidant vitamin C.
- If you have banned junk food from the house, but everyone gets hungry at 8pm, what do you want them to eat? Remember, snacking is healthy; the problem arises when the only available snacks are junk food. Consider buying healthy (low-fat, low-sugar) cereal bars, extra fruit or some pots of low-fat yoghurt.

Your shopping list

MEAL FOODS

- Fresh salmon (enough for one dinner)
- Mackerel or another type of oily fish, such as swordfish, fresh tuna or herring (enough for one dinner)
- Five different cooking vegetables (two of them should be dark green, leafy types)
- Five different nibbling vegetables
- Salad greens
- Whole grain breads
- _____
- _____

LARDER STAPLES

- Olive oil
- Canned tuna
- Anchovies
- Dried fruit
- Onions

- Garlic
- Canned and dried beans
- Black or green tea
- Low-sodium or sodium-free soups, sauces and other processed or canned foods
- A bottle of red wine
- _____
- _____

REFRIGERATOR STAPLES

- Six different fruits (including apples)
- Live-culture yoghurt (any flavour)
- Bags of frozen vegetables
- Bags of frozen prawns (if no one is allergic to shellfish)
- Semi-skimmed or other low-fat milk
- Butter
- _____
- _____

continued

Task 4 (continued)

3 Eat according to the Breathe Easy Plan

Without further ado, here are the basic rules of healthy eating. These apply for promoting general health, weight loss and relief from allergies and asthma.

1 Cook only with **olive oil and other mono-unsaturated fats**.

2 Use **butter**, not margarine, when you need a spread. Or choose a cholesterol-lowering spread such as Benecol.

3 Have one meal a day that consists mainly of **vegetables**, with a small amount of lean protein. This could be canned chicken mixed into dark salad greens, ratatouille over wholewheat pasta with grated Parmesan cheese, or vegetable lasagne.

4 Include **beans or pulses** at least three times a week.

5 **Have fish** at least three times a week. Canned tuna counts, as does spaghetti sauce with plenty of omega-3–rich anchovies. If you have no adverse reaction to shellfish, make prawns a weekly dinner staple. If you simply can't eat fish, begin taking daily fish-oil supplements to provide at least 1g of omega-3 fatty acids a day or look out for the new varieties of milk that contain omega-3 fats.

6 **Avoid any food that lists sugar** among the first four ingredients on the label. Look out for sugar-free varieties of foods such as ketchup, mayonnaise and salad dressing in the diabetic foods section of supermarkets.

7 Choose foods that are as **close to their natural state** as possible: fresh fruit and vegetables; fresh meat, fish, chicken and eggs; raw nuts and seeds; and fresh salad greens. Work on the assumption that the more preparation and packaging that were done at a factory, the more healthy ingredients have been removed and unhealthy ingredients added.

8 Choose **whole grain breads and pasta**. Make sure the first ingredient listed on the label is whole grain flour or whole wheat flour. You will know it is really whole grain bread if it has at least 3 or 4 grams of fibre per slice. Don't be fooled by colour, either: Some companies use molasses or artificial colourings to make their breads look like 'whole wheat' even if they are not.

9 For snacks choose fresh **vegetables** and **fruit**, raw **nuts**, low-fat **cheeses** and other healthy foods.

10 **Cut your salt intake** Substitute herbs and spices to provide flavour or use 'lite' salt. Don't add salt at the table.

11 At least three times a week, eat a portion of **live-culture yoghurt** for its beneficial acidophilus bacteria. If you can't bear yoghurt, take acidophilus supplements, widely available in drugstores and health food stores.

12 At breakfast, drink natural fruit juice, low-fat milk, tea or coffee, but for the rest of the day **focus on water** (you should aim to drink eight glasses a day). For a treat, have a glass of wine with dinner.

Increase your resistance

In simple terms, allergies – and in many cases, asthma – are caused by flawed responses by your immune system. It would make sense, then, to infer that taking good care of your immune system can have a beneficial effect on your condition.

In fact, that is true. Research shows that having an inefficient immune system increases your chances of allergic reactions or asthma attacks. While it is impossible to transform it and make your allergies or asthma go away, you can certainly reduce the chances of attacks if you have a balanced immune system.

There are various strategies you can adopt to help put your immune system into balance and increase its efficiency. The supplements suggested in step 2 can do it, as can the healthy diet outlined in step 4. But here in step 5, we will focus on a few other key strategies, namely reducing stress, increasing physical activity and bolstering your attitude.

Stress reduction is one of those topics that can often make people more stressed. Who has time to relax in today's world? But we are sure that after completing the worksheets and absorbing the tips in the following pages, you will be pleasantly surprised at how easy it can be to defuse the stress that is harming your body.

What you will be doing

There are eight phases to this step. The first is easy. It is simply a lesson you need to read and absorb. The rest require you to fill out a form or take at least one action. We suggest that you take a week or two to give each phase an honest effort. Habits require about three weeks to take hold, so keep up with your chosen actions as best you can.

How you should prepare

Reread the section in chapter 10 on relaxation techniques. Make note of any that appeal to you more than others.

What to have on hand

A blank journal, copies of the questions and logs in this step, and writing implements.

Lesson: the stress-immunity connection

Have you ever caught a cold just after meeting a tight deadline at work? At the end of a week in which the children were especially trying, have you ever gone down with flu or digestive trouble?

If you answered yes to either question, you have experienced firsthand the effects of stress on your immune system and your health. Research shows that each year 12 million adults see their GPs with mental health problems. Most suffer from anxiety and depression, and much of it is stress related. About 45 million working days are lost each year in the UK through anxiety and stress-related conditions, costing industry more than £3,000 million.

Numerous studies have also found that chronic stress can exacerbate both allergies and asthma. The more stress you are exposed to, the more difficult it is to control your asthma and the more likely you are to have allergy-caused eczema.

Now, when we say stress, we don't mean the kind of acute stress that you experience when you are involved in a car accident (although acute stress may well bring on an asthma attack). Rather, it's the kind of grinding, daily stress that may have become so much a part of your life that you barely even notice it any more. This type of chronic stress arises from stressors such as living from pay cheque to pay cheque, coping with a chronic health condition (such as asthma), dealing with challenging children, arguing regularly with your spouse, starting a new job or continuing in one that you hate.

Each time you are confronted with a stressor, your body releases a cascade of stress hormones such as adrenaline and cortisol. They in turn send a volley of signals to various parts of your body to prepare it for action. For instance, your liver releases glucose to provide instant energy to muscle cells. Your lungs expand to take in more oxygen, your heart beats faster, your blood pressure rises to send more oxygen-rich blood throughout your body, and your bowel and intestinal muscles contract.

It is a strong reaction, based on ancient wiring that says your response to stress should be physical: fighting, running or threatening. If this reaction takes place day in and day out without physical release, it leads to common stress-related conditions ranging from chronic high blood pressure, angina and gastric reflux to constipation.

Research by Asthma UK shows that 69 per cent of people with asthma say that stress triggers their symptoms. There is also evidence that children exposed to domestic violence and those with high levels of traumatic stress have a higher risk of asthma and other diseases; that psychological stress can affect respiratory sensation and perceptions of breathlessness; and that among college students the stress associated with final examinations increases asthma severity.

A recent Cochrane review of a number of studies concludes that emotional stress can either precipitate or exacerbate both acute and chronic asthma, and that stress-relieving relaxation therapy can be beneficial.

Identify your anxiety triggers

A. How stressful is your life?

Before you can begin to reduce the stress in your life or moderate how you react to stress, you need to pinpoint the triggers. Take a few minutes to work through the following questions.

1 The worst part of my day is:
- [ ] a. None; I love all parts of my day
- [ ] b. Daytime, dealing with work
- [ ] c. Morning or evening, dealing with home and family

2 I can feel the muscles in the back of my neck and shoulders tense up:
- [ ] a. Rarely
- [ ] b. Whenever something goes wrong
- [ ] c. When I'm feeling under lots of pressure

3 I would describe our financial situation as:
- [ ] a. Comfortable
- [ ] b. Tenuous
- [ ] c. Frightening

4 I find myself yelling at my children:
- [ ] a. Never
- [ ] b. At least once a week
- [ ] c. Several times a day

5 My spouse and I:
- [ ] a. Have a solid, close relationship
- [ ] b. Coexist, with little in common any more besides the children and bills
- [ ] c. Fight nearly every day

6 Every day when I walk into work, I:
- [ ] a. Am happy to be there
- [ ] b. Get a sinking feeling in my stomach
- [ ] c. Inevitably get a headache or stomach ache

7 When it comes to my job, I:
- [ ] a. Feel as if I have a fair amount of control over what I do and when I do it
- [ ] b. Feel as if I'm constantly up against one deadline after another
- [ ] c. Feel that I'm entirely at the mercy of others' needs and wants

8 When I look at myself in the mirror, I feel:
- [ ] a. Pretty good; I'm not doing badly for someone my age
- [ ] b. That I could lose about a stone
- [ ] c. As if I'm looking at a stranger

9 I am caring for:
- [ ] a. My spouse and children
- [ ] b. Just myself
- [ ] c. My spouse, children and ageing parents or other relatives, not to mention the neighbourhood children and several-needy friends

10 My weekends are spent:
- [ ] a. Relaxing and doing things I enjoy
- [ ] b. Running errands, cleaning the house, and taxi-ing the children
- [ ] c. Catching up on all the office work that I didn't manage to get done during the week, plus doing the ironing, cleaning the house and shopping

THE RESULTS The more 'b' and 'c' answers you have, the more likely it is that stress is having an effect on your health, including your asthma or allergies. Optimally, you should have at least seven 'a' answers.

continued

Task 2 (continued)

B. And how is the stress affecting you?

We all have to face challenges during our lives. The question is, how do we deal with them? Do we face them with confidence, or do they get us down? Listed below are various psychological and physical signs of stress. How many do you have? Answer truthfully.

Psychological signs of stress

1 Are you often nervous or anxious?
   YES ☐   NO ☐

2 Do you often feel depressed or sad?
   YES ☐   NO ☐

3 Are you often irritable or moody?
   YES ☐   NO ☐

4 Do you often become frustrated?
   YES ☐   NO ☐

5 Are you forgetful?   YES ☐   NO ☐

6 Do you have trouble thinking clearly?
   YES ☐   NO ☐

7 Can you make decisions without agonizing?
   YES ☐   NO ☐

8 Is it difficult to learn new information?
   YES ☐   NO ☐

9 Do you have insomnia?   YES ☐   NO ☐

10 Are you often plagued by negative
    thoughts?   YES ☐   NO ☐

11 Are you fidgety?   YES ☐   NO ☐

12 Are you accident-prone?   YES ☐   NO ☐

13 Do you bite your fingernails or cuticles?
    YES ☐   NO ☐

THE RESULTS Again, there is no rigorous scale here. Generally, the more *yes* answers you ticked, the more likely it is that stress is having a bad effect on your life. You should be concerned if you had more than three *yes* answers.

Physical signs of stress

The following physical symptoms, if chronic, may be signs of ongoing anxiety or stress problems. If your answers to the previous quizzes show that stress is a big issue in your life, and you are experiencing any of the following, it may be time to ask your doctor if the two are indeed related.

- Back pain
- Muscle tension
- Headaches
- Tremor of hands
- Diarrhoea
- Constipation
- Pounding heart
- Chest pain

- Sweaty, cold hands
- Shortness of breath
- Indigestion or gas pains
- Constant burping
- A burning sensation in your chest
- Feeling faint or dizzy
- A lingering head cold

- Ringing in the ears
- Grinding your teeth
- Hives or skin rashes
- Loss of appetite
- Feeling nauseated or vomiting
- Stomach pain

Identify your stress busters

What do you do when you're feeling stressed? Reach for a cigarette or a glass of wine? Go for a jog? Take a nap? Do you get depressed or find yourself energized to get twice as much done? How you react to your stress is an important clue to whether you are handling the stress or the stress is handling you. For the next week or two, complete this log to achieve a sense of what you are doing to cope with the stress in your life.

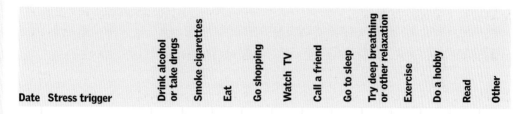

Date	Stress trigger	Drink alcohol or take drugs	Smoke cigarettes	Eat	Go shopping	Watch TV	Call a friend	Go to sleep	Try deep breathing or other relaxation	Exercise	Do a hobby	Read	Other

THE RESULTS If there are more ticks in the first five coping technique columns, your stress is handling you. These are not constructive ways to deal with stress; instead, they are unhealthy masking techniques. Read on to discover healthier ways to handle stress, as well as some simple steps you can take to reduce the most common stressors in your life.

Exercise

Your task is to integrate at least 10 minutes of high-energy movement into your day. Every day. Without exception.

Why? Study after study has shown the health benefits of moderate physical activity, including increased resistance to infectious disease. Even if exercise triggers your asthma, there are plenty of ways to get your body moving without causing attacks.

If you read health books and magazines, you will know that most health experts recommend taking 30 minutes of exercise a day if you want measurable improvements in muscle tone and cardiovascular function. And they are right. But in order to achieve 30 minutes a day, you must first be active for 10 minutes – and for most people, getting to those first 10 minutes is the most difficult part of all.

The topic of exercise can become enormously complicated. There are so many types, so many muscles, so much gear, so much sweat, so much spandex, and so many excuses. We prefer to reduce all this down to a few simple edicts.

- **There are no excuses** Just get moving.
- **There are no rules** Do whatever gets you moving. Wear whatever you feel comfortable in. Exercise wherever you like.
- **There are no measurements** You should simply exercise so that you breathe a little harder than normal, but not so hard that you can't talk.

Your simple goal is to move actively for at least 10 minutes a day. Out of that, an exercise habit or a hobby or even a passion could be born in time. Until then, don't complicate things. Here are a few suggestions to help you to get started.

Go for a walk There is no better choice than taking an energetic walk after lunch, for an afternoon break, or after dinner. For people who aren't interested in rigorous exercise programmes, walking is perfect.

Do a stretching routine Find a health book with a thorough, full-body stretching routine and practise it until you have it memorized. Pilates exercises are a good choice to help posture, chest expansion and abdominal muscles. Do the routine in the morning, before dinner or before bed.

Work out with stretch bands A pair of exercise-grade stretch bands is excellent for strengthening muscles, stretching your body and burning calories – and they are so much more fun than weights.

Dance Most of us listen to music at home. Commit to dancing to at least two songs every day. Dancing alone is also fun.

Do calisthenics in front of the TV Watch the evening news standing up. Do stretches, jumping jacks, simulated weight lifts, marching on the spot or shadow boxing.

Relax

This is where the techniques described in chapter 10 come in handy. Pick one technique from the list below, then find a class, practitioner, video or book and commit to doing it at least once a week.

- Yoga
- Tai chi
- Professional massage
- Biofeedback
- Meditation
- Progressive relaxation
- Hypnosis

If none of the above techniques appeal to you, make a commitment to do much more of the following each day. Although there are no studies directly linking them to a reduction in allergy or asthma symptoms, they have been shown to reduce stress hormones.

Sing Studies have found that singing, particularly choral singing, results in lower levels of the stress hormone cortisol.

Laugh It costs nothing, and it really works. When researchers divided 33 healthy adult women into two groups and had one watch a humorous video while the other viewed a tourism video, not only did those who laughed experience a drop in their stress levels, but their immune function increased when compared with that of the women watching the tourism video.

Enjoy your pet Numerous studies attest to the stress-relieving benefits of pets. In one, researchers evaluated the heart health of 240 couples, half of whom owned a pet. People with pets had significantly lower heart rates and blood pressure levels when exposed to stressors than those who were petless. In fact, pets worked even better than spouses at buffering stress. If you are allergic to dogs or cats, try a turtle or even a fish.

Whatever pet you decide on, test it out on a trial basis first to ensure that it doesn't aggravate your allergies or asthma.

Find inner calm Studies suggest that people who attend church regularly have stronger immune systems. This is one reason, researchers suggest, that other studies have found regular churchgoers to have better physical health overall. It makes sense when you think about it: sitting in a church or temple is like meditating. It is quiet and peaceful.

Love We're not talking about sex here, but about hugging, holding hands, giving compliments, playing with children, looking at the stars together, eating out together, forgiving, teasing, pillow fighting, sharing. Isn't this what really matters most? If you find you can share warmth and love with your family and friends, then you will have made a major step towards conquering stress.

Keep a journal

You wouldn't think that the simple act of writing down your thoughts for 10 minutes or so a day could affect your health, but it does. A 1999 study published in the *Journal of the American Medical Association* found that people with asthma who wrote about their most stressful life event showed a 19 per cent improvement on a lung function test, an improvement that lasted up to four months after the experiment ended.

You don't have to be a Hemingway to write in your journal. You simply have to find a quiet spot, uncap your pen (or start up your computer) and begin. Write about your day, listing not only what you did but also how you felt about what you did. Write about your dream last night. Write about your plans for the weekend, your fears about work and your hopes for your children. If you find that you have writer's block, try the following phrases to get started.

I am eager to

I am worried about

I did well at

I'm proud of myself because

The best thing that happened today was

I am so grateful for

I can solve a problem by

I feel my aim should be to

In my dreams, I

I believe in myself because

I wish I could

I am happiest when

I hope to

Develop a positive attitude

Are you a glass-half-full or a glass-half-empty kind of person? If you're the latter, you are probably exposing your body to far greater levels of stress hormones than if you're the former. This final phase of the Breathe Easy stress-busting plan concentrates on how you can develop a positive view of the world around you.

The whole idea of positive psychology (a fancy name for optimism and personal resilience) is a relatively new concept in the mental health field, but it is one with a growing body of evidence to support it. In a nutshell, researchers find that people with inner resilience – that is, an ability to cope with and overcome the many challenges that life throws at them – can form a shield against the harmful effects of stress.

Developing resilience is an extremely personal matter, and not something that lends itself to a formal programme. All we can ask is that you work at it – constantly. After all, being happy is better than being sad, isn't it? Not only does resilience help your life to become more important, more hallowed, more uplifting, but indirectly it helps your allergies and asthma.

Listed below are some thoughts that will help you to develop your personal resilience *before* a crisis hits you.

- **Appreciate all you do** instead of worrying about all that remains to be done.
- **Foster your sense of humour** If you can laugh at a situation rather than getting angry, you will automatically reduce your stress hormone levels.
- **Realize that you have choices** in your life and that there are always second chances. You don't have to handle everything perfectly the first time.
- **Remind yourself** that even the very worst situation, event or feeling eventually passes.
- **Reframe reality, don't ignore it** That means considering yourself to be a capable person, even if you have made mistakes or have constraints. The vision of yourself as strong empowers you, enabling you to feel less stressed and overwhelmed when crises or problems do occur and thus protecting your health. One study found that how women *perceive* stress can affect health as much as major stressors such as poverty. The researchers asked women to rank themselves on a picture of a ladder representing where people stood in society economically, with those who were best off at the top and those who were worst off at the bottom. Women who perceived themselves as being lower on the ladder, regardless of their actual socio-economic status, had more stress hormones than women at the same socio-economic level who perceived themselves as being higher.

So there you have it: a plan to not only reduce the stress *in* your life but also to modify how you react to that stress and arm yourself against its adverse effects on your health. All of this will greatly help to alleviate your allergies and asthma – and bring many additional benefits.

Live to beat allergies and asthma

We have covered plenty of ground so far in the Breathe Easy Plan, from medications and diet to home cleaning and stress relief. In this step, we provide advice to help you to cope with your allergies and asthma 365 days a year, 24 hours a day, no matter where you are or what time of year it is. We also point you towards tried and tested allergy-related products that could help to improve your quality of life.

What you will be doing

This step is similar to step 3, in which we asked you to go through your home room by room and make changes to help your condition. This time, though, we focus on six scenarios or locations beyond your daily life at home. They are your garden, your car, your workplace, travel, the Christmas holidays and the seasons. For each of these areas, we offer the best tips we know for managing your allergies or asthma. Find the ones most appropriate to your situation, then act on them.

How you should prepare

Rethink where you spend your time and where allergies and asthma tend to flare up most. You may wish to review some of the forms you filled out in part 1 to help you focus on the most problematic areas. Then, be prepared to do some cleaning and purging and perhaps buy some new products to help you to manage your condition.

What to have on hand

You will need no special equipment for this step. Each of the following sections is independent, so unlike in previous steps in the plan, you may be able to skip a section or sections if they are not relevant to your condition or lifestyle.

Make your world safe from allergens

The following pages contain a wealth of tips and advice on managing allergies and asthma outside your home. Remember: it's up to you to take action and do whatever is required to help you to manage your allergies and asthma effectively.

In the garden

If you are allergic to pollens, it is impossible, regardless of what any book may tell you, to plant an entirely 'allergy-free' garden. Pollens can drift hundreds of miles from their original sources as well as a short distance from the garden next door. However, there are some steps you can take so that you can continue to garden in relative comfort.

Take the right medication That means a daily non-sedating antihistamine such as fexofenadine (Telfast), mitolastine, cetirizine or loratidine. During the gardening season, take it even if you have no symptoms so that you will be protected from pollen every day not just when you have an urge to weed. You could also ask your doctor whether immunotherapy might help you.

Wear the right equipment That means a face mask to filter pollen grains from the air before they hit your nose and mouth. You may feel silly, but wear it anyhow (consider it the same way as wearing a bike helmet – unflattering, perhaps, but a mandatory safety practice). Comfortable and effective face masks are available online and from Allergy UK. If your eyes bother you, wear goggles or wraparound sunglasses. And try smearing petroleum jelly inside your nose. It sounds unpleasant, but it can help to prevent pollen and mould spores from settling on the lining of your nose.

Watch the clock Pollens are at their worst in the afternoon during spring and in the morning during autumn. Do your gardening when they are at their lowest levels.

Check the map Before you plan to spend a day in the garden, check the pollen map at **www.bbc.co.uk/weather/pollen/** or **www.pollen.co.uk** to see what is in store for your area.

Keep an eye on the weather If it's windy and dry, stay inside. You are better off gardening on still, even sultry, days when there is less airborne pollen. Best of all are misty days, with a little drizzle to keep down the dust and pollen.

Clean up properly When you have finished gardening, leave your shoes by the back door, immediately strip off your clothing and shower. Don't forget to wash your hair; otherwise you could transfer pollens to your pillow when you go to bed. Toss your dirty clothes into the wash straight away to avoid spreading pollens and other airborne allergens around the house.

Reduce moulds Substitute gravel, other rocks, or black plastic mulch for wood and leaf mulch to reduce the number of mould spores you come in contact with while you are gardening.

Keep it airy Heavy hedges can trap dust, pollen and mould. Opt for a fence instead.

continued

Opt for low-allergy plants Thomas Leo Ogren, author of *Allergy-Free Gardening* (the gardening bible for people with allergies), created the Ogren Plant-Allergy Scale (OPALS), which ranks plants according to their allergen potential. Among his suggestions for a garden that should reduce sneezing and itching are:

- **Stick to plants that have both male and female parts** (such as apple trees and roses). These pollens don't have to travel far, so they are less likely to invade your nose and eyes. So-called monoecious-flowered plants, such as maize, also have separate male and female flowers on the same plant.
- **Or go for female only** Ogren recommends creating a 'female-only' landscape, focusing on cleaner trees such as ash, willow, mulberry, juniper and maple. 'Female' plants produce more seeds, flowers and/or fruit and thus are messier to care for, but they are receivers of pollen rather than generators, so Ogren notes, such a garden would not release a single grain of pollen. The problem is that with no males around for pollination, you won't have any fruit from your trees. Low-allergen gardens designed by Lucy Huntington can be seen at Capel Manor, Bullsmoor Lane, Enfield, Middlesex EN1 4RQ and Probus Gardens, Probus, Truro, TR2 4HQ.

Choose flowers, not bushes, in your garden. Thanks to its large size, the pollen in flowers rarely causes allergies. It is the microscopic wind-borne pollens from many bushes and trees that are the culprits, so build a fence if you need privacy, and plant some bulbs.

Plants to avoid Allergy UK advice is to avoid heavily scented flowers (lillies, carnations, jasmine, wisteria, freesia and hyacinths), which can trigger asthma attacks, and members of the daisy family. Climbing plants near bedroom windows may transfer pollen into the house.

While travelling

Having asthma or allergies should not confine you to your home, but they can pose some unique challenges when you are travelling. To ensure a healthy, sneeze-free holiday or business trip, follow this advice.

On the plane

Ask about pets on board Ask the airline about its 'pets on board' policy. If it allows passengers to bring small dogs and cats into the cabin, insist that you be seated as far as possible from anyone carrying an animal. Some airlines also have a peanut-free policy.

Leave early Book the first flight of the day; you will travel on a freshly cleaned plane.

Consider an upgrade The fabric seats in economy class are havens for dust mites and other allergens. Often, seats in business class are leather and less hospitable to allergens.

Consider a filtering face mask If the highly processed and recycled air on a plane has triggered responses before, forget about what people may think and wear a mask. This can greatly reduce the allergens you breathe.

Have your medications with you at all times. This is particularly important in these days of airline delays and long waits. And premedicate: take antihistamines the morning of your flight and a puff of your inhaler before boarding.

Carry extra drinking water Having a large bottle of water on a plane trip is always useful. Even when flight attendants are diligent about serving water, they give you small cups, so you may end up feeling dehydrated.

- **Take your own food** Contact the airline and confirm that you can take your own food on board the flight to ensure wellbeing.
- **Pack properly** Add your own pillow and rug to your carry-on bag for long flights, and take an emergency phone number for your doctor. Allergy UK can supply translation cards with allergy alert messages in several languages.

At your destination

- **Consider the season** Just as weather varies widely around the globe, so do regional allergy seasons. Check the average pollen counts for your destination before booking your trip.
- **See the medical sights** Make sure you know where the closest emergency medical facility is located – just in case.
- **Pick the right lodging** You are probably better off at a modern, albeit sterile, hotel than at a cosy (and probably allergen heavy) bed-and-breakfast or inn. It is also advisable to stay in

a hotel than in a friend's or relative's home. Some hotels even have special allergy-free rooms or provide allergy packs, including face masks, special pillows and mattress covers. See if you can find a room without carpeting in a hotel that forbids pets.

- **Pick the right destination** Exploring damp, musty caves or touring old, historic houses is probably not the best holiday for you. A better choice would be the beach or the mountains, where the air is clearer, or a cruise on the pollen-free open seas.
- **Use housekeeping services** To save water and energy, many hotels now ask if they can change the sheets every other day or when you leave instead of daily. That may be appropriate for many people, but someone with allergies needs clean sheets daily.
- **Pack your own** If you are wary of your hotel's cleaning practices, pack a queen or king-size sheet to throw over the bedspread so that you will be less exposed to the dust mites and other allergens lurking in the cover.

In the car

We spend an average of 36 minutes a day in our cars – and often treat them as extensions of our homes and offices. We eat and drink and even take naps in them. Since most cars spend their lives exposed to the elements, they can quickly become minefields when it comes to allergies and asthma. To keep your car as allergen-free as possible, follow the advice below.

- **Sniff the air** If your car smells musty, you may have a mould problem. Check the airconditioning coil, which may harbour mould; the carpet in the interior and the boot; and that wet blanket you threw in the back seat after your son's soccer game last weekend.
- **Avoid air fresheners** The perfume used in air fresheners can exacerbate your asthma.
- **Clean your car regularly** You should steam-clean the carpet and upholstery

(unless the seats are leather), wipe down the interior with a damp cloth once a fortnight, and throw out any rubbish daily.

- **Time your commute** If possible, avoid rush-hour congestion with its high levels of exhaust fumes that can aggravate your asthma.

continued

Keep the inside dry Wet feet, spilled drinks and a window left open over a rainy night can all be catalysts for some serious mould, thanks to the absorbent fabrics found on so many car seats and floors nowadays. If your car's interior does get wet, do what you can to dry it quickly. Use towels to sop up as much moisture as possible and consider using a fan to dry up any remaining dampness. Remember to lift any rubber mats.

Avoid eating in your car A car that is full of crumbs, shrivelled chips and apple cores in the ashtray is a car full of mould and bacteria.

Use the air conditioning even on cool days, and set the airflow switch to 'recirculate'. This combination minimizes the amount of external pollen and dust that comes into the car.

Consider a car with a pollen filter Check the Allergy UK website (www.allergyuk.org) for one that carries their seal of approval.

At work

As you will learn in chapter 15, numerous chemicals and odours in office buildings can trigger allergy or asthma attacks, particularly given today's sealed-tight office environments. In addition, office equipment, such as photocopiers, computers, fax machines and printers, gives off ozone and other irritants that can exacerbate asthma. Yet a British Allergy Foundation survey found that 94 per cent of office workers don't even know that the equipment that surrounds them gives off ozone.

Asthma is Britain's most frequently reported occupational respiratory disease, ruining lives and costing society up to £1.1 billion over 10 years. The Health and Safety Executive (HSE) has set a target to reduce asthma caused by substances at work by 30 per cent by the year 2010, mainly through preventing or controlling exposure. Adapting the environment, providing respiratory protective equipment and arranging job transfers from problem areas are among the options for employers, who are obliged by law to report cases of occupational asthma. As part of the Breathe Easy Plan, here are some steps you can take to make your work environment healthier. For more advice, see chapter 15.

Treat your work space like your home Go back to step 3 of the Breathe Easy Plan and apply the same worksheets and advice you used for improving your living room or den to your work space. Identify the most likely sources of allergens and irritants and make as many improvements as your boss will allow.

Keep it clean Piles of paper, books, tools and product samples cause two problems. First, they attract dust and allergens and they also prevent the cleaning staff from doing their job. If you can't manage to keep yourself organized and neat for professional reasons, do it for health reasons.

Develop green fingers Live plants around the office can help to absorb chemical emissions. A study conducted by researchers from NASA and the Associated Landscape Contractors of America found that philodendron, spider plant and golden pothos were those most effective at removing formaldehyde molecules, while flowering plants such as gerbera daisy and chrysanthemum were best at removing benzene. But be sure to water plants properly, keep the leaves dust-free and insect-free, and change the soil or compost regularly. Plants and their soil can generate their own host of allergens and moulds if you aren't careful.

Choose the right spot Ask if you can sit in a part of the building that has solid-surface flooring close to a window that opens. If your allergies or asthma are serious, ask your doctor to provide documentation of your medical condition to strengthen your case.

Minimize food and drink in your work space Unwashed coffee cups, crumbs on the floor, a half-eaten sandwich left on your desk: all these contribute to dirt, mould and an unhealthy atmosphere. Turn over your keyboard and give it a gentle shake. If crumbs fall out, you need to change your snacking and meal habits.

Speak up Don't be afraid to talk to your boss if your office environment makes you wheeze. The Control of Substances Hazardous to Health (COSHH) Regulations, which form part of the Health and Safety at Work legislation, set out measures employers must take to protect employees. And once a substance is identified as a cause of occupational asthma controls must be put in place to protect employees from developing the disease.

Track it Use the symptom tracking log on page 86 to track your asthma/allergy symptoms in the workplace and identify specific triggers. This will provide valuable information that you can share with both your boss and your doctor.

Work in the right section If you work in a retail business, such as a department store, arrange to cover a section of the store that does not include toiletries, perfumes, scented candles or potpourri. The electrical appliances or kitchen and housewares departments would be appropriate choices.

Get your orders straight If you work in a restaurant and have allergies or asthma, at least cigarette smoke should no longer be a potential problem, thanks to government plans to ban smoking in cafes, restaurants and other public places by 2008. Yet if you are allergic to certain foods, simply touching them or even breathing in their vapours can trigger an allergic reaction. So if you have allergies to any foods that your guests order, ask another server to swap tables with you.

During the Christmas holidays

Christmas can be the season for major asthma and allergy attacks, if you're not careful. With live evergreens heading indoors to deck the halls amid potpourri-scented air, the Christmas holidays can make the most cheerful allergy/asthma sufferer miserable. But preparing ahead can guarantee a better time for all.

Get the right tree Go for an artificial one. Today, these trees are so realistic that you have to pinch the needles between your fingers to convince yourself they are not alive. The artificial rule also goes for wreaths and staircase decorations. Even if you're not allergic to pine or other types of evergreens, fresh trees have to be kept damp for weeks between the time they are cut and when they are sold, so they can often harbour mould.

Clean the decorations They may have been up in your attic all year. Make sure you wipe them well with a damp cloth to remove any dust, and throw away any that show signs of mould.

Handle the stress Now you need to make sure you are following the advice in step 5 of the Breathe Easy Plan. Christmas, with its parties, family tensions, travel, decorating and financial strains, can send stress levels soaring. Take extra time away from the bustle just for you.

continued

Have a quiet lunch in an out-of-the-way pub, go to a concert, or for a walk in the snowy woods. Take a day off from work to go shopping in the middle of the week when shops are less crowded and salespeople less surly. Hire some help. For instance, you could arrange to have your groceries delivered to your door. Housekeeping services come in handy at this time of year, and most super-markets these days stock an enticing array of prepared foods that work quite well as part or all of a company meal.

Scent your home naturally Instead of using scented candles and potpourri or scented sprays, simmer a couple of cinnamon sticks and some orange peel in water over a low heat on the back of your stove. Or put out small bowls of vanilla-soaked cotton balls to absorb odours.

Decorate the fireplace No matter how attractive and welcoming it may be, a blazing log fire won't help your asthma or allergies, so you are better off using the fireplace to display a dried flower arrangement or covering it with a decorative screen.

Watch what you eat If you have food allergies, you should be especially vigilant over the holiday period. Traditional plum pudding, mince pies and Christmas cake may contain nuts, as may other festive offerings. And be wary of food passed round at drinks parties.

Through the seasons

As you probably know all too well, weather conditions can mean the difference between a productive, energetic day and one in which you can do little more than reach for your inhaler and swallow antihistamines. You also know that many forms of allergies and asthma are seasonal, occurring at around the same time each year.

We have already given you plenty of advice about managing particular allergens and environmental issues, but there's more to be said on the topic. In this part of the Breathe Easy Plan, we ask that you be mindful of seasonal weather issues that might affect your condition – and then take action.

General guidelines

Monitor the weather If you have allergies or asthma, check the forecast on the website **www.met-office.gov.uk** or the Weather Channel, **http://uk.weather.com** There are also continuous weather forecasts on digital TV. Knowing the temperature, the humidity and the chance of rain or snow ahead of time gives you the information you need to take medication preemptively and prepare yourself for a potential flare-up of symptoms.

Make sure you have your medication People with allergies or asthma have to be especially careful about transferring medications and other assorted items from coat to coat according to the season. Once you have decided your coat strategy, stock the pockets of each with the items you need to manage your condition during that season: tissues, rescue medications, scarves, sun-glasses, throat lozenges, and so on.

Winter

Wrap up your face Wear a scarf or face mask over your nose and mouth on very cold days to warm the air you breathe. And wrap your face *before* you head outside. All it takes is a few full breaths of raw, cold air to bring on an attack. If cold air is a trigger for your asthma, try taking a dose of your inhaler 10 minutes before you go outside.

Take it slowly If you live in a snowy northern location, just walking outside in winter can be tough exercise. If you are susceptible to exercise-induced asthma attacks, be particularly careful as you walk, shovel snow or play. Start slowly and increase exertion only if your body has responded without any sign of stress after at least 15 minutes of activity.

Spring

Watch for lightning If thunderstorms are predicted, stay indoors, in air conditioning if possible. At the very least, keep all your windows closed. As we discussed in chapter 4, studies have found that airborne fungal spores nearly double during thunderstorms, significantly aggravating asthma.

Clear out any garden rot No matter how well you cleaned up four months earlier, spring – particularly in snowy areas – reveals the remains of the past autumn in all its allergy-inducing glory: rotted leaves, crumpled flower remains, broken branches, fallen pine cones and so on. Rain and warmer weather can turn all that organic waste into a haven for mould and mildew. While every good garden needs compost, you should clear out the waste that is not going to contribute to your prize-winning roses and tomatoes come the summer.

Summer

Pay attention to ozone Ozone tends to be worst during the May-to-October smog season, so try to limit outdoor activities on bad ozone days. Nowadays smog or ozone alerts are issued during the summer when the air is particularly bad. On those days, stay inside in air conditioning as much as possible. If you don't have air conditioning, go to a library or shopping centre during the afternoon – the worst part of the day for ozone.

Wear black Or at least stick to solid colours in neutral tones. Bright colours that mimic the colours of flowers entice stinging insects.

Beware the hot air For some people, hot, dry air can be as irritating to the lungs as icy air. If the temperature exceeds 30°C (85°F), be wary as you go about your outdoor business. If you start to wheeze, go back inside.

Autumn

Hands off the leaves Ideally, ask someone else to rake and pick up your leaves, which harbour mould and other allergens. Don't be tempted to use a leaf blower: it will blow allergens into the air around you as it does its work.

Clear the garden Cut back old perennials and rake out dead leaves and plants. The more air circulates, the less mould will grow.

Do an autumn clean indoors The days are shorter, the weather is less inviting – autumn begins the 'indoors' season. Why wait until spring to do a thorough houseclean? Instead, do a pre-emptive top-to-bottom cleaning of your home each October. Get the house into the best possible shape for several months of comfortable, allergen-free nesting.

Breathe to beat allergies and asthma

Most of us don't normally think much about breathing. After all, it's a reflex, something we perform as unconsciously as sleeping. If you have asthma or allergies, however, you probably stopped taking breathing for granted long ago. In this final step of the Breathe Easy Plan, you will learn how to focus on the way you breathe and strengthen your diaphragm to improve your breathing.

As any athlete knows, lung power can be developed. After all, breathing is controlled by muscles that – like any other muscles – can be exercised, strengthened and conditioned. An easy way to do that is with Breathing Coordination – a method based on the fact that with asthma, the problem is not so much getting air into your lungs as it is getting rid of the air completely. As airways narrow and fill with mucus, your body struggles to exhale all the air you have inhaled. Thus, carbon dioxide-laden air builds up in your lungs as you take in less oxygen with each breath.

To help people to move more carbon dioxide out of their lungs, US researcher Carl Stough created the Breathing Coordination process. The goal is to strengthen your diaphragm muscle so you can move air out of and into your lungs more efficiently. Also, by teaching you to extend your exhale, the exercise can reduce the panic that often occurs with an asthma attack, helping you to self-limit the attack and its severity.

'The most common problem I see among people with asthma is that they're over-inhaling,' says Lynn Martin, a Breathing Coordination instructor in New York City who also lectures to anatomy students at New York University. 'They're working too hard to try to pull more air into the lungs, using musculature that isn't appropriate for this use,' she says. This could be one reason why people with asthma often complain of a sore back after an attack.

By systematically developing the diaphragm using the following exercise, Martin says, you will be able to exhale air from your lungs more easily, preventing the shortness of breath and shallow breathing so common in those with asthma.

What you will be doing	How you should prepare	What to have on hand
Learning the Breathing Coordination technique to strengthen your diaphragm and improve your breathing.	Pick a time when you will have no interruptions, choose a quiet place and wear comfortable, loose clothing.	Two pillows, plus whatever else you need to lie comfortably on the floor.

The breathing coordination exercise

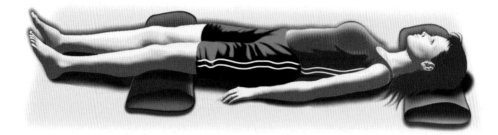

1 Although you can do this exercise while sitting or standing, the most relaxing position is **lying on your back with a pillow under your knees and another under your head**. In this position, your diaphragm doesn't work against gravity, and you don't need to bring any voluntary muscles into play in order to balance and support your body. Remember, you are not supposed to work at inhaling or exhaling.

2 Make sure that your **jaw is loose and your mouth** is open when you inhale. This doesn't mean that you do all mouth breathing, but at this point, it helps to keep your throat open.

3 Inhale, and then as you exhale **count without sound**, with easy jaw and tongue movements. Build the silent count in **continuous rounds of the numbers** from 1 to 10 (1-2-3-4-5-6-7-8-9-10-1-2-3-4-5-6-7-8-9-10). You have to speak the numbers, but you can do it very softly, below the level of an audible whisper. This tricks the space between the vocal folds to stay open and extends the exhale without any pressure.

4 Continue the relaxed exhale **as long as possible** in order to cause a reflex inhale. Make sure that your jaw is still loose and your mouth is open as you inhale. Repeat the process of exhaling with extended silent counting for a few minutes.

5 Continue the process but **start to make audible sound** in your larynx. This challenges the diaphragm slightly more by providing a progressive resistance exercise for the diaphragm to work against as you exhale. Start the audible counting very simply, with only five digits at a time (1-2-3-4-5). Once you start, remember that you want to be heard. Don't make a special effort to be loud, but think of projecting the sound so the air will continue to flow out freely while you count.

6 Repeat the process of exhaling with extended audible counting for a few minutes.

continued

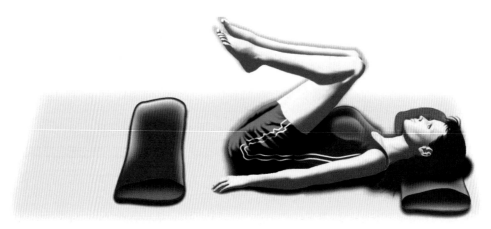

7 Occasionally during the breathing exercise, while lying down and continuing to count as you exhale, **bring your knees up** towards your chest and, with your feet off the floor, **gently swing your legs** from side to side, keeping your arms on the floor beside you.

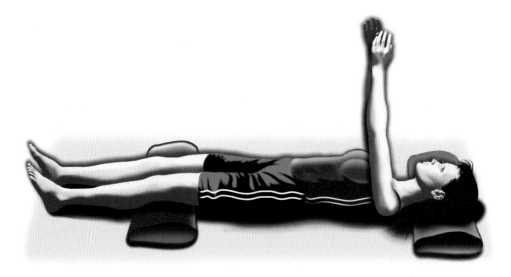

8 After swinging your legs, and while still continuing the breathing exercise, **raise your arms** towards the ceiling and **let them swing** from side to side to loosen your shoulders. These leg and arm movements reduce tension in the lower back and shoulder girdle, which is important because these muscles often interfere with the diaphragm's freedom of movement and with the freedom of the ribs to move in response to the diaphragm. Be sure that the swinging motions **occur as you exhale**, and keep counting quietly to keep the exhale going.

9 Do this exercise for **10 minutes a day**, either in a single session or in smaller increments.

Additional tips

- Once you feel comfortable with the Breathing Coordination exercise, you can **practise wherever you like** – maybe while driving your car or taking a shower or cooking dinner. In particular, you can do the silent portion of the breathing exercise anywhere, at any time. If you do the exercise daily for the prescribed time, Martin says you should feel an improvement in your breathing strength in about two weeks.

- **Never force either inhaling or exhaling**. You may be able to achieve an exhale count of 40 or 50 without rushing, but keep your diaphragm moving by doing it in a sing-song. If your count is too precise, your diaphragm may not move as smoothly.

- While counting, **make sure your diaphragm rises**. If the count goes too long and your diaphragm begins to tense, you will feel pressure in your lower abdomen between your hip bones. This means that your abdomen is not contracting but is dropping inwards when your diaphragm rises. Don't push past that. When your diaphragm rises, everything above it and below it releases, so that you can feel your chest and lower abdomen drop towards your spine. That's what you want to feel.

- As this exercise becomes easier, you should be able to accomplish the same thing **sitting or standing**, with a similar sensation.

- The best times to practise are **first thing in the morning** and **last thing at night**. You should also prime your breathing before you start by making physical demands on your body, such as going for a walk or doing some calisthenics. If you do the breathing exercise just before going to bed, it should be very relaxing and provide you with a better night's sleep.

- The more you practise, the faster your muscles will develop. But make sure that all practice is **done in a relaxed way**. The length of the practice session depends on your success. If it's going very well and you have the time, continue. If it's not going well, stop and try again later.

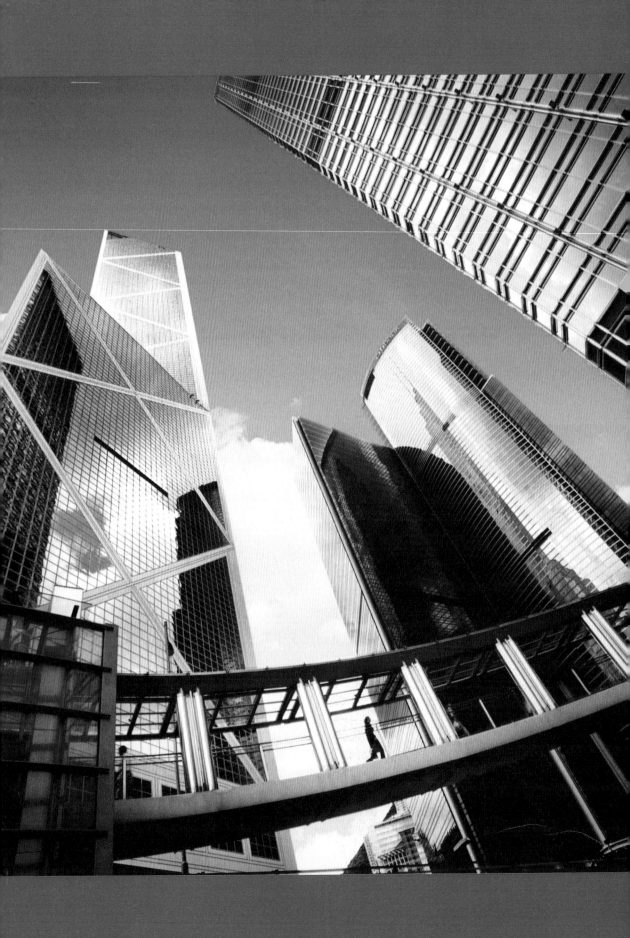

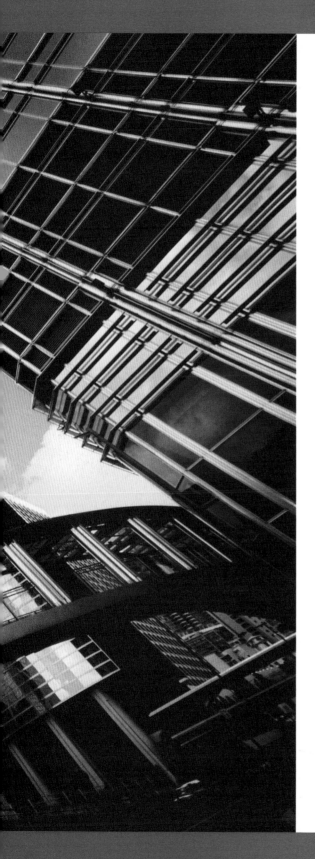

PART FOUR

Special
situations

The Breathe Easy Plan was designed to be effective for most types of allergies and asthma, but some forms of these conditions require more specialized advice. The following pages contain strategies for coping with skin and insect allergies, 'sick buildings' and exercise-induced asthma. And, most importantly, there is guidance for parents of children with allergies or asthma.

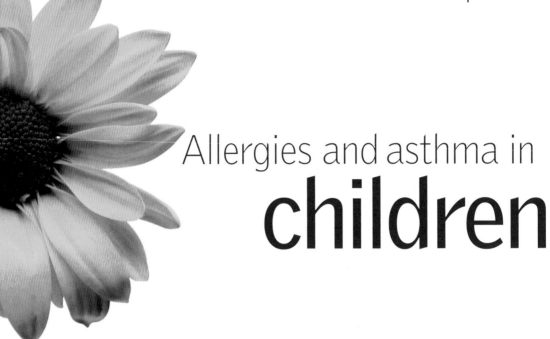

Chapter twelve

Allergies and asthma in
children

The opening pages of this book discussed the allergy and asthma epidemic in the UK, which affects people of all ages, of all backgrounds and in all locations. Although recent studies show that asthma rates in children have stabilized for the first time in decades, consider the following statistics:

- Respiratory disease is the most commonly reported chronic childhood illness, accounting for over 40 per cent of all long-term illnesses
- One in 8 children are living with asthma, as opposed to one in 12 adults
- Some 1.4 million children are receiving treatment for their asthma
- Children are more likely than adults to require hospital care for asthma
- Out of 56 countries worldwide, the International Study of Asthma and Allergies in Childhood reported that, in children aged between 13 and 14 years, the UK has the highest prevalence of severe wheeze.
- The annual cost to the NHS of diagnosed asthma in childhood is estimated at around £254 million.

Chapter 1 discussed many possible reasons for the dramatic increase in asthma and allergies, including an over-sanitized 'too-clean' environment, diet, actions a woman takes during her pregnancy and environmental exposure. This chapter looks at how allergies and asthma may differ between children and adults; it explains how to recognize these conditions in your child and perhaps prevent an inherited tendency to asthma from becoming full-blown and how to handle the everyday issues of having a child with allergies or asthma, and provides easy-to-use charts with notes on a selection of children's medications.

Signs to watch for

If you notice a scaly red patch on your baby's arm or chest, you should watch it closely. It could be atopic dermatitis, better known as eczema, a chronic itch that develops into a rash. It can be quite uncomfortable, making your baby fussy and irritable. Don't dismiss the problem as merely the sensitive skin of a child. Eczema is a sign that your child may have a tendency to allergies and/or asthma. Some 40 per cent of infants with eczema develop asthma by the age of four, and about 30 per cent of all eczema cases in toddlers are linked to an allergy, of which one-third are food related. So, if you see red, dry patches on your child's skin, talk to your doctor about allergy testing. The earlier allergies

Recognizing asthma and allergies in children

Although 50 to 80 per cent of children with asthma develop symptoms before the age of five, the vast majority of their asthma symptoms are triggered by viral infections, not allergies. That's one reason why symptoms of early asthma often mimic those of other childhood diseases, such as respiratory infections or stomach flu, and are often ignored by doctors. If you find that your child has periodic or persistent coughing, wheezing, shortness of breath, rapid breathing or chest tightness, and if these symptoms become worse during the evening or early morning or are associated with triggers such as exercise or allergen exposure, ask your doctor to evaluate your child for asthma.

Bear in mind that your child does not necessarily have to be wheezing to have asthma; not all children with asthma wheeze. Conversely, not all children who wheeze have asthma. Other causes of wheezing include respiratory infections, rhinitis, sinusitis and vocal cord dysfunction.

Allergic rhinitis strikes a little later, usually at the age of nine or ten, so if your child has already been diagnosed with asthma and then develops nasal symptoms that suggest allergies, you should be concerned. Expect the first two or three years of coping with childhood allergies to be the worst; after that, symptoms usually level off and may even improve by the time your child turns into an adult. In fact, about 20 per cent of children with allergic rhinitis find that their symptoms disappear as they enter adulthood.

Like asthma, allergic rhinitis often goes undiagnosed and untreated in children. Signs to look out for include 'allergic shiners' (dark circles under your child's eyes), an 'allergic crease' on his or her nose from constant rubbing, a nasal voice, constant mouth breathing and chapped lips, frequent snoring, coughing from postnasal drainage, frequent sneezing and gaping of the mouth. Other possible symptoms include fatigue, weakness, irritability and a poor appetite.

are identified and treated, the less likely they are to become more severe. Identifying and treating asthma early can prevent long-term lung damage that can make the condition worse.

Increasing numbers of infants are allergic to cow's milk, egg and, less commonly, fish, grains and nuts; excessive vomiting of these foods, a skin rash after eating them, chest tightness, 'vacancy' or 'droopiness' are all signs. Food allergies in children are strongly associated with the development of allergic rhinitis, asthma and eczema. Such allergies can be the first sign of what researchers call the allergic march, a constellation of clues in early life that signal a child's increased risk for these associated disorders.

The allergic march begins with a genetic predisposition, that is parents, siblings or other close relatives who have allergies or asthma. It continues with

Beyond a spoonful of sugar

It is not always easy to persuade a recalcitrant toddler to take medicine, especially if that medicine involves putting on a mask. Even older children can be loth to swallow pills or use their inhalers. So what is a parent to do?

Inhalers and medications

Most paediatricians in the UK recommend a metered-dose inhaler (MDI) and spacer for a child's routine asthma treatment attached to a face mask for very young children. (In the USA, nebulizers are widely recommended but here home use of nebulizers is generally discouraged.) Even in acute, severe asthma, an MDI, spacer and face mask is considered as effective as a nebulizer for emergency treatment.

Both devices can be ineffective if incorrectly used. Studies have found that even when children manage to master MDIs, only 10 to 15 per cent of the medicine reaches the lungs. The operation is generally much more successful if your child is prescribed a spacer with the MDI. This holds the 'puff' of medicine between the patient and the MDI so that it can be inhaled slowly and more completely. (See Delivering the medicine to your lungs, on pages 112-113.)

Another possibility for children aged five and above is a dry-powder inhaler, which gets more medicine to the lungs. Again, make sure that you and your child know how to use it or the medicine will be wasted. Here are more ideas for encouraging your child to take medication.

Use a sticker programme Each time your child takes the medicine without complaining, award a sticker. When 10 stickers have been earned, offer a reward.

Make it taste good If your child's medicine tastes bad, ask at your local pharmacy about adding appealing flavours to liquid medicines.

Make it easier to swallow Relatively few children in the UK have to take pills regularly for asthma, though they may need a short course of steroid tablets for flare-ups. These come as soluble tablets which may make them easier to take. Alternatively, ask your doctor if you can put oral medication in a cup of juice or mash it into yoghurt or ice cream.

Ask if you can give it less frequently Ask your doctor if there are longer-acting dosages that your child can take or if it would be OK to give a twice-a-day medicine all at once. Both options will reduce the stress of 'medicine time'.

the skin rashes and stomach upsets described above and progresses to recurrent ear infections (up to 79 per cent of children with chronic ear infections have confirmed allergic rhinitis), nasal congestion and asthma. GPs may not readily link these symptoms and recognize the signs of the allergic march. But if you are aware of the clues they will help you to monitor your child's health, avoiding treatments that won't work in favour of those that will, and possibly even preventing further stages on the march, such as development of asthma.

For instance, some research suggests that early use of inhaled corticosteroids may prevent the early development of asthma in at-risk children. A large US study sponsored by the National Institutes of Health called Prevention of Early Asthma in Kids (PEAK) hopes to have more definitive information on that hypothesis in a few years' time. (UK readers may associate PEAK with something quite different – holidays run by Asthma UK for children with severe asthma with or without eczema. For more information see the website at: **www.asthma.org.uk/kidszone/peak.php**).

In another research project, the ETAC study, one and two-year-olds who already had atopic dermatitis were given the antihistamine cetirizine (Zirtec). Eighteen months after treatment, researchers found that children who received Zirtec who were allergic to grass and/or dust mites were significantly less likely to develop asthma than those who did not receive the drug. The benefit continued for up to 18 months after the children stopped taking the medicine. However, it is still not certain whether the ETAC study reflects 'prevention' of asthma or simply inhibition of symptoms.

Early treatment also helps a child to avoid the psychosocial effects of allergies and asthma. Children with allergic rhinitis, for instance, are more likely to be shy, depressed, anxious and fearful than other children. Sleep problems and missed school days can interfere with academic development and their self-esteem.

Your first step should be to take a child to the doctor. If the GP finds evidence of allergies or asthma, discuss what you can do to minimize their effects on your child's health. This may include environmental changes, starting medications or removing any allergy-causing foods from your child's diet. In fact, the Breathe Easy Plan is as appropriate and effective for a child as it is for an adult. And if the whole family follows the plan everyone's health will benefit.

Finally, you might consider allergy injections for your child. Studies suggest that an early course of immunotherapy in children with allergic rhinitis significantly reduces their risk of developing asthma. Here, immunotherapy may be used in children over 5 years for severe allergic rhinitis and occasionally for severe animal allergies. In pollen-allergic children it does appear to 'prevent' asthma (or at least reduce the expression of symptoms) and there is some evidence that it limits sensitization to new allergens. It is a rigorous, difficult treatment for a child to undergo, but the payoff may last for years.

It's different for children

In recent decades, it has become clearer that many children who wheeze in infancy and early childhood do not go on to develop asthma. Often, viral chest infections cause temporary wheezing which then resolves. The evidence suggests that different combinations of genes and environment influence the risk of a child developing asthma. Thus if you have one of several genes linked to asthma and are exposed to certain factors in the environment, such as tobacco smoke, then your chances of having asthma are substantially increased. Alternatively, if you are not exposed to the environmental factor you may not develop asthma even if you have the gene.

In one study researchers looked at 243 children at different ages and asked parents to record whether their child wheezed before or after the age of six years; children were grouped depending on whether they wheezed at one, neither or both of these ages. At 11 years of age, there were differences in breathing and allergy tests between these groups. The researchers came to the conclusion that different patterns of wheezing are present in childhood, some of which are linked with allergy and the changes in lung function associated with asthma, and some of which are not. These findings have been reported in other countries including the USA and Italy.

'Many children experience severe wheezing in infancy, which is often only associated with colds,' says study author Dr Stephen Turner of Royal Aberdeen Children's Hospital, 'many of these children stop wheezing between the ages of three and six and do not develop asthma. In contrast, some children continue to wheeze beyond the age of six and go on to develop asthma.'

The major challenge, he says, is predicting which children will go on to develop asthma. A new 'breathalyser' test may prove useful for both monitoring and diagnosing asthma in school-aged children. Dr Turner is currently developing the technique for use in younger children to see whether it can help predict which wheezy young children go on to become asthmatic. If the studies in Aberdeen and elsewhere in the world are positive, the test will become more widely available across the UK.

Asthma and gender differences

What is certain is that a child's chances of having asthma are higher if they have a co-existing allergic condition such as food allergy or eczema or if they have parents with asthma or who smoke. There are also several differences between asthma in adults and children. One difference is that, in children, boys are more much more likely to have asthma than girls (three-year-old boys are at least twice as likely to have asthma), but, after puberty, the situation changes and females are more likely to have asthma. The reasons for this are not fully known, but one theory is that, generally speaking, boys exercise more and therefore their asthma symptoms, which can be brought on by exercise, may be more obvious. A second is that oestrogen and progesterone (the female sex hormones) may play some role in the increased rates of asthma.

Explaining asthma to your child

You have just learned that your seven-year-old son's chronic cough and wheezing are due not to a viral infection but to asthma. He has to take medicine every day, learn to use a peak flow meter, and remain aware of things that most children never think about, such as whether his friends have pets in their homes. How do you explain all this?

■ **Use simple language** Describe what the lungs do and how they fill with air when you breathe, and then explain what happens when you have asthma and how they can feel clogged and just don't work as well.

■ **Use visual aids** Asthma UK is an excellent resource for parents of children with asthma and has a children's website at: **kickasthma.org.uk** There are also many children's books that explain how our bodies work, and several specifically targeted at children with asthma. Your doctor may also have pamphlets or colouring books.

■ **Be honest** Don't pretend that the medicine is a sweet or a 'cure'. Instead, tell your child that luckily there is now medicine to help his or her lungs work better, but that it's important to take it every day. And don't minimize the seriousness of the condition. Make sure that your child understands what to do if he or she can't breathe.

■ **Involve your child** Depending on age, encourage your child to

parents **ask**

Is immunotherapy safe for my child?

Although a collaborative committee of the three major allergy and immunology medical societies in the USA found that immunotherapy for children is effective and often well tolerated, it is generally not recommended in the UK. However, this may change if emerging evidence that immunotherapy can prevent the development of asthma and limit the development of allergies to other allergens becomes clearer.

Certainly, it could be used for extreme hay fever and if, despite the best attempts at avoidance, a child has severe reactions to animals such as cats, says Dr Chris Corrigan, Consultant Physician in the Department of Asthma, Allergy & Respiratory Science at Guy's, King's and St Thomas' School of Medicine. But for insect venom allergy, it would probably be considered suitable for only a handful of children, he adds, as reactions tend to be milder and there is a very high spontaneous remission rate.

participate in managing the condition. For instance, the child can fill in the peak flow meter chart every day or keep a journal to track how he or she feels. If the child is too young to write, *you* should set aside a few minutes each day to find out how he or she is feeling and then write it in the journal.

Explain the warning signs It is vital that your child knows what to do if feeling 'funny' or 'weird'. The child must recognize that this is a warning sign of an asthma or allergy attack, and tell you, the teacher or another adult.

Building a support team

Generally speaking, GPs and pediatricians are not as aware of the latest treatments and recommendations as allergy specialists are. For instance, initial data from a large study of children found that many who end up in hospital casualty wards are not using preventer medications or are using them inappropriately. The vast majority did not have asthma action plans or use peak flow meters, suggesting that they were being undertreated. Furthermore, a study published in the *British Medical Journal* in 2002 reported that of 1,444 children using asthma inhalers, 35 per cent used an inappropriate inhaler device. Both children and parents overestimated the child's ability to use the inhaler, and researchers concluded that large numbers of children are given inhalers that they cannot use.

If your child has mild asthma or allergies that are easily controlled, you probably don't need to see a specialist. But if your child's condition results in missed school days, visits to casualty, hospitalizations and a noticeable effect on his or her quality of life, ask your GP for a referral to a specialist. The chances are, you will find that your child's condition will be better managed.

Whether you consult a GP or specialist, remember that managing your child's condition is a team effort. You need to enlist all of the following to make sure your child is getting the best support possible.

Your child's GP and the surgery staff Not only is your GP crucial, but so are the nurses, the receptionist who makes the appointments and the staff of the surgery's asthma clinic, if it has one. Even printed material is important: the surgery should be a major source of information on the treatments provided.

Your child's school Remember that school is to children as work is to you – that is, the place where they spend a lot of time and where they have a unique set of people with whom they interact daily. If your child has asthma, contact the school and highlight your concerns. As soon as you believe there is a problem, make an appointment to see your child's form or class teacher. If you want to speak to someone more senior, contact the head teacher or the special educational needs (SEN) co-ordinator. You have a right to know which school governor is responsible for SEN and to see the school's SEN policy. Asthma UK has a fact sheet that summarizes the five stages that a child with severe asthma may encounter in establishing special educational needs.

Other adults in your child's life From the parents of your child's friends to his or her piano teacher, swimming instructor or football coach, each adult should be aware of his or her unique health needs. It is important to have that short conversation and let them know the essentials of your child's condition.

Your family The golden rule of health care today is to take responsibility. Managing the condition is a family commitment for you, your spouse or partner and your child; it is not your doctor's or anyone else's job. Reading this book is a good start. Exploring the resources listed on page 277 will also help. Most of all, talking extensively with each other is crucial. If there are other children in the family who don't have allergies or asthma, tell them about their sibling's health and how they can help. Encourage them to ask questions and explain any special equipment.

Asthma-friendly schools

You have torn up your carpets, thrown out your six-year-old's stuffed animals, encased the bed in mattress and pillow covers and invested in HEPA vacuum cleaners and filters. But have you thought about what awaits your child at school?

Although Ofsted school inspectors check that schools conform to all their obligations under the Health and Safety Act, the Department for Education and Skills is working on new guidelines for air quality in school, to be published in 2006 – an initiative triggered by increasing concern over air quality prompted by studies in the USA, which showed that children in half the nation's 115,000 schools have health problems that are linked to poor indoor air quality.

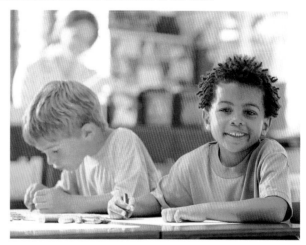

If you have a child with asthma or allergies, no matter how carefully you have modified your home environment, going to school could well exacerbate the condition. In fact, almost 75 per cent of the children who responded to a survey on the impact of asthma missed school during the past year because

You may need to campaign to improve the air quality at your child's school but it will take time and effort.

of their asthma, and one-third of those surveyed had taken at least a week off school. In a 1999 survey, many children reported missing some PE lessons (45 per cent) and having to stay in at playtime (34 per cent).

There are three key steps to take when your child goes to school: first, enlist the support of teachers and classroom assistants in monitoring and helping your child; second, make sure that your child's asthma is adequately treated; exercise-induced symptoms are often an indication of generally poor asthma control; and third, try to ensure that the environment is as healthy as possible.

To determine how environmentally healthy your child's school is, you could ask about the school's health, environmental and cleaning policies and whether you might walk through during school hours to assess the situation. Asthma triggers often found in schools include furry or feathery animals, chemicals or fumes, mould, chalk dust, pollen and grass. Asthma UK recommends that schools take the following steps to help to prevent asthma attacks in pupils.

- Do not keep furry or feathered pets in classrooms or in the school.
- As far as possible avoid fumes that trigger pupils's asthma in science and craft lessons. Use fume cupboards in science lessons if possible. If fumes are known to trigger a child or young person's asthma, allow them to leave the room until the fumes are no longer in the classroom.
- Avoid condensation as this will help to reduce house-dust mites and mould spores.
- Remove any newspaper piles in classrooms. They can harbour mould and dust mites.
- Damp-dust chalk boards.
- Ensure that classrooms are well aired.
- Ensure that rooms are regularly damp-dusted and cleaned to reduce dust and house-dust mites.
- Use HEPA vacuum cleaners and filters to clean the school.
- Check that the school heating and ventilation systems/filters are cleaned or replaced regularly.
- Remove any damp and mould in the school quickly.
- Avoid keeping pollinating plants in the classroom or playground areas.
- Close windows during thunderstorms as they can release large quantities of pollen into the air and trigger asthma attacks.
- Be aware that some chemicals in cleaning products may trigger asthma symptoms for some pupils. Check the list of triggers on the school asthma cards and stop using those identified.
- Vacuuming and cleaning with chemical solutions should be done out of normal school hours.
- Ensure that sporting fields are mown out of school hours.

Ensure that piles of autumn leaves (which can contain mould spores) are kept away from pupils and regularly removed from the school grounds.

These guidelines are in line with recommendations made in 2000 by the European Federation of Asthma and Allergy Associations, in its survey of indoor air quality in nursery, primary and secondary schools. Its report, summarized in a booklet *The Right to Breathe Healthy Indoor Air in Schools*, proposes that as well as avoiding tobacco smoke, allergen sources and moisture or mould, schools ensure adequate cleaning and maintenance, good heating and ventilation control and maintenance, regular monitoring of indoor air quality and training of those responsible for management, maintenance and cleaning. It calls for the right to breathe clean air in school to be recognized as a fundamental health right, and recommends a European programme on indoor air quality in schools.

You have the right to ask the head about your child's school environment and to have access to your child's classroom to see if the environment is healthy. If you are not satisfied with the response make your dissatisfaction known to the school's governors, who will discuss your concerns and take appropriate action.

While it may take time and effort to change a school's environmental policies, enlisting people to help monitor and care for your child needs just a few well chosen words. Make an appointment with your child's teacher and, if possible, the school nurse, before the start of the school year to make them aware of his or her condition. Offer to visit the class and talk about asthma so that other children understand why your child sometimes needs an inhaler or gets out of breath quickly.

parents **ask**

Should my child stay at home today?

If your child is in the midst of a major asthma or allergy attack, going to school is clearly out of the question. But what if he or she has a cold or was coughing more than usual last night? The following guidelines may help you to decide what to do.

Your child can go to school with:
- A stuffy nose but no wheezing
- Mild wheezing that clears after medication
- The ability to do usual daily activities
- No difficulty breathing

Keep your child at home with:
- Evidence of infection, sore throat or swollen, painful neck glands
- A fever over 37.8 °C (100°F), measured orally; a hot, flushed face
- Breathing that continues to be laboured 1 hour after medicine is given
- Weakness or tiredness that makes it hard to take part in normal daily activities
- Difficulty breathing

You should also keep a close watch on your child's peak flow meter readings. If they are lower than normal, and your child has signs of infection or simply seems out of sort, you may want to keep him or her home for a day just in case an attack is imminent.

Talk to other parents of asthmatic children, who may provide support if any issues arise. Asthma UK has produced a comprehensive school pack, called School Asthma Policy Guide, that provides information on asthma, asthma in PE and sports, what to do when a child with asthma joins the class, asthma medications, and how to develop a good school asthma policy, with an example. To obtain a free copy, telephone 020 7704 5888; it is also available online at **www.asthma.org.uk/about/resource07.php**

Talk to the school about allowing your child to keep an inhaler with him or her at all times. (But warn your child that it is not a toy; and should not be taken out as a distraction to show to friends and play with.) Teachers should be notified: March 2005 guidance documents called 'Managing Medicines in Schools and Early Years Settings', published by the Department of Health and Department for Education and Skills, include practical advice on asthma and anaphylaxis and on medicines. The head is responsible for ensuring that all medicines are stored safely. Children should know where their medicines are stored and who holds the key. All emergency medicines such as asthma inhalers and adrenaline pens, should be readily available.

You also need to make sure your child's coaches and gym teachers have a list of emergency phone numbers and step-by-step instructions for what to do in an emergency. If exercise is a trigger (as it is for most children with asthma), be sure they know that your child needs to use an inhaler before activities. Stress that asthma is not a reason to cut out exercise or keep a child off a team.

Safe drugs for children

National guidelines on the treatment of asthma in children call for doctors to start with the therapy needed to achieve control, then gradually 'step down' medication dosages and types to the minimal therapy that will maintain control. Choosing the right medication is a little more complicated for children than for adults because not all medications have been officially approved for use in children. Don't worry if your doctor prescribes a medication for your six-year-old that is labelled for children aged 12 years or above. This is often just a case of licensing, rather than a reflection of a particular problem with the medication in this age group. An experienced GP or paediatrician will know which medicines are safe and helpful.

For allergic rhinitis
As sedating antihistamines can cause drowsiness, it is generally better to ask your GP for a prescription for one of the newer, non-sedating antihistamines. Tablets are often best as they treat symptoms in the eyes as well. As in adults,

antihistamine nasal sprays are available but tablets are often better as they treat symptoms in the eyes as well. A regular corticosteroid nasal spray is the best preventative treatment for allergic rhinitis in children.

Your doctor may prescribe an alternative such as a mast cell stabilizer if your child is receiving corticosteroids from other sources (such as an asthma inhaler or eczema cream). Doctors recommend that children receiving regular nasal steroids should have their height monitored regularly.

Antihistamines (prescription)

Brand/generic name	MHRA-approved for ages	Comments
Cetirizine	Over 2 years	Dose recommendation by age; tablets or solution
Neoclarityn (desloratadine)	Over 1 year	Dose recommendation by age; tablets or syrup
Telfast (fexofenadine)	Over 6 years	Dose recommendation by age; tablets only
Mizollen (mizolastine)	Over 12 years	Tablets only
Xyzal (levocetirizine)	Over 6 years	Tablets only
Loratadine	Over 2 years	Tablets only

Antihistamines (over the counter)

Brand/generic name	MHRA-approved for ages	Comments
Benadryl Allergy Relief (acrivastine)	Over 12 years	Tablets only; must be taken 3 times daily
Allertek, Benadryl One a Day, Piriteze Allergy, Zirtek Allergy, Zirtek Allergy Relief (cetirizine)	Over 2 years	Dose recommendation by age; tablets or oral solution
Boots Hayfever and Allergy Relief All Day Boots Hayfever and Allergy Relief Fast Melting Tablets (loratadine)	Over 2 years	Dose recommendation by age; tablets or syrup

Nasal antihistamines (prescription)

Brand/generic name	MHRA-approved for ages	Comments
Rhinolast (azelastine) nasal spray	Over 5 years	Also available OTC as Aller-eze
Livostin (levocabastine)	Over 9 years	Also OTC as Livostin Direct Nasal Spray (for children aged 12 and over)

Nasal mast cell stabilizers

Brand/generic name	MHRA-approved for ages	Comments
Rynacrom (sodium cromoglicate)	All ages	To be taken at least twice, preferably 4 times daily
Vividrin (sodium cromoglicate)	All ages	To be taken at least 4 times daily and, preferably, 6 times daily

Nasal corticosteroids (prescription)

Brand/generic name	MHRA-approved for ages	Comments
Beconase (beclometasone)	Over 6 years	OTC brands only for over-18s.
Budesonide	Over 12 years	OTC brands only for over-18s.
Flixonase (fluticasone)	Over 4 years	Dose recommendation by age
Nasonex (mometasone)	Over 6 years	Dose recommendation by age
Syntaris (flunisolide)	Over 5 years	Dose recommendation by age

For asthma

Mast cell stabilizer drugs may be effective for mild, intermittent asthma but if your child needs stronger anti-inflammatory medicine, do not hesitate to use inhaled corticosteroids. Studies show that they can safely be used even in infants and young children, and evidence is strong that they improve the long-term condition of children of all ages with mild to moderate persistent asthma more effectively than using beta2-agonists alone during asthma attacks.

Research also shows that asthmatic children who are started late after onset of their disease on inhaled corticosteroids have trouble 'catching up' perhaps reflecting early changes in the lungs caused by asthma which may later become difficult to reverse. Leukotriene receptor modifiers may provide additional benefit (and also help rhinitis) but as in adults would normally be used only as an optional 'add on' to inhaled corticosteroids. In some cases corticosteroids may cause some temporary decrease in the rate of bone growth, but children taking inhaled corticosteroids still reach their normal predicted adult height – severe uncontrolled asthma is a more more common cause of growth delay.

Mast cell stabilizers (inhalers)

Brand/generic name	MHRA-approved for ages	Comments
Sodium cromoglicate	All ages	Take regularly at least 4 times daily and additionally before exercise. Dry powder, metered dose and nebulizable preparations available
Intal (sodium cromoglicate)	All ages	Available as metered dose inhaler with spacer device (Syncroner or Fisonair), dry powder inhaler (Spincaps for Spinhaler) or nebulizer solution.
Tilade (nedocromil sodium)	Over 6 years	Metered dose inhaler with spacer device (Syncroner). Use regularly at least 4 times daily

Leukotriene receptor modifiers

Brand/generic name	MHRA-approved for ages	Comments
Accolate (zafirlukast)	Over 12 years	Must be taken twice daily; helpful adjunct to regular inhaled corticosteroid therapy in some adolescents
Singulair (montelukast)	Over 6 months	Available in regular 10mg tablets and chewable 4mg and 5mg tablets and dissolvable granules (4mg); dose recommendation by age

Inhaled corticosteroids

Brand/generic name	MHRA-approved for ages	Comments
Becalazone, Filair, Cyclocaps, Pulvinal (beclometasone)	All ages (low dose inhalers only)	Must be used regularly (with spacer device and mask for under-5s).
Asmabec Clickhaler, Beclazone Easi-breathe (beclometasone)	All ages	Breath activated aerosol (not appropriate for very young children)
QVAR (beclometasone)	all ages	also available as Autohaler and Easi-breathe breath-activated versions

Brand/generic name	MHRA-approved for ages	Comments
Novolizer, Cyclo Caps (budesonide)	Over 6 years	Higher dose generic preparations
Pulmicort Turbohaler (budesonide)	All ages	Not suitable for young children
Pulmicort LS aerosol (budesonide)	All ages	Low dosage inhaler available for children under 6.
Flixotide Accuhaler, Fixotide Diskhaler (fluticasone)	Over 4 years	Dry powder inhalers not suitable for infants

Compound preparations

Brand/generic name	MHRA-approved for ages	Comments
Symbicort Turbohaler (budesonide + formoterol)	Over 6 years	For children not controlled on low doses of inhaled coricosteroids alone; regular use essential; different steroid doses available according to age of child and severity of disease
Seretide Evohaler (fluticasone + salmeterol)	Over 4 years	Metered dose inhaler; can be given with a spacer and mask if necessary
Seretide Accuhaler	Over 4 years	Dry powder inhaler

Short-acting bronchodilators – a selection

Brand/generic name	MHRA-approved for ages	Comments
Airomir (salbutamol)	All ages	Can be used with a spacer and mask
Asmasal Clickhaler (salbutamol)	All ages	Breath activated device
Bricanyl Aerosol (terbutaline)	All ages	Can be used with spacer and mask if necessary
Bricanyl Turbohaler (terbutaline)	All ages	Dry powder inhaler, less suitable for very young children

Long-acting bronchodilators – a selection

Brand/generic name	MHRA-approved for ages	Comments
Foradil (formoterol)	Over 5 years	Must be used with regular inhaled corticosteroid dry powder inhaler
Oxis Turbohaler (formoterol)	Over 6 years	Dry powder inhaler usually used with regular inhaled corticosteroid therapy; may be used intermittently prior to exercise to relieve exercise-induced asthma
Serevent Aerosol Inhalation (salmeterol)	Over 4 years	Metered dose inhaler; may be used with spacer
Severent Accuhaler (salmeterol)	Over 4 years	Dry powder inhaler

Oral steroids

Brand/generic name	MHRA-approved for ages	Comments
Nuelin SA (theophylline)	Over 6 years	Third line medicines for asthma generally tried
Slo-Phyllin (theophylline)	Over 2 years	only if moderate doses of inhaled corticosteroids
Uniphyllin Continus (theophylline)	All ages	together with regular long-acting bronchodilators
Phyllocontin continus (ammophylline	All ages	are ineffective; dose must be adjusted for age and blood concentrations monitored regularly

Oral steroids

Brand/generic name	MHRA-approved for ages	Comments
Prednisolone	All ages	May be necessary intermittently for acute severe asthma; inhaled and add-on therapy should be continued; dosage adjusted for age and asthma severity; soluble tablets available

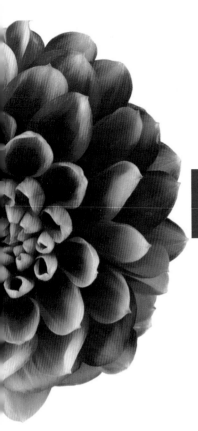

Chapter thirteen

Exercise-induced asthma

Watching children run and play outside – seemingly tireless and packed with energy – is one of the great joys in life. They appear to move so effortlessly – racing around, jumping, diving for the ball. But for a child – or an adult – with asthma, exercise is all too often an enemy rather than a friend. It triggers attacks in 80 to 90 per cent of people with asthma.

Exercise-induced asthma is chronic asthma. It is not a type of asthma, an 'asthma-like' condition or a separate disease. It is diagnosed when you have an asthma attack 5 to 15 minutes after beginning or ending physical exertion. Although frequent attacks may be a sign of inadequate asthma control, the main cause of exercise-induced asthma is not really known. Researchers suspect that it is related to the loss of heat, water or both from the lungs during exercise. This occurs because of the common tendency to breathe through your mouth when you are exercising, so that you take in cooler, drier air that has not had a chance to pass through your nose (which warms and moistens the air).

Confusingly, exercise may also trigger exercise-induced bronchospasm (EIB), a common but frequently undiagnosed problem that often affects athletes, in which the bronchial airways temporarily go into spasm 5 to 10 minutes after starting vigorous exertion. Unlike exercise-induced asthma, however, EIB has no inflammatory element. Both amateur and professional athletes have particularly high rates of EIB, with studies finding that between 11 and 50 per cent are affected. The breathlessness and wheezing that you experience after exercise may be the only symptom of EIB, leading people to think that they simply get out of breath easily. That may also explain why one study found unrecognized exercise-induced bronchospasm in as many as 29 per cent of the athletes studied.

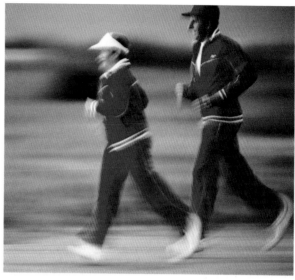

By contrast, asthma is a chronic disease that requires treatment on a regular basis, not only when symptoms occur. When you take exercise, watch out for shortness of breath or wheezing, decreased exercise endurance, chest pain or tight-ness, cough, sore throat, and upset stomach or stomach ache.

Researchers suspect that exercise-induced asthma is related to the loss of heat, water or both from the lungs during exercise.

If you experience any of these symptoms, you should stop exercising and allow your breathing and heart rate to return to normal. Generally, the 'attack' will last only a few minutes, but it can be as scary as any other kind of asthma attack, often leading otherwise healthy people to avoid exercise altogether.

The only way to know for sure if your symptoms are related to asthma is to consult an asthma specialist, who may conduct an 'exercise challenge' test to confirm a diagnosis. The test usually involves evaluating your lung function before and after you have run on a treadmill or used an exercise bicycle for about 10 minutes.

Preventative strategies

As with any form of asthma, medication plays a major role in controlling your symptoms, but there are also several non-medical steps that you can take to avoid exercise-induced asthma.

Improve your overall physical condition. The better shape you are in, the stronger your lungs are, the less sensitive they will be to the cool, dry air you take in while exercising.

Warm up for at least 10 minutes before you start exercising.

Try not to exercise outside in cold weather. If you do, cover your mouth and nose with a scarf or mask (as when skiing) to warm and moisten the air.

Exercise in warm, humid places. Swimming in an indoor pool (if not heavily chlorinated) is often good for people with exercise-induced asthma.

Try not to exercise outside in areas of high pollution or at times when the air quality is poor. For example, don't run alongside a busy road or go cycling on hot days when ozone levels are high.

Wait at least 2 hours after eating before exercising. This ensures that your stomach has emptied and reduces the risk of gastric reflux, or heartburn, which could lead to aspirating bits of food into your lungs if you have an asthma attack.

Try to breathe through your nose, not your mouth.

It is also worthwhile thinking about what sport is best for you and changing your current sport if necessary. Asthma UK recommends sports that are not continuous but have with only intermittent periods of activity such as football or hockey. Long-distance or cross-country running are particularly strong triggers as they are undertaken outside in cold air without short breaks. Swimming in cold water or heavily chlorinated pools may also trigger asthma; the warm, humid air of a heated indoor pool is less likely to trigger symptoms. Yoga is a good form of exercise for people with asthma as it relaxes the body and may help with breathing. You should monitor your condition with a peak flow meter. If your readings indicate that your asthma is getting worse, don't take strenuous exercise.

When exercise becomes dangerous

Exercise-induced anaphylaxis is a rare condition in which intense exercise leads to a life-threatening systemic reaction. Symptoms range from relatively mild, such as hives, to severe, such as a sudden drop in blood pressure, loss of consciousness, and even death. But since the condition was first identified in the 1970s, only one death has been reported. Either most people have mild symptoms, or doctors fail to recognize it as a cause of death.

If you have ever had a dramatic reaction to exercise, such as breaking out in hives or becoming dizzy (a sign of low blood pressure), you should talk to your doctor about it, and from now on, never exercise alone. Make sure that you always have an EpiPen with you and that you are with someone who knows how to administer the adrenaline. At the first sign of flushing or hives, stop exercising and use the EpiPen.

Taking the following precautions will help to reduce the risk of exercise-induced anaphylaxis: wait 4 to 6 hours after eating before exercising; don't take aspirin or other nonsteroidal anti-inflammatory drugs, such as ibuprofen, before exercising; and, if you are female, don't exercise just before or during menstruation. Studies have found that taking an antihistamine before exercising may also help to reduce problems.

Medications

Most asthma medications control exercise-induced asthma reasonably well. The type and dosage you will need depend on a variety of factors, such as whether exercise is the only trigger for your asthma, how often you exercise and your fitness level. For instance, if you work out only a couple of times a week and have a reaction once in a while, you may only require a short-acting bronchodilator (rescue medication), which can prevent symptoms if you take it 15 minutes before exercising. It lasts for 4 to 6 hours – more than enough time for a good workout. Other pre-workout medications include the mast cell stabilizers cromolyn sodium and nedocromil sodium.

If, however, you are an athlete – a competitive runner, for instance, or a bicyclist – your doctor may put you on a more aggressive regimen that includes long-acting bronchodilators and inhaled corticosteroids.

asthma **sufferers ask**

Can I exercise if I have asthma?

You certainly can. In fact, it's a myth that you can't or shouldn't exercise if you have asthma. Unfortunately, too many children with asthma stay in during school break and are forbidden to participate in team sports. Just consider that several studies have found that children with asthma are 'unfit' not as a result of their disease but because of their lack of physical activity. Given today's growing epidemic of obesity among children, regular exercise and a healthy diet to maintain a sensible weight are particularly important.

As this chapter explains, proper treatment of asthma, along with taking a few sensible precautions before you head out onto the playing field, will enable you to run, jump and roll with the best of them, with no adverse effects on your health.

The bottom line

You need a healthy body to cope with asthma (even if exercise can sometimes prompt attacks). The trick is to identify the types of exercise and other physical activities you can take part in without triggering symptoms, to be prepared by pre-treating your asthma before exercise according to your doctor's instructions, and to follow the guidelines outlined above. Don't let your asthma stand in the way of a healthy body or a good workout. Done correctly, exercise will greatly help your condition.

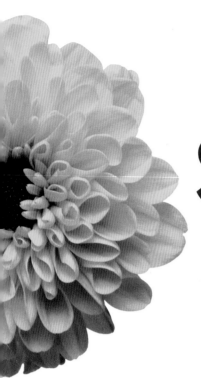

Chapter fourteen

Skin
and insect
allergies

No one wants to be stung by a bee. But if you knew that the potential result of a bee sting was widespread swelling, cardiac arrest and even death, you'd be justifiably terrified; that's how serious an insect allergy can be.

Skin allergies, on the other hand, are generally more benign, but that doesn't make them easy or insubstantial. Just ask the thousands of people who wear long-sleeved shirts in summer solely to keep scaly patches on their arms hidden from sight. With their incessant itchiness and high visibility, skin allergies can be as frustrating and debilitating as any other form of allergy.

This chapter explores both skin allergies and insect allergies – and explains how you can minimize their interference with your life by avoiding the causes or recognizing and treating reactions if you are not able to prevent them.

Skin allergies

Hear that scratching sound? The sound of fingernails on skin? That may be the first sign of allergies and asthma. It often transpires that one of the earliest indications of both conditions is not sneezing, coughing or wheezing but a skin rash called atopic dermatitis, or atopic eczema. The condition, which affects as many as one in five children and one in 12 adults in Britain, has increased threefold over the past three decades.

The name *atopic dermatitis* actually defines the condition. *Dermatitis* means 'inflammation of the skin', and *atopic* refers to an inherited tendency to develop allergic conditions. Put it together, it means that your skin reacts when you eat or inhale a substance to which your body is allergic.

This is an important point. A common misconception is that an allergic reaction on the skin has to be caused by something touching the skin. And indeed, there is a type of eczema, called allergic contact dermatitis, in which your skin has an immune system reaction to direct contact with an allergen, such as certain plants or various preservatives in creams and lotions. But that is not true in most cases of skin allergy. Rather, atopic dermatitis (or atopic eczema) is usually an external reaction to an internal trigger, such as food.

In either case, skin allergies are not life-threatening, but they can seriously affect your quality of life. One study found that people with eczema reported a worse quality of life than those with heart disease or high blood pressure.

It makes sense when you think about it. After all, no one needs to know that you have high blood pressure, and certainly no one can tell by looking at you. But with eczema – or any skin condition, for that matter – your situation is

Eczema defined

The terms *dermatitis* and *eczema* are often used interchangeably. But in fact atopic dermatitis is one type of eczema, albeit the most common one: it is endogenous – a reaction to something internal. Here are the other forms.

Irritant contact dermatitis A localized reaction that includes redness, itching and burning where the skin has been in contact with an acid, a cleaning agent, or other chemical.

Allergic contact dermatitis An allergic skin reaction to something external, for example nickel allergy.

Dyshidrotic eczema Irritation of the skin on the palms of the hands and soles of the feet characterized by clear, deep blisters that itch and burn. The causes are not known, but stress and ingestion of certain minerals (such as nickel, chromium or cobalt) may be factors. It is most common in adolescents and young adults.

Neurodermatitis Chronic, itchy inflammation of the top layer of the skin, usually caused by chronic scratching. Sometimes the itch has no apparent cause; at other times, an insect bite or irritant can launch the itch-scratch-itch cycle.

Discoid (nummular) eczema Coin-shaped patches of irritated skin that may be crusted, scaly and extremely itchy. They are most common on the arms, back, buttocks and lower legs. The coin shape of the spots makes this eczema distinct, but its causes are unknown.

Seborrhoeic eczema Yellowish, oily, scaly patches on the scalp, face and occasionally other parts of the body. Its cause is unknown, although it may be due to the pityrosporum yeast.

Stasis dermatitis (incorrectly called varicose eczema) Irritated skin on the lower legs that is generally related to circulatory problems, such as pooling of blood or other fluids in the leg veins.

Skin allergy glossary

If you are coping with any form of dermatitis you may come across confusing words. Here's a glossary to help you to better understand what your doctor says and what you read about your condition.

Allergic shiners Dark shadows under and around the inner corners of the eyelids.

Cheilitis Inflammation of the skin on and around the lips.

Dennie-Morgan fold An extra fold of skin that develops under the eyes and points to a tendency towards asthma and allergies.

Hyperlinear palms Extra skin creases on palms.

Hyperpigmented eyelids Eyelids that have darkened in colour due to inflammation or hay fever.

Ichthyosis Dry, rectangular scales on the skin.

Keratosis pilaris Small, rough bumps, generally on the face, upper arms and thighs.

Lichenification Thick leathery skin due to constant scratching and rubbing.

Papules Small bumps that may open when scratched and become crusty and infected.

Urticaria Hives (red bumps) that may occur after exposure to an allergen, at the beginning of flare-ups, or after taking exercise or a hot bath.

highlighted for the world to see. That can lead to embarrassment, shyness and general withdrawal from public life. Children with eczema, for instance, often refuse to wear shorts or short-sleeved shirts. Then there's the constant itching and scratching, which can lead to redness, swelling, cracking, 'weeping' of clear fluid and crusting and scaling of the skin.

The disease itself tends to ebb and flow; sometimes it's worse (often due to stress) and sometimes it vanishes altogether. It's generally present before the age of five and in some instances may disappear with age; in other cases, it is a lifelong condition.

There is no single test to diagnose atopic dermatitis. Even allergy tests are not always accurate, because people with eczema are generally sensitive to a variety of substances. Food allergies often exacerbate eczema in infants and these should be identified. There is less good evidence in adults that any sort of diet improves eczema although patients should avoid foods to which they have allergic reactions and may benefit from avoiding perennial domestic allergens, such as house dust mites or pet dander.

Treating atopic dermatitis

Traditionally, eczema has been treated with corticosteroid ointments and creams that help by keeping the immune response that causes it in check. But steroids bring with them their own problems, including thinning of the skin, dilated blood vessels, stretch marks and infection.

In recent years, however, two new nonsteroidal drugs known as topical immunomodulators have been licensed: tacrolimus (Protopic) ointment and pimecrolimus (Elidel) cream. Although researchers don't know exactly how these medications work, they are thought to block immune cells from creating the chemical messages that lead to eczema. Both drugs have been approved for use in children aged two and older, as well as adults. The main side effect of both is that they increase your skin's sensitivity to sunlight and other UV light, so it is important to cover up the part of your body on which you're using either product when you are outside.

If neither of these treatments is effective, you may need systemic steroids to suppress your immune system and prevent flare-ups. These drugs are given only in very serious cases, and then only for a short time. Other immune-suppressing drugs, such as methotrexate and cyclosporin, may be prescribed, again for a short time. Your doctor may also recommend antibiotics to prevent infection if your skin is severely scratched, along with antihistamines to reduce itching at night and to help you to sleep.

Phototherapy, or the use of ultra-violet A or B light waves, alone or in combination, is also used to treat atopic dermatitis. But your doctor must monitor this treatment carefully as it may increase your risk of skin cancer later in life. *Don't* self-treat by going to a tanning salon. There is also weak evidence that as a cream, St. John's wort, best known as a herbal treatment for depression, can treat atopic dermatitis.

Meanwhile, there are precautions you can take to reduce the incidence and severity of flare-ups.

▨ **Treat your skin kindly** In particular, avoid irritants that may aggravate your condition, such as scratchy fabrics, perfumes and dyes in laundry detergents, soaps and body creams, and exposure to smoke and chemicals.

▨ **Dress in light, loose layers** Natural fibres such as cotton are most gentle on the skin. In fact, 100 per cent cotton is best for clothes and bed linen as well. Wash new clothes before wearing to soften them and cut out labels that may further irritate your skin.

revealing **research**

Piercing and metal allergies

The trend towards piercing numerous parts of the body – ears, nose, tongue, navel, breasts and genitalia – is probably the key to dramatically increasing rates of metal allergies as well as an increase in latex allergies.

Studies show that the more piercings you have, the more likely you are to be allergic to metal – generally nickel, which accounts for more cases of allergic reaction than all other metals combined. A major source of sensitization to nickel among adolescents is ear piercing, and a recent Finnish study found that 31 per cent of young people with pierced ears had nickel allergy. The allergy may cause redness, watery blisters, hives or eczema. Often the symptoms are only at the site of contact, but in some cases, they spread over the entire body.

Simply removing the body jewellery is no solution, because once you have a metal allergy, you have it for life. And nickel is everywhere, including in many coins and everyday alloys. In Europe, for instance, Euro coins have such high nickel levels that some people develop reactions from handling their money.

Even gold or silver studs may not be a safe option because many of them also contain nickel. A European study that tested 66 earrings found that 25 exceeded EU limits on the amount of nickel they could safely contain. The safest body jewellery to choose is that made from titanium and surgical-grade stainless steel – the kind used for implants.

Stay cool Sweating, as well as sudden temperature changes, can aggravate atopic dermatitis. If you are in the midst of an outbreak, avoid the gym or just do some light stretching. Keep the temperature cool in your home and office.

Avoid regular soaps Scented soaps can exacerbate the condition; if the skin is inflamed, try cleansing it with aqueous cream rather than soap and water.

Try cool baths to help the itching Avoid water above room temperature, as heat dilates the blood vessels in your skin, causing even worse itching. After bathing, gently pat your skin with a soft towel and apply a non-scented cream or lotion to seal in moisture. Use emollient lotions to soothe and soften the skin.

Divert your hands If you can't seem to stop scratching the itch, try to keep your hands busy with activities such as knitting or crossword puzzles. Also, keep your nails short to avoid tearing the skin when you do scratch. If possible, 'scratch' with a flat hand, rubbing the itchy spot rather than scratching it. Wearing cotton gloves, expecially for infants and small children at night, can also prevent the worse effects of scratching.

Reduce stress in your life Or at least moderate how you react to it. Stress, while not a cause of atopic dermatitis as once thought, can definitely make it worse. Follow the stress-relieving guidelines in step 5 of the Breathe Easy Plan.

Dip into the yoghurt If you have an infant with eczema, try adding probiotics to his or her diet with either yoghurt or supplements. A Finnish study found that consumption of the probiotic *Lactobacillus acidophilus* (safe to use at an early age) halved the incidence of infant eczema, compared with infants receiving a placebo. You could add a container of live-culture yoghurt to your own daily diet, too, as long as you're not allergic to dairy foods. Although no studies have yet been done to prove its efficacy, yoghurt may work just as well for adults as for babies.

Latex allergies

In 1985, as a direct consequence of the AIDS epidemic, health authorities implemented the use of universal health precautions to protect against transmission of HIV and hepatitis C. Basically, that meant that all health care and emergency workers – anyone who could conceivably come into contact with blood or other body fluids – began wearing protective gear, including surgical gloves, which are typically made from natural rubber, or latex.

Today, most large hospitals get through some 100,000 rubber gloves a year, resulting in a significant increase in latex allergies. An estimated 1 to 5 per cent of the general population is affected and at least 8 per cent of health care workers (some studies show that up to 17 per cent are at risk of reactions to latex), which in some cases can lead to anaphylaxis. Yet until 1979 only two cases of latex allergy had been reported. The National Patient Safety Agency (NPSA) has advised all the NHS organizations in England and Wales to take steps to better protect patients with latex allergy. A survey by the NPSA, in conjunction with the Latex Allergy Support Group (LASG) and the National Association of Theatre Nurses (NATN), found that 40 per cent of NHS trusts and primary care organizations do not have local policies on managing latex which could put sensitized patients at risk from harm.

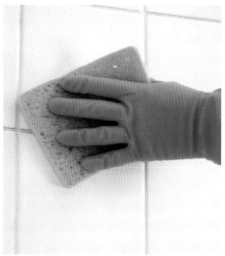

The occurrence of the allergy is directly proportional to the frequency and degree of exposure to latex. That wouldn't be so bad, except that latex is everywhere. It is found not only in surgical gloves but also in condoms and diaphragms, surgical masks, adhesive strips, balloons, nappies, incontinence pads, baby feeding teats, underwear elastic, rubber bands, sports equipment and athletic shoes, water toys and equipment, carpets, adhesives and even in zipper-seal plastic storage bags.

The occurrence of a latex allergy depends on the frequency and degree of exposure. The problem is that latex is everywhere.

One major problem for those allergic to latex is that latex proteins can become fastened to the lubricant powder used in some gloves to make them easier to put on and take off. When workers change gloves, the protein/powder particles become airborne and can be inhaled.

Symptoms of true latex allergy (that is IgE-mediated latex reactions) are instant but may be relatively mild, such as itchy, red, watery eyes; sneezing or runny nose; coughing; and a rash or hives. Or they may be severe, including anaphylactic shock. More commonly, people develop localized itchy rashes after wearing latex gloves which are usually caused by an allergy to the chemicals in latex that are used to make it polymerize – this is a form of allergic dermatitis, which does not lead to generalized allergic reactions.

If you suspect that you are allergic or sensitive to latex, you must try to avoid any products that contain natural rubber latex, or NRL. Read labels carefully, ask questions, and, if you're in any doubt, don't touch it. Also, if you need to be examined by health care professionals, inform them of your allergy so they don't use latex gloves and masks. You should also wear a medical alert bracelet in case you are injured and unable to communicate.

If you work in an industry that uses latex products, you should take the following precautions to reduce your risk of developing an allergy.

Change your gloves Use non-latex gloves for activities that are not likely to involve contact with infectious materials, such as food preparation, routine housework and general home and garden maintenance tasks.

Go powder-free If you use latex gloves when handling infectious material, choose powder-free gloves with reduced protein content, which lessen exposure to latex protein and reduce the risk of latex allergy.

Be wary of marketing claims So-called hypoallergenic latex gloves do not reduce the risk of latex allergy, although they may reduce allergic reactions to chemical additives in the latex.

Skip the lotion When wearing latex gloves, don't use oil-based hand creams or lotions, which can cause glove deterioration.

Wash after use After removing latex gloves, wash your hands with mild soap and dry them thoroughly.

Practise good housekeeping Frequently clean areas and equipment contaminated with latex-containing dust.

Be watchful Learn to recognize the symptoms of latex allergy: skin rash; hives; flushing; itching; nasal, eye or sinus symptoms; asthma; and (rarely) shock.

Insect allergies

If you are allergic to wasp or bee stings, navigating your way through the summer can be more dangerous than cycling through London. According to estimates, up to 3 per cent of people in the UK have such allergies, which in rare instances can be fatal. If you suspect that you may be allergic, ask your doctor to do a skin test.

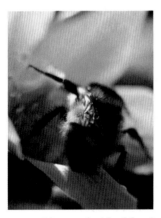

Almost half of fatal reactions occur in people who have no history of insect allergies.

In the UK, only bee and wasp stings can cause severe, generalized, allergic reactions. Some people have large local swellings when bitten by other types of insect but these are not normally serious nor strictly 'allergic' reactions unless accompanied by other symptoms.

You will know that you are allergic to one of them if, after being stung or bitten, you develop hives, itchiness, swelling in areas other than the sting site, difficulty breathing, dizziness, a hoarse voice, and/or swelling of the tongue. In the most severe reactions, it is possible to lose consciousness and have a cardiac arrest as the body becomes overwhelmed and goes into anaphylactic shock. The more severe reactions tend to occur only with bee or wasp stings. Surprisingly, in some cases, symptoms strike several hours after the initial encounter and gradually worsen before dissipating.

Once you have had a systemic reaction to an insect sting, such as hives or swelling, there is a chance of experiencing a further reaction if you are stung again. That is why people who know they are allergic should *never* be without

Finding a pest-control specialist

Most councils provide pest control services to residents at subsidized rates or free of charge depending on the risk to health, the cost of treatment and the extent to which the infestation may be attributed to an individual premise. Contact your local council to arrange treatment or for more information. Alternatively, visit the British Pest Control Association website **www.bpca.org.uk** to find a private pest controller. All pest controllers must comply with the Control of Pesticides Regulations 1986, the Control of Substances Hazardous to Health Regulations 1999 and other relevant legislation. Follow the advice below when choosing a pest-control service.

Shop around Ask friends, neighbours or work colleagues for names of firms with which they have had positive experiences. Obtain two or three written estimates, but make your selection based on the value of their service, not the price. The lowest price may not be the best value if the company cuts corners on safety.

Be wary of special deals and high-pressure sales tactics Avoid any company claiming that its treatments include 'secret' chemicals or offering you a special discount on condition that you have the work done immediately.

Choose a company that meets your needs Competent pest-management companies will carry out a survey, and produce a written report that identifies the pests to be controlled, the extent of the infestation, the specific pesticides they intend to use, and the steps you can take to minimize the chance of future infestation. The initial inspection may even indicate that pesticides are not necessary.

Check licensing Any pest controller who is on the Professional Register of Managers and Pest Technicians (PROMPT) has a recognized industry qualification, has agreed to abide by the code of professional ethics, and will have up-to-date technical knowledge.

Ask for references A contractor should be able to provide evidence of length of experience in pest control and be prepared to supply names and addresses of at least six clients from whom references may be sought.

Discuss Integrated Pest Management (IPM) options IPM techniques involve the use of monitoring devices, formulations, insect growth regulators (IGRP), sanitation, cultural practices and other physical steps to avoid or reduce problems. The company should be able to explain your pest problem and how best to solve it.

---

an emergency kit containing adrenaline (epinephrine). The good news is that your risk of a severe reaction tends to decrease with time, down to 25 per cent 10 or more years after the initial reaction. Also, reactions generally don't become more severe with successive stings.

There is really no way to know if you are allergic to an insect until you have been stung, since this is one of the few allergies in which there is no clear family history. Just because your mother is allergic to bee stings doesn't mean that you will be; conversely, just because no one in your family dating back three generations has had an insect allergy doesn't mean that you won't.

If you are stung, try applying cold compresses and/or an over-the-counter hydrocortisone cream to reduce the stinging and swelling. If you experience more widespread symptoms, talk to your GP and make sure you see an allergist.

Not only do you need a doctor's prescription for the adrenaline kit, you should also ask if you are, perhaps, a suitable candidate for venom immunotherapy, or allergy injections, which can desensitize you to bee and wasp stings. Some studies have found that immunotherapy is more than 97 per cent effective in protecting allergic people from potentially life-threatening reactions to insect stings. However, the injections may carry a higher risk of adverse reactions than allergy injections given for airborne allergens.

The other critical step you need to take is avoiding contact with these insects in the first place. Forget insect repellents, though; they don't work against stinging insects such as bees. Instead:

Avoid the beeline When honey bees are foraging for pollen, they fly a direct route (the 'beeline') from the food source to the hive. So, if possible, try to work out their beeline and make sure that you are not caught in the middle.

Don't keep bees If you are a bee-keeper, consider another hobby. Most allergic reactions to bee stings occur in people regularly stung by bees, whereas wasps are more ubiquitous.

If you're stung, don't slap Fast hand motions combined with the scent released from a stinging bee can bring more bees. Remove the sting as soon as possible by scraping it out with a fingernail or hard object such as a credit card. Don't pull it out with tweezers or attempt to squeeze it out because more venom might be released. Apply an ice pack to alleviate the pain.

Wear a hat Furry animals steal honey from bees, so if bees see anything that looks like fur, they become nervous and generally stay away.

Stay still The worst thing you can do if you see bees approaching is to wave your arms and run away. It's the rapid movement that startles the bee and encourages stinging. Instead, be as still as a statue.

Blow gently Try this if a bee lands on you; it can encourage the bee to move on while not startling it.

Wear shoes It is much easier to step on and crush a bee when you are wearing a pair of trainers than when you are barefoot or in flip-flops.

Avoid scented soaps and loud clothing If you smell or even look like a flower (by dressing in bright colours and floral prints), you will attract bees.

Picnic properly That means keeping food covered when you are eating outdoors, and never drinking from soft drink or juice cans. Stinging insects are attracted to the sweetness and may crawl inside a can. Even if you use a cup, always check the contents before sipping.

Maintain your home Make sure your outside dustbins or wheelie bins have tight-fitting lids; don't leave kitchen wastebins uncovered in summer.

Drive safely That means with the car windows closed. Also check for any stinging insects before you climb in.

Hire a gardener If you love gardening but are allergic to bees or wasps, you might consider hiring someone else to do the maintenance jobs, such as cutting grass or weeding, and save your own time outdoors for the most rewarding work, such as planting new flowers and harvesting herbs and vegetables.

Hire an exterminator When the first roses begin to bloom, arrange for a professional pest controller (see page 263) to check your property for bee and wasp nests. If any are found, give very specific instructions to get rid of them. If you employ a pest-control contractor, you will probably only need to ask him to visit a two or three times a year. When taking quotes for the work be wary of any pest controller who gives you a price over the telephone to use pesticides without first carrying out a thorough inspection of your home.

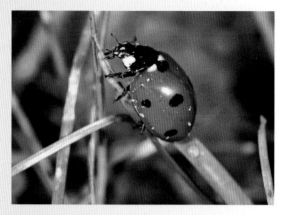

Beware the gentle ladybirds

As more gardeners turn to non-toxic methods of pest control, the ladybird, star of the children's rhyme exhorting it to 'fly away home', has become a predator of choice to vanquish aphids from the garden. As the numbers of ladybirds proliferate in some areas, doctors have begun noticing that some patients are allergic to the red-and-black bugs. If your allergy symptoms worsen (or appear for the first time) soon after introducing ladybirds to your garden, you should consider an alternative approach to aphid control.

Mosquitoes: beyond West Nile

Not only do mosquitoes carry the potentially deadly West Nile virus; they can also cause an allergic reaction in susceptible people. If you have a mosquito allergy, you will experience far worse than the typical itchy reactions that last for a few hours. Because of your increased antibody reaction to mosquito saliva, you can expect a large red swelling, skin blisters, bruises or even hives, all lasting for a week or more. But fortunately systemic reactions (anaphylactic shock) are very rare with mosquito allergies.

Although no cases of West Nile virus have been reported in the UK, 264 people in the USA died from the disease in 2003 and recent outbreaks have occurred in Romania and Russia. The UK Department of Health has drawn up plans for dealing with an outbreak of the West Nile virus. Even if you are not allergic, you should take the following steps to reduce your exposure to mosquitoes when travelling abroad.

Avoid sitting outside at dusk Mosquitoes are at their most active around the time when the sun sets and during the first half-hour or so of darkness.

■ **Drain all standing water around your house or holiday home** Mosquitoes lay their eggs in standing water. So after any summer rainfall be sure to empty out any watering cans, flower pots and other receptacles.

■ **Use insect repellent** In particular, you should use repellent containing DEET when you are outside during mosquito season. DEET is considered to be safe for children and adults of all ages when used according to the instructions on the package.

■ **Wear protective clothing when outdoors** To minimize the skin area exposed to mosquitoes, wear long-sleeved shirts, long trousers, socks and closed shoes (no sandals or clogs). Add a hat and gloves when you are gardening.

■ **Don't use perfumes** They could attract the blood-sucking bugs to you.

Bedbugs: numbers are rising

Bedbugs, or *Cimex Lectularius*, are tiny wingless insects with oval-shaped bodies that live inside bedding and mattresses, and also in furniture, cracks and crevices around the bed, and come out at night to feed on human blood – and also on the blood of any pets that sleep in your bedroom. Bedbugs don't carry disease and their bites, which resemble small red bumps, cause itchiness but don't hurt. However, if you are allergic to them bed bug bites have been known to cause anaphylaxis.

According to the British Pest Control Association, bedbugs are staging a resurgence in many parts of the country. Pest-control companies are reporting a surge in calls about them and expect the numbers to keep rising. To avoid elimination, the bugs have developed formidable strategies. They can survive up to a year without a feed and are capable of transferring food to each other. They reproduce fast and there is strong evidence of tolerance to some of the available insecticidal treatments. Eradication of bedbugs is best left to the professionals.

With no immunotherapy treatment available for bedbug bites, your best strategy is avoidance. Here's what to do.

■ **Clean your luggage and clothes** Bedbugs often enter a home via clothing or luggage. After travelling, vacuum your luggage on your return, and wash all your travel clothes in very hot water, whether you wore them or not.

■ **Manage your laundry** Always wash clothes soon after wearing, and don't leave dirty clothes near your bed. This applies to the whole family, particularly children, who can pick up bedbugs from contact with other children at school.

■ **Be watchful** Bedbugs resemble tiny lentils: flat, oval, brown and 5mm (¼ in) long. They come out at night and congregate where people sleep, since their only food is blood. Typically, they are found in the seams of a mattress (during the day they tend to rest inside it). An infested area has a faint cucumber smell.

React fast If you spot bedbugs, get rid of your mattress, wash your bedding and clothes in hot, soapy water and call a pest-control expert. Bedbugs are virtually impossible to get rid of on your own; you need an expert.

A pristine home won't deter them Unlike many other insects, bedbugs are not drawn to dirt or repelled by cleanliness. What they seek is blood.

Remove clutter from your bedroom This limits their hiding places.

Don't let pets sleep in your bedroom Bed bugs will suck your pets' blood as well. Pet dander is also best avoided.

Sleep in long-legged, long-sleeved pyjamas and socks Since the bugs bite only bare skin, the less you have exposed, the less likely you are to be bitten.

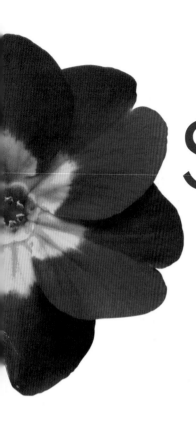

Chapter fifteen

Sick buildings
the truth and the response

There is increasing concern that buildings in which we live and work could be making us ill. In the United States mould is considered to be the chief culprit and it has become a major cause of concern for many home-owners. According to recent media reports, American families have been rendered nearly insensible by its toxic effects and some multimillion-dollar homes have had to be stripped down to the foundation to eradicate it, sparking a crisis in the home insurance industry.

By contrast, in the UK, recent media reports have focused more on office buildings with so-called sick building syndrome (SBS), in which symptoms such as headaches and dry coughs can be linked to poor ventilation, toxic fumes from building materials and poorly managed heating and air-conditioning systems rather than to mould.

In one high-profile case, explosives were used to destroy the entire 19-storey St John's House in Bootle, Merseyside, because it was said to have SBS after 2,000 Inland Revenue workers there developed flu-like symptoms.

'There was obviously a problem with staff falling ill in the old building' explained an Inland Revenue spokesman. 'They were always treated sympathetically but it got to the stage where we had to get a new building.'

SBS defined

The term *sick building syndrome* describes a building – typically a modern office with mechanical ventilation or air-conditioning – in which the occupants experience a range of symptoms causing discomfort and a sense of being unwell, rather than specific illnesses. It should not be confused with a building-related illness, in which symptoms of diagnosable illnesses such as asthma and allergies can be directly attributed to airborne contaminants in a building, such as dust mites, animal dander and pollen.

The World Health Organization (WHO), which first recognized SBS in 1982, summarizes the range of symptoms that may occur for no readily identifiable reason as: eye, nose and throat irritation; sensitization of mucus membrane and skin; erythema (reddening of the skin); headaches; high frequency of airway infection and cough; hoarseness; wheezing; itching; nausea; dizziness; and unspecified hypersensitivity.

A 1987 study of 4,373 people working in 46 buildings, found that 80 per cent had symptoms that they associated with their place of work, and 29 per cent had five or more symptoms; people in clerical or secretarial jobs had 50 per cent more symptoms than those with managerial posts; and workers in public sector buildings had higher rates of building-related sickness than those in the private sector. Other studies show that women report symptoms more frequently than men, and that people working in air-conditioned buildings consistently show higher rates of sickness than those working in naturally ventilated buildings or those with mechanical ventilation systems.

SBS is a complex problem and much of the evidence for it is inconclusive and circumstantial. Both physical and psychological causes have been suggested and it remains controversial in medical circles. However, the real issue is: if you *think* that something in your office building is causing your symptoms, and you *know* these symptoms are interfering with your ability to work or live your normal life, does it matter if the building is really 'sick'? The bottom line is that you want the problem solved and your symptoms relieved.

Pinning the blame

There are a number of different elements that can affect the air in your office. With Sick Building Syndrome the most likely suspects include the following:

Volatile organic compounds (VOCs) These are chemical irritants released by sources inside the building, such as adhesives, carpeting, upholstery, manufactured wood products such as plasterboard, copying machines,

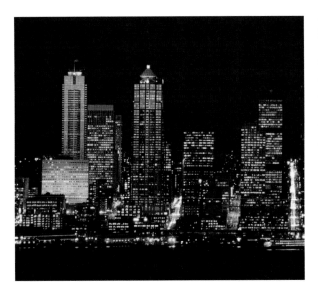

pesticides and cleaning agents. They also include formaldehyde (contained in MDF furniture), which, according to the British Lung Foundation, can cause nausea, headaches, dizziness, rashes and irritation to eyes, nose and throat.

Carbon monoxide This odourless gas is regulated in the outdoor environment but not indoors, where it can cause major health problems. The American Lung Association reports that in some US offices, afternoon levels of carbon monoxide can be 10 to 20 times greater than the daily standard for outdoor air quality. Major sources include improperly vented garages and loading docks and leaks in ductwork that enable the gas to seep into offices. It causes symptoms including fatigue, confusion, headache, dizziness and nausea. Poorly maintained heating appliances can also cause a potentially fatal build-up of the gas; in the UK around 50 people a year die of carbon monoxide poisoning.

Less fresh air filters into buildings these days, as we have become more reliant on complex automated heating and cooling systems.

Inadequate ventilation This is probably a major cause of SBS symptoms in the UK. By law, under the 1992 Management of Health, Safety and Welfare Regulations, 'effective and suitable provision shall be made to ensure that every enclosed workspace is ventilated by a sufficient quantity of fresh or purified air'. There is no standard requirement for indoor air quality in the UK, but a guideline for office building ventilation is 8 litres of fresh air per second per person.

Under the Health and Safety at Work Act, employers are obliged to provide a safe working environment. Rooms housing office machinery such as photocopiers or workshop machinery producing dust or fumes, should have separate extract ventilation systems. Air inlets for the ventilation system should be sited to avoid introducing pollution from outside the building. If there is a general exhaust ventilation system, in which the air in an office or factory is replaced with pure air, EC guidelines are three complete changes of air per hour. More guidance on air flow rates is available from the Health and Safety Executive.

Outdoor chemical contaminants Although many buildings today are well sealed (perhaps too well sealed), outdoor contaminants from motor vehicle and building exhausts can enter through poorly located intake vents, windows and other openings. If your office is above the parking area, take note. For more advice telephone Allergy UK's chemical sensitivity division: 01322 619898.

■ **Biological contaminants** These include mould, bacteria, pollen and viruses. For instance, the bacterium *Legionella pneumophila* causes Legionnaire's disease. In a recent case in Wales, there were two deaths from Legionnaire's disease because filters had not been fitted to a buffet unit's water tank.

■ **Climate control** Simple temperature problems – whether too warm or too cold – can cause common complaints such as headache, fatigue and dryness.

Breathing better at work

If the stale air in your office is getting to you, there are certain initiatives that you can take to clear the air. Step 6 of the Breathe Easy Plan explained what you can do to improve your personal work space. But what if you lack control over your work environment? Here's what you can do.

■ **Be proactive** Although you are not responsible for setting policies, you certainly have a right to know what they are. If you suspect that something in your workplace is triggering your asthma or allergies, politely ask questions. In all probability your boss won't know the answers, so ask his or her permission to talk to the building maintenance supervisor on behalf of yourself and your fellow workers. Find out when the heating and ventilation systems were last cleaned and repaired. Ask if the systems meet, at a minimum, building regulations for ventilation standards. Ask if all systems use HEPA filters. If storage areas have been turned into office space, ask if appropriate ventilation changes were made.

■ **Make a list** Have you noticed any water-stained ceiling tiles or damp patches on the carpet? Are volatile compounds (such as copy machine toner, pesticides and cleaning supplies) stored in unventilated areas? Compile a list of any such potential problems and send a memo (politely worded) to the maintenance supervisor.

■ **Walk around outside the building** Are extractor vents blocked by dirt or weeds? Are intake vents located close to the parking area? If so, add these problems to your list for the maintenance supervisor.

■ **Consider space planning** Are furniture and/or boxes blocking air vents? Is heat-generating equipment placed close to thermostats? Are too many desks crammed into too small a space? Notify the maintenance supervisor if you see any such contributors to poor air quality: they can be easily corrected.

Under the Health and Safety at Work Act employers are obliged to maintain a healthy and safe working environment which should be achieved through risk assessment. This means that the employer must look at potential hazards and remove or reduce any risks, including any causes of SBS, to an acceptable level.

Even if pollutants are below legal maximums, if they are believed to be causing ill health, employers have a duty to remove them. The Workplace Health, Safety and Welfare Regulations specify minimum standards on ventilation, temperature, lighting, cleanliness, space and room dimensions. However, they are of limited use – there is no maximum temperature at work, for example.

Mould: uncovering the truth

There is no doubt that mould can be a potent trigger for allergies and asthma. Yet there is little scientific evidence here or in the States that the much-maligned *Stachybotrys chartarum*, a greenish-black mould that grows on materials with a high cellulose content such as timber, dry linings and ceiling tiles poses a major health problem or need trouble us much in the UK. It is of only minor concern, says Stephen Lloyd of the Building Services Research and Information Association. But there is much that we do know about mould and its possible health effects.

▌ Mould is a fungus, of which there are thought to be more than 1.5 million species. Fewer than 100 are known to be infectious in humans or animals.

▌ You may have at least six types of mould spores in your house, no matter how well you clean or how dry the air is. They come inside on clothing or on your pets and they thrive on houseplants and their compost or soil. Contaminated air conditioners and humidifiers can also circulate indoor spores.

▌ There is no standardized method for accurately collecting, measuring and identifying mould spores in a home and no consensus on how to interpret the data. Thus, if you hire some air-quality inspector who tells you that you have high levels of mould, he or she is really not telling you anything.

▌ Unseen mould is no more dangerous than the mould on your bathroom shower curtain. Finding mould on your walls does not mean that your house has to be ripped apart; it is estimated that one in five homes in England suffer from dampness, condensation and mould growth.

▌ When it comes to *Stachybotrys* and other moulds, the concern is not so much the fungus itself but the toxins that the organism normally produces as a by-product of living. However, there has been no conclusive proof linking *Stachybotrys* to any specific health conditions.

▌ Foods contaminated with certain toxins that mould and other fungal products can cause have been linked to both liver and kidney cancer. Respiratory illnesses among workers attributed to mould exposure include hyper-sensitivity pneumonitis (called farmer's lung, woodworker's lung and malt worker's lung).

A healthy home

Whether you have allergies, asthma or other chemical sensitivities, one way to alleviate your symptoms is to live in a 'healthy home' – moving house or renovating using non-toxic materials. Nowadays you can find builders and architects who specialize in this type of work, creating homes and offices designed both to conserve resources and reduce indoor air pollutants.

If you are undertaking new construction work or renovating an existing building, you should consider incorporating the following tips into your building plans.

- Avoid wall-to-wall carpeting and synthetic flooring and choose natural, hard-surfaced materials such as tiles and wood.
- Choose low-odour paints, caulking and sealants that are designed to reduce exposure for people with chemical sensitivities.
- Use natural coloured plaster instead of paint.
- Choose a foundation that lifts the home off the ground in order to separate it from both radon and moisture.
- Choose nontoxic, nonallergenic insulation materials such as cork, cotton and even 'cementitious foam' insulation made from magnesium silicate.
- Stick to low-formaldehyde products for furniture, cabinets and finishes and steer clear of MDF.
- Use metal pipes for plumbing instead of plastic pipes, which allow organic matter to seep into the water.
- Consider opting for steel or other modern construction materials rather than the standard particle board.
- Make sure that rooms are well ventilated.

So what does this mean? Not only does mould exacerbate allergies and asthma, but people with compromised immune systems or underlying lung disease are particularly susceptible. Researchers at Manchester University have found that up to 70 per cent of the 1.1 million people who experience severe asthma symptoms are allergic to one or more common fungal spores in the air.

A research team from Wythenshawe Hospital, led by Dr Robert Niven, is studying the antifungal treatment of asthma triggered by fungal spores. They aim to find a treatment that will reduce steroid use and serious attacks for people with severe asthma. Antifungal drugs have been shown to benefit some people with asthma caused by Aspergillus mould (allergic bronchopulmonary aspergillosis), and the Manchester researchers hope to find a more common association between fungal allergy and severe asthma symptoms.

Volunteers, who have severe asthma and are allergic to one or more fungi, will be given the antifungal drug itraconazole or a placebo for eight months and the result analysed. Whether this is the reason for their asthma being more severe is unclear, but a trial of an appropriate antifungal treatment should help to answer that question.

So the search continues for answers and solutions to the problems of asthma and allergies. See the following pages for further organizations and resources that will help you and affected family members to tackle the issues now.

Glossary

ACTION PLAN A written set of directions or a chart that tells you what to do when asthma symptoms occur as well as preventive steps to take when you are not experiencing symptoms.

ADRENALINE (known in the USA as epinephrine) A form of medication used to treat severe allergic reactions, such as anaphylaxis.

ALLERGEN A substance that triggers an allergic reaction. Many allergens, such as dust mites, animal dander and mould, also trigger asthma.

ALLERGIC RHINITIS A condition that occurs when an allergen binds with IgE antibodies linked to cells that line the mucous membranes in the nose, causing the release of chemicals that lead to classic allergy symptoms: itchy, runny nose; watery eyes; sneezing; and so on. Also known as hay fever.

ALLERGIST A doctor with additional special training in the care of asthma, allergies and related conditions.

ALLERGY An inappropriate or exaggerated reaction of the immune system to substances that cause no symptoms in the majority of people.

ALVEOLI Tiny air sacs in the lungs where oxygen is transferred into the bloodstream and carbon dioxide waste enters the airways, from which it is exhaled.

ANAPHYLAXIS An allergic reaction that is severe, sudden and life-threatening. Although rare, it can occur after an insect sting or as a reaction to an injected drug, such as penicillin or anti-tetanus (horse) serum. Less commonly, it occurs after consumption of a particular food or drug. Also known as anaphylactic shock.

ANTIBODY A specialized defender protein that latches onto invaders and marks them so that other immune system cells can destroy them. Antibodies also send out chemical signals calling white blood cells into action.

ANTIGEN A substance, usually a protein, that the body perceives as foreign.

ANTIHISTAMINE A medication that prevents symptoms such as congestion, sneezing and itchy, runny nose by blocking histamine receptors.

ANTI-INFLAMMATORY A medication that reduces inflammation; used to reduce airway inflammation in asthma. See also *Inflammation*.

ASTHMA A chronic inflammatory disorder of the airways of the lungs.

ASTHMA ATTACK A period of coughing, wheezing, breathlessness and chest tightness.

ASTHMA MANAGEMENT A comprehensive approach to controlling asthma.

ATOPIC ECZEMA Most common type of eczema. An allergic-type skin reaction triggered by internal factors. Sometimes called atopic dermatitis.

ATOPY The propensity, usually genetic, to develop IgE-mediated responses to common environmental allergens.

BASOPHIL A white blood cell filled with granules of chemicals including histamine that is involved in allergic reactions.

BETA-AGONIST An asthma drug (bronchodilator) that relaxes the muscles around the bronchial tubes, thus opening the airways and helping to keep them open. There are two main types: long-acting, taken daily to prevent symptoms, often in combination with an inhaled steroid; and short-acting, used for quick relief of symptoms during an asthma attack.

B LYMPHOCYTE An immune cell that produces antibodies.

BRONCHIAL TUBES Airways in the lungs. One major branch goes into each lung, then divides into many smaller branches.

BRONCHIOLES The smallest airways in the lungs.

BRONCHOCONSTRICTION Constriction of the airways that occurs when the muscles that wrap them tighten forcefully, pinching them closed.

BRONCHODILATOR A medication used to relax and open the airways. See also *Beta-agonist*.

CONJUNCTIVITIS Allergic conjunctivitis is inflammation of the conjunctiva membrane covering the white of the eye and inner eyelid, causing swelling and itchy, watery, red eyes. Conjunctivitis is also commonly caused by bacterial or viral infection.

CONTACT DERMATITIS See *Dermatitis*.

CONTRIBUTING FACTOR A risk factor that adds to the likelihood of a medical condition developing with exposure to it or may increase susceptibility to that condition. For asthma, contributing factors include smoking, viral infections, small size at birth and environmental pollutants.

CORTICOSTEROID A type of medication used to reduce inflammation in people with asthma. The inhaled form is the most common and effective drug used for long-term daily control.

DANDER Tiny flakes of animal skin.

DECONGESTANT A medication that shrinks nasal tissues to reduce or relieve symptoms of swelling and congestion.

DERMATITIS Skin inflammation due to contact with an irritating substance (irritant contact dermatitis), an allergic reaction (allergic contact dermatitis) or an internal trigger, such as if you inhale or eat a substance to which you are allergic (atopic dermatitis/atopic eczema). Symptoms include redness, itching and a rash.

DRUG ALLERGY An allergic reaction to a specific medication. The most common cause of drug allergies is penicillin.

DRY-POWDER INHALER A small device similar to a metered-dose inhaler but in which the drug is in powder form and is breath activated instead of aerosol activated.

DUST MITES Microscopic creatures that survive on skin flakes and other dust components and are among the most common triggers for allergies.

ECZEMA Inflammation of the skin, usually causing itching and sometimes accompanied by crusting, oozing and scaling. See also *Atopic eczema*.

ELIMINATION DIET A diet in which certain foods are temporarily excluded to rule them out as possible causes of allergy symptoms.

ELISA (enzyme-linked immunosorbent assay) A blood test used to identify substances that cause allergy symptoms and to estimate a relative sensitivity.

ENVIRONMENTAL CONTROL The removal of risk factors and allergy and asthma triggers from the environment.

EOSINOPHIL A white blood cell that secretes chemicals that trigger the inflammatory process and helps to destroy foreign cells.

EXACERBATION Any worsening of asthma or allergy symptoms.

EXERCISE-INDUCED ASTHMA Asthma triggered by physical activity.

EXTRINSIC ASTHMA Asthma triggered by an allergic reaction, generally to something that is inhaled.

FOOD ALLERGY An allergic reaction to proteins in certain foods. The most common foods involved in food allergy include milk, eggs, seafood, peanuts, tree nuts and soy.

HAY FEVER See *Allergic rhinitis*.

HEPA FILTER (high-efficiency particulate air) A filter that removes particles from the air by forcing it through screens containing microscopic pores.

HISTAMINE A naturally occurring substance released by mast cells and basophils after exposure to an allergen. It attaches to receptors on blood vessels, causing them to dilate, and binds to other receptors in nasal tissues, causing redness, swelling, itching and changes in secretions.

HIVES Itchy, swollen, red bumps or patches on the skin that appear suddenly as a result of the body's adverse reaction to the release of histamine and other chemicals. Also known as urticaria.

HYPOALLERGENIC Formulated to contain the fewest possible allergens.

IgE Immunoglobulin E, a type of immunoglobulin that triggers the release of histamine from mast cells, resulting in an allergic reaction.

IMMUNOGLOBULIN See *Antibody*.

IMMUNOTHERAPY A series of injections to help build the immune system's tolerance to an asthma or allergy trigger.

INFLAMMATION The body's response to a host of insults, including invasion by bacteria or viruses, injury or reaction to your own tissues. When tissues are injured, they and the cells that flock to the injury release a barrage of chemicals, including histamine, bradykinin, serotonin and others that cause blood vessels to leak fluid into the tissues, leading to swelling, redness and heat.

INHALER A small plastic device used to deliver medication to the airways.

INTRINSIC ASTHMA Asthma with no apparent external cause.

IRRITANT Any substance that causes irritation of a body tissue and may set off an allergy or asthma attack.

LATEX ALLERGY An allergy that develops after sensitizing contact with latex (natural rubber).

LEUKOTRIENE MODIFIER A type of oral medication used to treat mild to moderate asthma and allergies.

MACROPHAGE A large immune cell that engulfs and destroys large particles such as bacteria, yeast and dying cells.

MAST CELL A type of cell present in most body tissues but particularly numerous in connective tissue lining the skin and airways. In an allergic response, an allergen stimulates the release of antibodies, which attach themselves to mast cells. Following subsequent allergen exposure, the mast cells release substances such as histamine into the tissue, triggering an allergic reaction.

METERED-DOSE INHALER The most common device used to deliver asthma medication, allowing inhalation of a specific amount (a metered dose) of medicine.

MUCOUS MEMBRANE Moist tissue that lines body cavities with an external opening, such as the respiratory, digestive and urinary tracts.

MUCUS The liquid secretions of the mucus glands found in body lining tissues, which can change according to allergic reactions.

NEBULIZER A device that creates a mist of an asthma drug, which can then be inhaled into the lungs.

NEUTROPHIL The most numerous type of white blood cell and the first to arrive on the scene after a body insult occurs, especially an infection.

PEAK FLOW A measurement of how well you can blow air out of your lungs. If your airways become narrow and blocked due to asthma, you can't blow air out as well, and your peak flow values drop.

PEAK FLOW METER A small, portable device that measures airflow from the lungs.

POLLEN AND MOULD COUNTS Measurements of the amount of allergens in the air.

PROSTAGLANDIN A chemical released during an allergic reaction that contributes to allergy symptoms.

RAST (radioallergosorbent test) A blood test used to identify specific antibodies associated with allergy symptoms and to estimate a relative sensitivity.

RESCUE MEDICATION A drug used as needed to alleviate symptoms during an allergy or asthma attack.

SINUSITIS Inflammation or infection of one or more of the sinuses, the hollow air spaces located around the nose and between and over the eyes.

SKIN TEST Injection of a small quantity of an allergen into the skin to determine which allergens trigger an allergic response.

SODIUM CROMOGLICATE A medicine used to prevent asthma and/or allergic rhinitis symptoms.

SPACER A device that works with a metered-dose inhaler to deliver medication more easily and effectively and reduce side effects. It holds the 'puff' of medicine between you and the inhaler so you can inhale it slowly and more completely.

SPIROMETRY The most important test used for diagnosing asthma. A spirometer measures the maximum volume of air you can exhale after breathing in as much as you can. The total volume you exhale is called forced vital capacity, or FVC. The spirometer also measures the volume of air you exhale in the first second, called forced expiratory volume in 1 second, or FEV1. In general, the more air you breathe out during the first second of a full exhalation, the better.

T LYMPHOCYTE An immune system cell that secretes potent substances to attract other immune system cells that destroy invaders. Some T lymphocytes also attack and destroy diseased cells. Also known as T cell.

THEOPHYLLINE A drug sometimes used to help control mild to moderate persistent asthma, especially to prevent night-time symptoms.

TRIGGER Any substance that either causes or exacerbates an allergy or asthma attack.

URTICARIA See *Hives*.

Resources

This book should be a starting point in your search for information and understanding about allergies and asthma. Here's how you can find out more.

Organizations

Action Against Allergy
Offers support, advice, information leaflets, self-help book list and a 'find a specialist' service.
www.actionagainstallergy.co.uk
PO Box 278, Twickenham TW1 4QQ
020 8892 2711

Allergy UK
Supplies information, advice and support for people with allergies and their carers plus leaflets on all aspects of allergies. Helpline directs you to nearest NHS allergy clinic and consultant.
www.allergyuk.org
3 Oak Square, London Road, Swanley,
Kent BR8 7AG
01322 619 898
Helpline 01322 619 864 (9am-5pm Mon-Fri)

Anaphylaxis Campaign
Guided by leading UK allergists, offers support and advice on peanut and other food allergy and anaphylaxis management, plus educational children's books, videos and news about latest food alerts. Also campaigns over issues of product labelling and allergy services.
www.anaphylaxis.org.uk
PO Box 275, Farnborough, GU14 6SX
01252 373793 Helpline 01252 542029

Asthma UK
Dedicated to improving health and well-being of people whose lives are affected by asthma and campaigns for their interests, funds research and supplies informative leaflets and publications.
www.asthma.org.uk
Summit House, 70 Wilson Street,
London EC2A 2DE
020 7786 4900
Helpline 08457 010 203 (9am-5pm Mon-Fri)

British Lung Foundation
Provides support for people living with a lung disease and their carers, with comprehensive information on 40-plus lung conditions.
www.lunguk.org
73-75 Goswell Road, London EC1V 7ER
08458 50 50 20

British Dietetic Association
Publishes fact sheets on nutrition and campaigns to raise awareness of how a balanced, varied diet contributes to a healthy lifestyle.
www.bda.uk.com
Charles House, 148-9 Great Charles Sreet,
Queensway, Birmingham B3 3HT
0121 200 8080

British Thoracic Society
For medical professionals with an interest in respiratory disease, society promotes highest standards of clinical care, supports research and disseminates findings.
www.brit-thoracic.org.uk
17 Doughty Street, London WC1N 2PL
020 7831 8778

Latex Allergy Support Group
Provides support for those with latex allergy, raises public awareness and encourages research.
www.lasg.co.uk
PO Box 27, Filey, YO14 9YH
Helpline 07071 225838 (7pm to 10pm)

Coeliac UK
Provides help for diagnosed coeliacs.
www.coeliac.co.uk
SuitesA-D, Octagon Court, High Wycombe,
Bucks HP11 2HS
01494 437 278
Helpline 0870 444 8804

European Academy of Allergy and Clinical Immunology
Umbrella organization of EU member state allergy organisations. Website has up-to-date allergy information for doctors and the public.
www.eaaci.net/site/homepage.php

Health and Safety Executive
Offers advice on occupational asthma.
www.hse.gov
Rose Court, 2 Southwark Bridge,
London SE1 9HS
uk/asthmainfoline: 08701 545500

Medic Alert Foundation
Emergency alert emblems and bracelets.
www.medicalert.org.uk
1 Bridge Wharf, 156 Caledonian Road,
London N1 9UU
Freephone 0800 581420

National Eczema Society
Provides help for people with eczema.
www.eczema.org
Hill House, Highgate Hill, London N19 5NA
020 7281 3553
Helpline 0870 241 3604

Surrey Allergy Clinic
Dr Adrian Morris of the Surrey Allergy Clinic and BBC Health Online explains common allergies and their treatment.
www.allergy-clinic.co.uk

Books

The Allergy Bible: Understanding, Diagnosing and Treating Allergies and Intolerances by Linda Gamlin and Jonathan Brostoff (Quadrille Publishing, 2005)
Asthma, A Simple Guide contributors Dr Eleanor Bull, Professor David Price *et al* (CSF Medical Communications, 2005)
Asthma Free Naturally: Everything You Need to Know About Taking Control of Your Asthma by Patrick McKeown (Harper Thorsons, 2005)
Beat Your Allergies: Find Relief, Feel Free by Dr Rob Hicks (The Infinite Ideas Company, 2005)
Rapid Reference Allergy by Dr Chris Corrigan and Dr Sabina Rak (Elsevier Moxby, 2004)

Coping with Childhood Asthma by Jill Eckersley (Sheldon Press, 2003)
Asthma and COPD by David Price, Juliet Foster *et al* (Churchill Livingstone, 2003)
Asthma at Your Fingertips by Mark Levey, Sean Hilton and Greta Barnes (Class Publishing, 2000)
The Complete Guide to Allergies by Pamela Brooks (Robinson, 2001)

Major asthma/allergy journals

You can view free abstracts from these journals at www.pubmed.gov *or on their websites. Some offer email delivery of their tables of contents.*

Lung
Publishes original articles, reviews and editorials on all aspects of healthy and diseased lungs, the airways and breathing.
www.springer.com

Thorax
A leading respiratory medicine journal with articles on clinical and experimental research in respiratory medicine, pediatrics, immunology, pharmacology, pathology and surgery.
thorax.bmjjournals.com

Clinical and Experimental Allergy
Official journal of the British Society for Allergy and Clinical Immunology. Publishes original research and review articles.
www.blackwell-synergy.com

Products for allergy sufferers

Allergymatters
Online allergy shop selling allergy prevention products. No catalogue, but a print-out of relevant pages on request.
www.allergymatters.com
020 8339 0029.

Healthy House
Allergy information and a wide range of allergy products. Free catalogue within UK.
www.healthy-house.co.uk
The Old Co-op, Lower Street, Ruscombe,
Stroud, Glos GL6 6BU
01453 752216

index

Allergy and Asthma Relief was published by
The Reader's Digest Association Limited
11 Westferry Circus, Canary Wharf
London E14 4HE

First UK edition copyright © 2006

Adapted from Allergy & Asthma Relief
© 2004 originated by the editorial team of
The Reader's Digest Association, Inc., USA

We are committed to both the quality of
our products and the service we provide to
our customers. We value your comments,
so please feel free to contact us on
08705 113366 or via our website at:
www.readersdigest.co.uk
If you have any comments or suggestions
about the content of our books, email us at:
gbeditorial@readersdigest.co.uk

Editor Rachel Warren Chadd
Assistant editor Liz Clasen
Designer Kate Harris
Researcher Angelika Romacker
Proofreader Ron Pankhurst
Indexer Hilary Bird

Reader's Digest, London

Editorial director Julian Browne
Art director Nick Clark
Head of book development Sarah Bloxham
Managing editor Alastair Holmes
Picture resource manager Martin Smith
Pre-press account manager Penelope Grose
Product production manager Claudette Bramble
Senior production controller Deborah Trott

Origination Colour Systems Limited, London
Printing and binding Cayfosa Quebecor,
Barcelona, Spain

Reader's Digest, USA
Editor-in-chief and publishing director Neil Wertheimer
Designer Rich Kershner
Illustrator Rod Little, Information Illustration

ISBN-13	978 0 276 44085 4
ISBN-10	0 276 44085 4
Book code	400-279-01
Oracle code	250008472S.00.24
Concept code	US 4422/IC